Y0-CCO-449

The Biochemistry and Physiology of Bone

SECOND EDITION

VOLUME II

Physiology and Pathology

Contributors

N. A. Barnicot

Geoffrey H. Bourne

D. Harold Copp

Robert J. Cousins

S. P. Datta

Hector F. DeLuca

Reuben Eisenstein

Frederic W. Rhinelander

Marshall R. Urist

Alfred Weinstock

The Biochemistry
and Physiology of Bone

SECOND EDITION

Edited by GEOFFREY H. BOURNE

Yerkes Regional Primate Research Center
Emory University
Atlanta, Georgia

VOLUME II
Physiology and Pathology

ACADEMIC PRESS New York and London   1972

COPYRIGHT © 1972 BY ACADEMIC PRESS, INC.

ALL RIGHTS RESERVED
NO PART OF THIS BOOK MAY BE REPRODUCED IN ANY FORM, BY
PHOTOSTAT, MICROFILM, RETRIEVAL SYSTEM, OR ANY OTHER
MEANS, WITHOUT WRITTEN PERMISSION FROM THE PUBLISHERS.

ACADEMIC PRESS, INC.
111 Fifth Avenue, New York, New York 10003

United Kingdom Edition published by
ACADEMIC PRESS, INC. (LONDON) LTD.
24/28 Oval Road, London NW1

LIBRARY OF CONGRESS CATALOG CARD NUMBER: 70 - 154375

PRINTED IN THE UNITED STATES OF AMERICA

Contents

Chapter 1. Circulation of Bone

Frederic W. Rhinelander

Chapter 2. Phosphatase and Calcification

G. H. Bourne

Chapter 3.   Elaboration of Enamel and Dentin Matrix Glycoproteins

Alfred Weinstock

Chapter 4.   Growth Hormone and Skeletal Tissue Metabolism

Marshall R. Urist

Chapter 5.   Vitamin A and Bone

N. A. Barnicot and S. P. Datta

Chapter 6.   Vitamin C and Bone

Geoffrey H. Bourne

Chapter 7.   Vitamin D and Bone

Robert J. Cousins and Hector F. DeLuca

Chapter 8.   Calcitonin

D. Harold Copp

Chapter 9.   Pathological Calcification

Reuben Eisenstein

List of Contributors

Numbers in parentheses indicate the pages on which the authors' contributions begin.

N. A. BARNICOT (197), Department of Anthropology, University College London, London, England

GEOFFREY H. BOURNE (79, 231), Yerkes Regional Primate Research Center, Emory University, Atlanta, Georgia

D. HAROLD COPP (337), Department of Physiology, University of British Columbia, Vancouver, British Columbia, Canada

ROBERT J. COUSINS (281),* Department of Biochemistry, University of Wisconsin, Madison, Wisconsin

S. P. DATTA (197), Department of Biochemistry, University College London, London, England

HECTOR F. DELUCA (281), Department of Biochemistry, University of Wisconsin, Madison, Wisconsin

REUBEN EISENSTEIN (357), Division of Pathology, Presbyterian-St. Luke's Hospital, Chicago, Illinois

FREDERIC W. RHINELANDER (1), Cleveland Metropolitan General Hospital, Cleveland, Ohio

* Present address: Department of Animal Science, Rutgers University, New Brunswick, New Jersey

MARSHALL R. URIST (155), Bone Research Laboratory, Rehabilitation Center, Los Angeles, California

ALFRED WEINSTOCK (121),* Department of Anatomy, McGill University, Montreal, Canada, and School of Dentistry, and Department of Anatomy, School of Medicine, University of California, Los Angeles, California

* Present address: Departments of Periodontology and Anatomy, Schools of Dentistry and Medicine, University of California, The Center for the Health Sciences, Los Angeles, California

Preface to Second Edition

The first edition of this treatise filled a long-existing gap. It found an immediate place on the library shelves of anatomists, orthopedists, biochemists, cell biologists, physiologists, biomedical engineers, and others who had anything to do with this hard but plastic, living, and contentious tissue. The book appealed to graduate students and professors, pathologists and clinicians, and in many places of the world became a standard work.

This second edition, appearing fifteen years after its predecessor, has expanded into a three-volume work, attesting to our growth of knowledge in many aspects of this field. Volume I, dealing with structure, covers the nature and behavior of bone cells, the structure of the organic matrix of bone, mineral organization, and bone strength. Volumes II and III deal with the blood vessels which nourish bone, the mechanisms of bone formation, bone growth, repair, and transplantation, and the role of hormones and vitamins in the formation and maintainance of bone. Pathological calcification and radiation effects on bone complete each of these volumes. We believe we have matched the first edition in interest and importance and hope it will appeal to as diversified an audience.

I would like to thank the contributors for their cooperation and courtesy and for their hard work and enthusiasm. To the staff of Academic Press I owe many years of cooperation, forebearance, and understanding.

GEOFFREY H. BOURNE

Preface to First Edition

In the last 25 years there has been a rapid development of new techniques and enthusiasm in their application to bone studies. A store of new knowledge has been accumulated about structure and function of bone and a growing appreciation of the skeleton as a plastic, actively metabolizing tissue. Papers dealing with these and other aspects of bone are published in an astonishingly wide range of journals throughout the world. The present treatise is the outgrowth of a belief that the time had come to collect these diverse studies into an integrated volume. Its comprehensiveness should make it of interest to many experts, in particular to histologists, to anatomists, to specialists in orthopedics and pediatrics, and to dentists; in addition I hope that many biologists, physiologists, biochemists, and pathologists will find a great deal of interest and value to them between its covers.

The study of bone has passed through a number of phases. Many of the older workers were well aware of the plastic nature and metabolic activity of bone, but later a tendency to regard bones as immutable structures that one could cut and shape and treat as inanimate building material became widespread.

Frey, in his manual of histology, published nearly 100 years ago, summarized what was until relatively recently thought to be the function of bones: "Owing to their hardness and solidity, the bones are peculiarly well adapted for the mechanical construction of the body. . . . They serve to protect internal organs, and form systems of levers." But Frey also goes on to say "The bones take part also, to a great extent, in the chemical occurrences of the organism, owing to the lively interchange of matter going on in them." This is, in fact, a modern outlook on bone.

To some extent it was the mechanical investigations of bones by engineers such as Carlmann and Kochlin which tended to emphasize their structural nature and to suggest a permanence which was illusory; in fact it has been said that Kochlin designed the struts for the Eiffel tower on the same plan as the trabeculae at the head of a long bone (first described by Meyer in 1873). The bone struts of course can do what those of the Eiffel tower cannot; they can be altered in shape, size, and direction with varying stresses and strains and this is one of the characters which most distinguishes bone from an inert supporting structure.

In the last hundred years investigation of bone has proceeded actively in a wide variety of fields and in the present century the development of biochemistry has contributed a good deal to our knowledge of the nature of the organic matrix, the problems involved in calcification, and so on. The influence of vitamin deficiency on bone is well known but recent research has helped towards an understanding of the mechanism by which such changes are brought about. More recently a great deal of attention has been paid to the role of hormones in bone formation and structure. The cells of bone and problems of bone development and repair have been extensively studied. Probably the most recent field is the application of radioisotopes to the study of bone structure and function.

It would be too great a feat to expect any one person to deal comprehensively with all these facets of bone study and therefore the best solution was found to be a composite book.

In such a book a certain amount of planned overlap of chapters is both inevitable and desirable. Chapters which deal, for example, with osteoblasts, phosphatases, and calcification must be expected to have a good deal in common; in the same way the growth of bone would naturally be discussed in chapters other than that bearing such a title. In fact, one can think of this book, in a sense, as a spectrum, each of the chapters representing a pure spectral color but shading indistinguishably into its neighbors.

The collecting together, on time, of 24 chapters by authors scattered over Europe, America, and the Middle East seemed an intimidating task but thanks to the cooperation and hard work of all who participated in this volume it proved to be by no means as difficult as it seemed at first.

My thanks are due to all, authors and staff of Academic Press, for their help in bringing together and getting into print so promptly the mass of material contained in this book.

GEOFFREY H. BOURNE

London Hospital Medical College
February, 1956

Contents of Other Volumes

CHAPTER 1

Circulation in Bone

FREDERIC W. RHINELANDER

1

I. Introduction

A. Importance of Knowledge of Bone Blood Supply

All of the physiologic processes within bone are dependent upon the presence of an adequate blood supply, and alterations in this blood supply can profoundly affect any of these processes. When a bone is injured, the vascular response is an essential consideration in treatment and it greatly affects the final result.

The chemical and cellular responses of bone's many constituents, under normal and under pathologic conditions, have been studied extensively. However, investigations of the essential blood supply have been relatively few. Those that have been carried out are well reviewed, with bibliographies, by Trueta (1964) and Brookes (1964). The review by Brookes will be drawn upon particularly in the ensuing presentation.

In discussions of bone blood supply, the so-called long bone is the generally used model because it is a fundamental component of the mammalian skeleton and it encompasses the chief types of osseous tissue. At the outset, a clear understanding of a long bone's basic anatomic features is essential for an analysis of its complex vascular patterns to be comprehensible.

B. Anatomy of a Long Bone

The long bone is the major unit of the appendicular skeleton. It consists basically of a shaft (diaphysis) with an expansion (metaphysis) at each end. An idealized long bone is illustrated in Fig. 1.

In an immature animal, each metaphysis is surmounted by an epiphysis which is united to its metaphysis by a cartilaginous growth plate (epiphyseal plate). At the extremity of each epiphysis, a specialized covering of articular cartilage forms the gliding surface of the joint (articulation) which provides motion between the particular long bone and the adjacent bone in the skeleton.

The diaphysis is a hollow tube. Its walls are composed of dense cortex

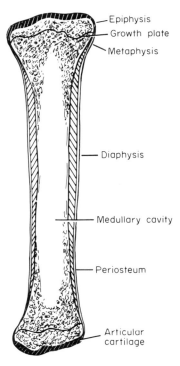

Epiphysis
Growth plate
Metaphysis

Diaphysis

Medullary cavity

Periosteum

Articular
cartilage

Fɪɢ. 1. Diagrammatic representation of the parts of a long bone.

(compactum) which is thick throughout the extent of the diaphysis but tapers off to become the thin shell of each metaphysis. The central space (medulla or medullary cavity) within the diaphysis contains the bone marrow—a hematopoietic organ residing in the skeleton. The medullary cavity is present only in the diaphysis.

In contrast to the diaphysis, which is composed of compact bone, the metaphyses consist entirely, except for the cortical shell, of thin osseous spicules (trabeculae) in a latticework of cancellous or spongy bone.

At the cessation of growth, the epiphyses, composed of cancellous bone, become fused with the adjacent metaphyses at the sites of the previous growth plates. The outer shell of the metaphyses and epiphyses is a thin layer of cortical bone continuous with the compactum of the diaphysis.

Covering the entire external surface of a mature long bone, except for the articulation, is the periosteum. This is composed of two layers. The inner or osteogenic layer contains the highly active cells which produce circumferential enlargement and remodeling of the growing long bone. After maturity, this layer consists chiefly of a capillary network. The outer layer is fibrous and supporting and comprises almost the entire periosteum of a mature bone. In the event of injury to a mature bone, some of the resting cells of the inner periosteal layer become osteogenic.

The intimacy of attachment of the periosteum to the surface of a mature long bone differs markedly in different portions of the bone, and this is of great significance where vascular connections are concerned. The periosteum covering most of the diaphysis is tenuous and loosely attached, and it can therefore convey only delicate capillaries. However, at the expanded ends of long bones, ligaments are attached firmly and can convey blood vessels of relatively large size to and from the bone. The same is true at the ridges along diaphyses where heavy fascial septa are attached, such as the ridge on the ulna for the interosseous membrane and the linea aspera of the femur.

II. Historical Concepts of the Overall Blood Supply of a Long Bone

A. ANATOMIC VASCULAR COMPONENTS

In simplest anatomic terms, a long bone has three basic circulations or blood supplies: (1) the nutrient, (2) the metaphyseal (combined with the epiphyseal[1] after closure of the growth plate), and (3) the periosteal. Figure 2 outlines the interrelationships between the three blood supplies as visualized by Brookes and Harrison (1957).

The nutrient blood supply emanates from the principal nutrient artery (marked 1 in Fig. 2), which arises directly from an artery of the systemic circulation and enters the diaphysis through a distinct foramen. Within the medulla it branches into ascending and descending medullary arteries. These subdivide into arterioles which penetrate the endosteal surface to supply the diaphyseal cortex.

The numerous metaphyseal arteries (marked 2 in Fig. 2) arise from periarticular plexuses and enter the expanded ends of the long bone to supply each metaphysis. They also anastomose with terminal branches of the ascending and descending medullary arteries.

The periosteal capillaries (marked 3 in Fig. 2), which are present on all smooth diaphyseal surfaces where muscles are not firmly attached, are considered by Brookes (1964) to be efferent from the cortex—as would be confirmed by surgeons who have noted the punctate bleeding that occurs when periosteum is stripped from such surfaces. The perios-

---

[1] The circulation of mature bone only will be presented. The changing circulation in growing bone is a subject unto itself.

plugging a bone's entire medulla or wrapping its outer surface in a plastic sheath in order to obliterate all endosteal or periosteal blood supply. However, before the studies on fracture healing are presented, a more detailed consideration of the intrinsic vascularization of diaphyseal cortex is indicated.

III. Blood Supply of Normal Compactum

Figure 3, from Ham's textbook, shows in diagrammatic form the internal structure of cortical bone as observed in man and also in the dog. The basic osseous unit is the Haversian system or osteon. Its central artery is connected, through transverse channels, with the major endosteal and periosteal vasculature. In an actual bone, of course, both the longitudinal and transverse channels run more or less obliquely. The transverse channels, called Volkmann's canals, probably do not represent a distinct functional entity. The osteogenic layer of periosteum applies primarily to growing bone. In mature periosteum, the osteogenic

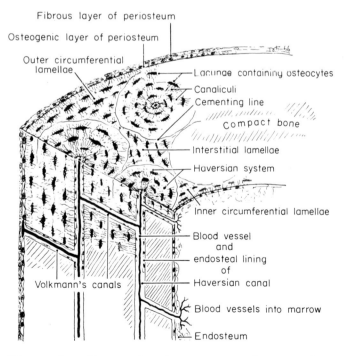

FIG. 3. Diagram from Ham to show basic structure of compact bone. Note its vascular channels. (Reproduced from Ham, 1969.)

properties appear only after injury. Normal adult periosteum is composed chiefly of an outer fibrous layer which contains few blood vessels, and a very thin inner layer consisting chiefly of a capillary network. That type of periosteum will be the author's only concern in this discussion of the blood supply of mature bone.

A. Experimental Techniques Used by Author

The studies on bone blood supply carried out in the author's laboratory are based on the technique of microangiography and correlated histology as described in various of its aspects by Barclay (1951), Bellman (1953), and Trueta *et al.* (1947). Their original techniques have been considerably amplified (Rhinelander and Baragry, 1962; Rhinelander *et al.*, 1968). In brief, the main artery of a dog's limb is perfused with a 30% by weight suspension of Micropaque[2] in physiologic saline solution, just after the administration of heparin and an overdose of Nembutal intravenously. The perfusion pressure is always 120 mm Hg, the low normal blood pressure of a dog. By this means, it is intended to have the vascular system in as physiologic a state as possible and to fill with Micropaque only those blood vessels which are functional at the time. Since the perfusion pressure is the same for all animals, the microangiograms from all experiments are comparable.

Only the afferent side of the circulation, down to and including the smallest capillaries,[3] is injected by this technique. Run-off from the veins is too fast; only the ghosts of veins are occasionally demonstrated. The experimental observations in the author's laboratory are made from correlated standard roentgenograms, microangiograms, and histologic preparations.

The microangiograms show the vascular pattern in a slice of decalcified bone 1 mm thick. Decalcification is necessary in order for the small injected vessels in dense cortex to be visible. These 1-mm slices are generally cut longitudinally, as shown disgrammatically in Fig. 4 from a report on fracture healing, but sometimes they are cut transversely to produce microangiographic cross sections. The microangiograms are made routinely in steroscopic pairs because of the enormous number of overlapping small blood vessels (see Fig. 12) which may be included in a 1-mm slice of tissue. Each 1-mm slice is then sectioned further

---

[2] Micropaque is finely and evenly divided barium sulfate produced by Damancy & Co., Ltd. of Ware, England, and imported into the United States by the Picker X-Ray Corporation. Only the white powdered form should be used. The saline solution should be thoroughly and frequently shaken. Gelatin should not be added because it can inhibit the filling of small blood vessels.

[3] See Fig. 11 for an illustration of the injectability of 7 μ capillaries.

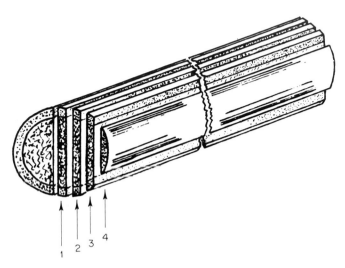

Fig. 4. Manner in which fixed and decalcified bone specimens are cut into 1-mm slices for microangiography.

on a microtome, and stained, to produce standard histologic sections of the identical tissue observed in the microangiogram. In this respect the author's technique differs from that of Trueta's laboratory, where alternating thick sections (for microangiography) and thin sections (for histology) were prepared. Also unlike Trueta, colored infusion fluids to demonstrate small vessels have not been used. Micropaque granules, slightly yellowish in color, are readily observed in standard hematoxylin and eosin (H & E) histologic sections. For photography under the microscope, these granules are accentuated by using somewhat oblique substage lighting. Such lighting obscures cellular detail, but these preparations are of value chiefly for demonstrating blood vessels which are injectable, and therefore actively functional, at the time of infusion. Sometimes, in the same histologic section, small vessels which contain Micropaque and others which contain only residual erythrocytes are observed, and this may occur in a single Haversian canal. Thus, the vascular patterns which are demonstrated in these experiments are a great deal more sparse than are those revealed by high pressure injection of plastic solutions (Wray and Lynch, 1959) which permeate all vascular channels whether actively functional or not.

Microangiography, of course, portrays only a static picture of blood supply. Blood flow through entire limbs and bones can be assessed by various techniques (Wray and Spencer, 1960; Kane, 1968; Shim, 1968). The actual movement of blood cells within small vessels of the marrow, close to the endosteum, has been observed in a tiny area under the microscope (Brånemark, 1959). But the functional status of blood vessels within large areas of cortex, and within fracture callus, can only be inferred by the injectability[4] of the vessels. It is granted that infusion under anesthesia, after a cannula has been tied into the main limb artery, is not a normal physiologic situation. However, when the infusions are made under the same conditions at the same pressure, as done in all the author's experiments, the situation is as close to the physiologic normal as can be obtained through currently available technology.

B. Experimental Results with Normal Canine Bones— Anatomic Findings

It has been demonstrated in the author's laboratory that the active blood supply of cortical bone varies greatly under different conditions. Figure 5 demonstrates the injectable afferent blood vessels in a 1-mm-thick slice from the midshaft of a radius of a completely normal mature dog.[5] Figure 6 contains the microangiograms of two serial 1-mm-thick longitudinal slices of the cortex of a dog's normal ulna, but the circulation in this bone has been physiologically stimulated by a minor fracture in the opposite forelimb 3 weeks previously, leading to more complete filling of the vascular channels of cortex than takes place under completely resting conditions.

[4] The smallest capillaries are filled by the technique employed when the pathway to them is open, as demonstrated in Fig. 11.

[5] All of the dogs used in these studies were mongrels and were mature, as judged radiologically by epiphyseal closure.

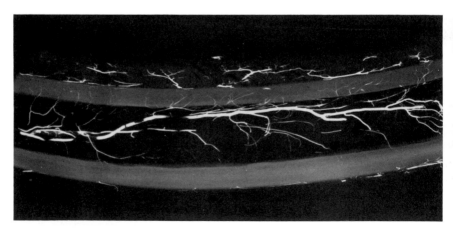

Fig. 5. Microangiogram of midshaft of a normal dog's radius to show the resting arterial blood supply (×2.8).

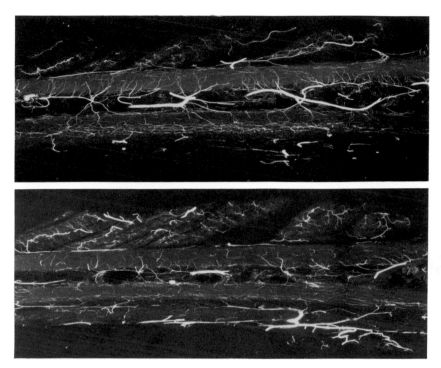

F<small>IG</small>. 6. Microangiograms of two adjacent 1-mm slices from the normal ulnar diaphysis of a mature dog. The circulation in this ulna had been stimulated physiologically by a fracture in the opposite forelimb (×3.2).

It would appear most unlikely that the large number of additional cortical blood vessels demonstrated in Fig. 6 are new vessels which formed secondarily to the fracture of the other leg. The formation of new vascular channels through cortex would require bone resorption, which would be a highly nonphysiologic response for a bone which was bearing increased stress by reason of the injury to its paired limb. Variation between radius and ulna, and individual variation between animals, may of course play some part. However, the differences observed in many comparable experiments in the author's laboratory appear to be much too great to be explainable solely on these bases. More likely, the greater vascular filling in the sound leg results from opening up of resting vessels in response to a physiologic stimulus.

An increased blood flow through the paired uninjured limb acutely after fracture has been demonstrated by Wray and Spencer (1960), and preliminary experiments in the author's laboratory with a square-wave electromagnetic flowmeter have suggested that this increased flow in the uninjured limb as a whole persists for some weeks. This could be attributable to muscular hypertrophy from increased use of this leg. However, there is no explanation of the greatly enhanced filling of the existing vascular channels of osseous cortex. And the mechanism by which the arterial blood supply is reduced and increased within cortex remains a mystery. Changes can be very profound, as has been demonstrated. Most of the cortical afferent channels of the radius depicted in Fig. 5 must be in a resting state insofar as transport of blood is concerned.

A comparison of the histologic sections which correspond, respectively, to Fig. 5 and Fig. 6 reveals that the bone with the stimulated circulation has a slight increase in remodeling activity but no increase in the number of vascular channels within cortex.

Figure 6, by virtue of a circulatory stimulation within physiologic limits, depicts in unusual detail what appears to be normal afferent vasculature of a mature dog's ulna. This can be taken as representative of canine, and probably of human, long bones. Observe how the curving principal medullary artery dips from one tissue slice into the next, giving the false impression of being interrupted. The arborization of the arteriolar branches of the medullary trunks within the inner two-thirds to three-quarters of the cortex, especially in the superior cortex, is well demonstrated. Differences with respect to the pattern of injected vessels, within the cortex's outer layers, are obvious between the superior and inferior cortices. These differences are relatable to differing periosteal attachments. Firm fascial attachments are able to convey blood vessels of larger caliber into bone than are the filamentous attachments which are present beneath loosely applied portions of muscles.

Observe the strands of muscle attached to the superior cortical surface of each tissue slice in Fig. 6, and note their independent blood supply. In the upper microangiogram, an occasional muscular arteriole appears to penetrate this surface, presumably along a fascial attachment; but in the lower microangiogram, the superior cortex is entered by no arterioles.

The inferior cortex is at the attachment of the interosseous membrane (which is very heavy in the dog) and is comparable to the linea aspera of the femur (see Section IV, F,4 below). Branches of the forelimb's interosseous artery, lying along this membrane in the lower microangiogram, are as large as the chief medullary artery. Observe, in the outer third of the inferior ulnar cortex, the abundant anastomoses between medullary and periosteal vessels. This becomes very significant when the medullary supply is blocked, as was the situation in the author's femoral studies.

C. Reports by Other Investigators—Flow of Blood through Cortex

No information concerning the direction of blood flow through cortex is given by Fig. 6 as is no information regarding the venous channels which must be injected retrograde to obtain adequate filling Brookes has studied these aspects extensively, and Figs. 2 and 7 depict his concept of them.

The flow of blood through cortex is very sluggish, as has been shown by Leriche and Policard (1926) and other workers. Brookes and co-authors (1961) have presented the concept that the direction of flow through normal cortex is centrifugal. This is supported by the observations of many investigators quoted by Brookes (1964): sulfate solutions enter the cortex from the marrow, but not from the periosteum, in perfusion experiments; intravital dyes pass slowly from marrow to periosteum following injection; there is a diminished intensity of radioactive ions from medulla to periosteum in radioautography studies; and India ink, which can readily traverse capillaries, does not enter cortex through available periosteal connections after the nutrient arterial system has been blocked.

The concept of a centrifugal flow of blood through normal cortex

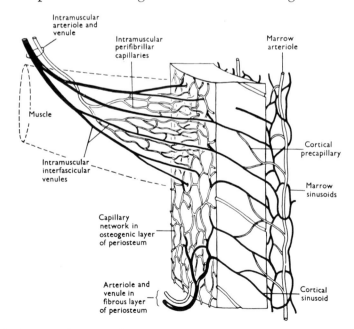

Fig. 7. Drawing from Brookes to show his concept of the microcirculation of cortical bone. (Reproduced from Brookes, 1964.)

is consistent with the classic experimental observations of Johnson (1927), and more recently of many others, that the periosteal arteries play only a minor part in the nutrition of mature cortex. The contrary observations are very few, and they are probably accounted for by immaturity of the experimental animals used. While an animal is immature, the osteogenic layer of the periosteum is constantly laying down new bone which continues to be nourished by the periosteal vascular system which is then highly active.

If the flow of blood through the entire thickness of mature cortex is indeed centrifugal under normal conditions, there must be an ultimate capillary network along the external cortical surface directly beneath the periosteum. Such a network is illustrated by Brookes (1964) in Fig. 7. He remarked that the junction between the blood vessels of the general periosteal circulation and the vessels of the cortical vascular network takes place along the external surface of cortex "almost exclusively at the capillary level" in a "profusion of gutters" which are "uniform in calibre and orderly in orientation." This is the situation where fleshy muscle bellies overlie bone, only a feeble periosteal attachment being present. The cortical surface appears grossly to be smooth, but observation at low magnification readily discloses the gutters. On the other hand, where strong fascial attachments exist, the cortical surface is macroscopically rough, and the vascular connections between muscle and bone are of greater than capillary size.

There are, thus, three types of blood vessels which connect the musculo-periosteal vascular system with the intracortical vascular channels of long bones. Venules, capillaries, and arterioles, in different areas, are all concerned. This observation will be discussed in more detail below.

Although Brookes believed that the flow of blood through mature cortex is normally centrifugal, he concluded from experiments on the rabbit's femur (Brookes, 1960) that this flow can in part be reversed when the nutrient arterial supply is intentionally suppressed. This observation will also be considered further.

D. Summary of Concepts of Normal Circulation in a Long Bone

The important concepts regarding the normal blood supply of mature mammalian tubular bones, based on the reports of other investigators, may be summarized as follows:

(1) The nutrient arterial system consists of branches of the nutrient artery and the metaphyseal arteries, in vigorous anastomosis with each

other, to become the medullary blood supply. This system is largely fed by arterial trunks derived from the systemic circulation of the animal.

(2) The periosteal arterial system is a component of the larger vascular system which also supplies the muscles that surround tubular bones.

(3) At least the inner two-thirds to three-quarters of the compactum are primarily supplied by ramifications of the nutrient (medullary) system.

(4) According to some investigators, the outer third or quarter of the compactum is primarily supplied by periosteal arterioles.

(5) According to Brookes, the direction of blood flow through the compactum as a whole is normally centrifugal—from medulla to periosteum.

(6) Also according to Brookes, in the rabbit, under the abnormal condition of blockade of the nutrient system, the periosteal system is able to reverse the usual centrifugal flow and convey blood supply to the compactum.

(7) The most peripheral capillary connections between the nutrient afferent and the periosteal efferent vessels lie in the deep layer of periosteum, in intimate association with the external cortical surface, where the periosteum is attached only loosely to most of the diaphyseal cortex.

(8) Larger vascular elements of the periosteal system (arterioles and venules) penetrate the cortical surface in the limited areas where fascial structures are firmly attached to the diaphysis.

The author's investigations substantiate these concepts except for (4) and (6) in part. He would conclude, from the experiments on medullary reaming and nailing of dogs' femora described below, that periosteal arterioles supply the outer third or quarter of the compactum in only localized areas (related to fascial attachments), and that these periosteal arterioles become more active when the medullary supply is blocked, but that there is no major reversal in the direction of flow of blood supplied by the so-called periosteal circulation (see Section IV, F,4).

IV. Blood Supply of Healing Compactum

A. UNDISPLACED CLOSED FRACTURES

1. Necrosis of Cortex at Fracture Site and New-Bone Formation

When the diaphysis of a long bone is fractured, an area of cortex on either side of the fracture line necessarily becomes devascularized—as described by Ham and Harris, Chapter 10, this volume. The devascu-

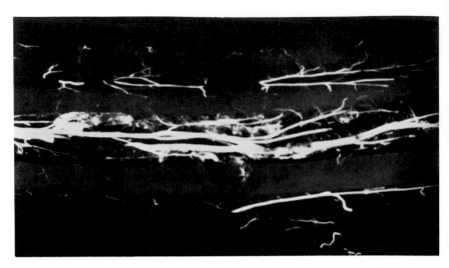

Fɪɢ. 8. Microangiogram of 1-day undisplaced fracture of canine radius showing enhancement of the medullary blood supply over the resting level (×2.1).

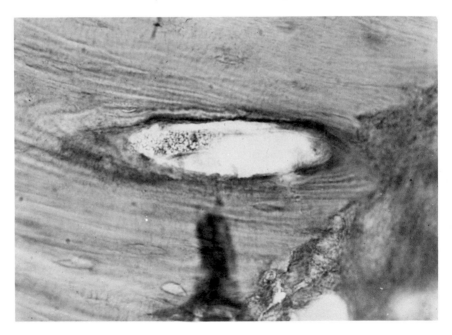

Fɪɢ. 9. Photomicrograph of 1-day radial fracture showing Micropaque-filled capillary in a bone canal very close to the cortical fracture site. The fracture, visible at the lower right, contains debris (H & E, ×359).

larized zone varies in width, depending on the local configuration of
the ruptured vessels which were supplying the area of injury.

Figure 8 is the microangiogram of a dog's radius 1 day following
an undisplaced closed fracture produced by the controlled force of a
hydraulic press, with the animal under intravenous nembutal anesthesia
(Rhinelander and Baragry, 1962). A cast was applied immediately. The
medullary circulation remained basically intact. In comparison with the
resting blood supply (Fig. 5), the arteries in the medulla have opened
up markedly; but as yet the periosteal vessels, and the major intracortical
vessels, show no significant change. Histologically (Fig. 9) an injected
capillary is observed in a bone canal which lies 30 μ from the fracture
site (as measured on the original histologic section). The Micropaque
granules in the capillary are definite. This is evidently a Haversian
vessel, cut obliquely, which remained connected with the nutrient arterial system. Cortex closely bordering a fracture can thus continue to
be vascularized. This does not mean, however, that all the osteocytes
in the vicinity of such an active capillary will continue to be nourished.
Microfractures are always present close to the actual fracture line, and
these can interrupt the canaliculi through which osteocytes obtain their
nourishment.

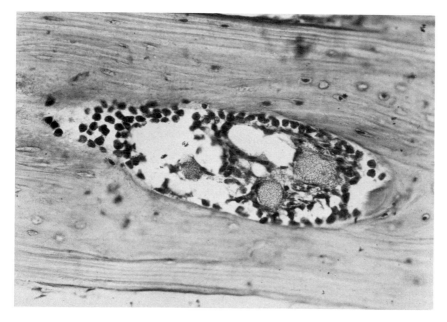

Fig. 10. Photomicrograph of 4-day fracture of radius, showing injected capillaries
and osteoblasts in a bone canal near the fracture site (H & E, ×175).

The bone canal of the 4-day fracture portrayed in Fig. 10 is situated 350 μ from the fracture site. It is lined by osteoblasts and contains three injected capillaries. The lacunae lying between this canal and the fracture, which is out of the microscope's field to the left, are empty while many of the lacunae situated away from the fracture contain osteocytes that appear viable.

In the series of experiments on undisplaced closed fractures carried out in the author's laboratory (Rhinelander and Baragry, 1962), periosteal new-bone formation supported by injected capillaries was observed on the third day, and new bone formation along the endosteum on the fourth day. By 5 days, both the periosteal and medullary circulations had proliferated greatly, and the abundant periosteal capillaries shown in Fig. 11 were supporting new-bone formation. Capillaries of minimal size are injected when they are functional.

2. Proliferation of Medullary and Periosteal Circulations

The extreme degree of vascularity of the callus within the fracture site is demonstrated in Fig. 12 from a 2-week undisplaced fracture of

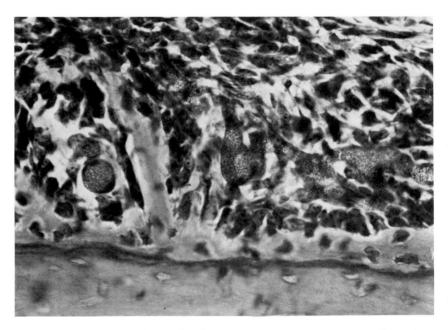

Fig. 11. Photomicrograph of 5-day fracture of radius, showing periosteal new-bone formation and abundant capillaries injected with Micropaque. The largest capillary, cut in cross section, measures 11 μ in diameter, and the smaller ones measure 7 μ (H & E, ×289).

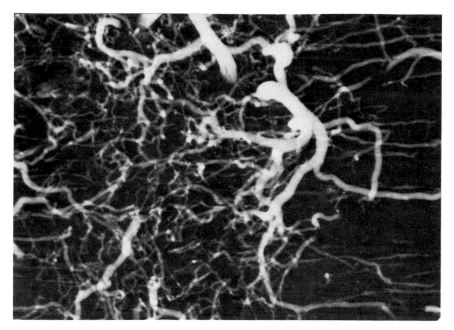

Fig. 12. Enlarged microangiogram of 2-week undisplaced fracture of radius, to demonstrate the enormous number of injected vessels at the cortical fracture site (×24.5).

the radius. This microangiographic enlargement provides almost a three-dimensional concept of the vast number of vessels that lie within a thickness of 1 mm. The tiny longitudinal vessels to both sides of the healing area are the Haversian capillaries of adjacent cortex. They are active but have not yet significantly enlarged. Both the periosteal and medullary circulations of this fractured bone had proliferated greatly and were supplying the area of cortical repair.

3. Dominant Role of Medullary Circulation

The persistent local increase in the number of medulla-derived vessels within cortex at 5 weeks after undisplaced radial fracture (Fig. 13) is the chief indication of the original fracture site. Note that even the external callus is now supplied by medullary vessels which traverse the full thickness of cortex. Histologically, this fracture was solidly united and remodeling was in progress.

By 8 weeks (Fig. 14) the vascular pattern of normal resting bone has almost been restored. A few arterioles of medullary origin still traverse the cortex to supply the thin zone of external callus which remains.

From this series of experiments it is evident that in undisplaced frac-

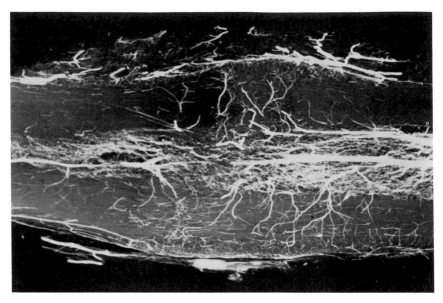

FIG. 13. Microangiogram of 5-week undisplaced radial fracture showing advanced healing of cortex. Note the penetration of medullary arterioles to supply the external callus (×4.9).

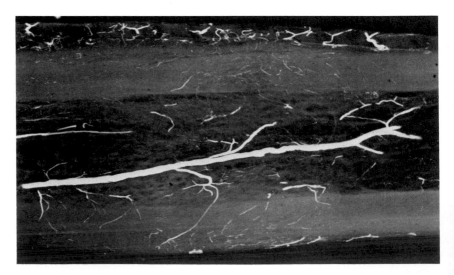

FIG. 14. Microangiogram of radius of 8-week undisplaced fracture which has almost completely healed. The exuberant blood supply of the active healing processes has disappeared, but medullary vessels still supply the remnants of periosteal callus (×5.6).

tures of canine forelimb bones, immobilized by plaster casts, the intact medullary supply dominates all stages of healing. The limited role of the periosteal afferent circulation does not appear until the repair of displaced fractures is considered.

B. DISPLACED CLOSED FRACTURES

1. Early Enhancement of Periosteal Circulation

Displaced fractures were also made with a hydraulic press, but more force was used (Rhinelander *et al.*, 1968). After fracture, the bones were manipulated to assure disruption of the medullary circulation; then they were reduced and a cast was applied. Dogs walk immediately on their casts; thus, immobilization of the fracture fragments is less adequate than can be obtained with man. In the microangiogram of the ulna from a 3-week experiment (Fig. 15) the medullary arterial supply is seen to have proliferated in each fracture fragment. However, it has not yet been able to bridge the fracture gap, which remains filled with avascular debris. The periosteal afferent circulation also shows great enhancement and is supplying the external callus.

The origin of the increased external blood supply has been shown by Göthman (1961) to be the arteries of the surrounding soft tissues. His studies on the rabbit and monkey substantiate the author's findings that the periosteal afferent circulation is only important early in fracture healing when it supplies the initial external callus. He observed that it gave off only a few sprouting branches toward the fracture hematoma itself.

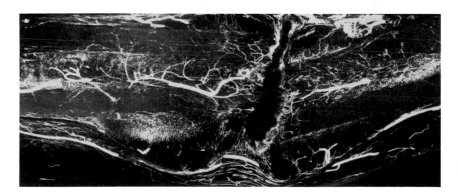

Fig. 15. Microangiogram of 3-week dispaced fracture of ulna. The medullary circulation is active in each major fragment but it remains disrupted at the fracture site and there has been no medullary or intercortical healing. The extraosseous blood supply has greatly increased (×2.8).

2. Effect of Immobilization on Vascular Regeneration and Osseous Healing

In another 3-week experiment, as shown in the microangiogram of Fig. 16, the effect of better immobilization in the treatment of the fracture is demonstrated. A spike of one main fracture fragment was locked into the medulla of the other main fragment. As a result, a large medullary artery has been able to bridge the fracture, and osseous union is present in the medulla. The abundant external callus appears largely to be supplied by the periosteal afferent circulation at this stage of fracture healing. Note especially that the arteriolar vessels of this periosteal callus are directed perpendicularly to the external surface of the cortex. That is the angiographic hallmark of early periosteal callus.

Histologically (Fig. 17) it is observed that medullary bridging callus is uniting the tip of the invaginating cortical spike of the right-hand fracture fragment to the endosteal cortical surface of the left-hand fracture fragment. At the base of the invaginating spike, avascular cortical surfaces are in contact and there is no healing. Significantly, the abundant periosteal callus at this fracture site has not yet been able to bridge the fracture gap. This is in keeping with the constant observation in these studies that the first osseous union to develop is always by means of medullary callus.

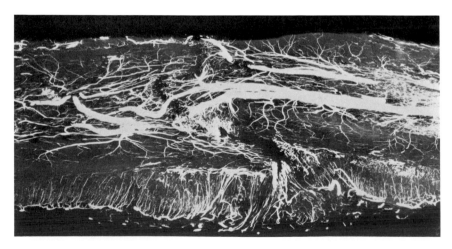

FIG. 16. Microangiogram of another 3-week displaced fracture, involving the radius, with interlocked bone fragments. The medullary circulation has been reconstituted across the fracture site. Note the characteristic vascular pattern of early periosteal callus, below, with blood vessels perpendicular to the cortical surface ($\times 3.85$).

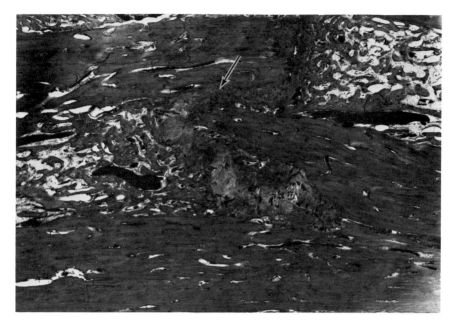

Fig. 17. Photomicrograph of fracture site in Fig. 16. Fibrous and cartilaginous union predominate, but true bone union is present (arrow) between the endosteal surface of the spicule projecting into the medulla and the endosteal surface of the adjacent cortex (H & E, ×8.75).

3. Fibrocartilaginous Delayed Union

The continuing effect of inadequate immobilization is demonstrated in a 6-week experiment. Figure 18 shows the familiar radiologic picture of delayed union in a fracture which appears united clinically. The large masses of external callus have built up in an effort to improve stability, but they and the fracture lines are still crossed by radiolucent gaps. By microangiography (Fig. 19) these radiolucent gaps are seen to correspond to avascular zones—the typical angiographic picture of fibrocartilage, which forms when the abundant capillaries required to nourish osseous callus are constantly being ruptured. If fibrocartilage, rather than merely fibrous tissue, is able to form, as occurred in this case, then sufficient stabilization is present for the cartilage to be able to ossify. The brush borders of terminal capillary loops, shown here, advance into the cartilage from each side. The histologic appearance of this process is demonstrated in Fig. 20. Observe the tufts of injected capillaries invading the cartilage along the osteogenic front. This is fibrocartilaginous delayed union.

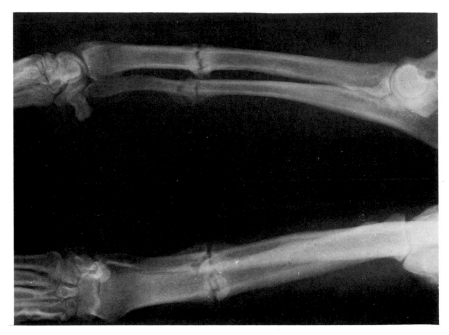

Fig. 18. Final roentgenograms of 6-week displaced fracture of canine radius and ulna. Although excellent position of the fragments was maintained, both fractures are surrounded by heaped-up external callus traversed by a zone of radiolucency—the typical picture of delayed union.

In contrast to the orderly microvascular pattern of fibrocartilaginous delayed union, which will always progress to osseous union if the zone of fibrocartilage is not disrupted, the disordered vascular picture of fibrous nonunion, which requires surgical intervention, is striking. For this, however, one must turn to an osteotomy experiment (see Section IV, C,4 below).

4. Final Dominance of Medullary Circulation

The extreme degree to which the medullary circulation can proliferate, as it provides the major blood supply to external callus, is shown in Fig. 21, a microangiogram from a 12-week displaced fracture of the radius which remained well reduced but was evidently not completely immobilized when the dog walked on its cast. Endosteal osseous union is only in the early stages, and the enormous mass of periosteal callus is still not fully ossified. Nevertheless, the periosteal afferent circulation has receded almost to a resting level. All of the healing areas are supplied by vessels of medullary origin.

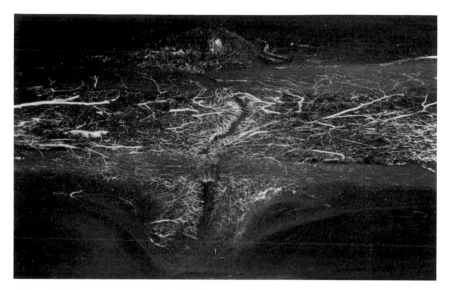

FIG. 19. Microangiogram of radial fracture shown in Fig. 18. Note the avascular zone corresponding to the radiolucency. This represents a plate of fibrocartilage with a brush border of invading capillaries on either side (×4.2).

5. Regeneration of Osteon across Fracture Cleft

Figure 22, from a 16-week displaced fracture experiment, demonstrates a type of healing which may develop at a crevice between two tightly compressed avascular bone fragments.[6] A bridge of new-bone, containing an injected capillary, has traversed the crevice in the same manner that osteons traverse an osteotomy cleft following compression fixation (see Figs. 32 and 34). The difference is that in this 16-week fracture experiment, the process is one of late remodeling of segments of apposed cortex totally devitalized by the injury, whereas following compression fixation of an osteotomy performed with great care to spare blood supply, the process occurs within 4 weeks between viable bone fragments.

6. Summary of Vascular Effects

The studies on displaced closed fractures carried out in the author's laboratory (Rhinelander *et al.*, 1968) may be summarized as follows. The periosteal afferent circulation, derived from overlying soft tissues, is initially highly important in that it supplies the external callus which attempts to bridge the fracture gap. However, this periosteal bridging callus never produces primary osseous union. It always contains an early

[6] For further illustrations from this experiment, see Figs. 19–21 of Rhinelander *et al.* (1968).

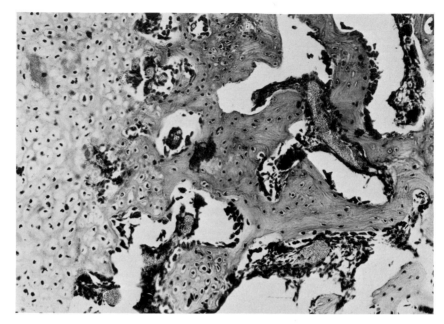

FIG. 20. Photomicrograph demonstrating replacement of fibrocartilage by new-bone, as shown microangiographically in Fig. 19 (H & E, ×8.75).

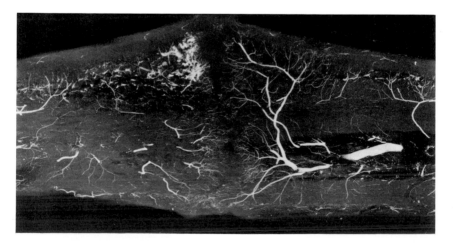

FIG. 21. Microangiogram of 12-week displaced fracture of radius with delayed union. Note the complete dominance of the medullary circulation (×4.2).

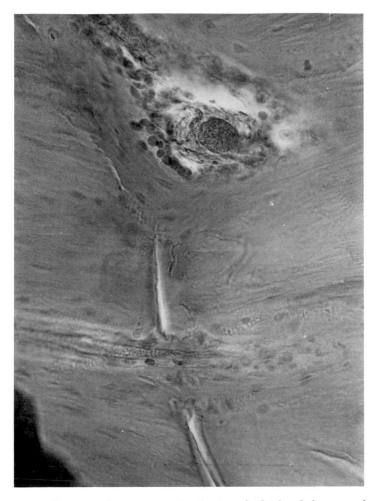

Fig. 22. High-power photomicrograph of 16-week displaced fracture of radius, showing two devitalized segments of cortical bone facing each other across a remnant of the fracture line. Observe the new osteon that has advanced through dead cortex to bridge the fissure which was too narrow for blood vessels and osteoclasts to enter from the ends (H & E, ×330.5).

zone of fibrocartilage. The disrupted medullary circulation also proliferates at once in each main fracture fragment and mediates the production of endosteal osseous callus. In a canine fracture which is well reduced and stabilized, this endosteal osseous callus can bridge the fracture gap within 3 weeks without the intermediate production of fibrocartilage. Arteries derived from the medulla permeate the cortex of both fracture fragments, rendering it extremely porotic, and by 6 weeks they traverse it completely to afford the major blood supply even to the external callus. This is further evidence that the blood supply of cortex is functionally centrifugal in direction of flow.

When major fracture fragments remain widely displaced, as observed in the author's experiments (Rhinelander *et al.*, 1968), or when there is extensive comminution, as demonstrated in the rat by Wray and Spencer (1960), the periosteal afferent circulation persists much longer in the important function of supplying the chief areas of bone repair. It appears, however, that the endosteal circulation makes every attempt to assume the major function of afferent blood supply as soon as possible. Concomitantly, the periosteal efferent circulation, being at the termination of the centrifugal flow through cortex, plays the equally important role of mediating the vascular efflux—from healing bone just as it does from normal bone.

C. OSTEOTOMY AND STANDARD PLATE FIXATION

1. Early Regeneration of Medullary Circulation

The great regenerative powers of the medullary circulation are demonstrated by a 1-week osteotomy experiment in which the radius was securely fixed by a four-hole plate and screws. The medullary blood supply was, of course, severed completely by the transverse osteotomy. The microangiogram, Fig. 23, reveals that fine medullary vessels are already spanning the gap. These are the characteristic arterioles and capillaries of medullary bridging callus which, as stated previously, always produce the first osseous union.

2. Effect on Cortical Blood Supply of Tight and Loose Plate

The microangiogram of Fig. 24 is from a canine experiment in which a transverse osteotomy of the radial shaft had been fixed internally by a standard four-hole plate and screws 3 weeks previously. To the left of the osteotomy, where the plate had remained securely fixed to the bone, the full thickness of cortex is avascular even though the subjacent medullary circulation is intact and should anatomically be supplying at least the inner two-thirds of this segment of cortex.

To the right of the osteotomy, both screws have loosened, and the bone has become depressed by the thickness of one cortex. Vascular granulation tissue has grown beneath the elevated plate, and blood vessels course through the cortical hole provided by one loosened screw. Most significantly, however, the cortex in contact with this granulation tissue is vascularized normally throughout. The periosteal vessels here

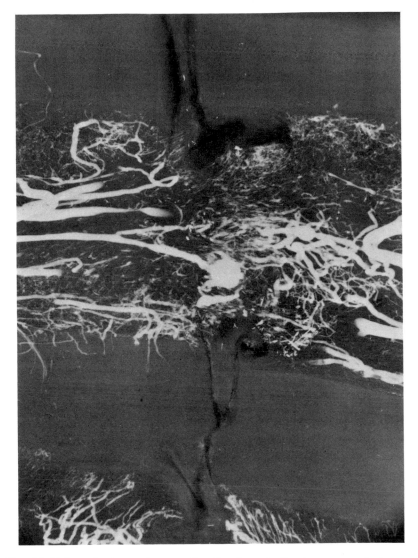

Fig. 23. Enlarged microangiogram of radius 1 week after transverse osteotomy and secure fixation by a standard four-hole bone plate. Observe the reconstitution of medullary vessels that has already taken place (×22.5).

must once have been blocked—when the plate in that area was initially tight. Then there would have existed the situation now observed to the left of the osteotomy—no inflow of blood at all. Thus, on the right, the reestablishment of periosteal vascular connections has apparently permitted the medullary blood supply to function again. The findings

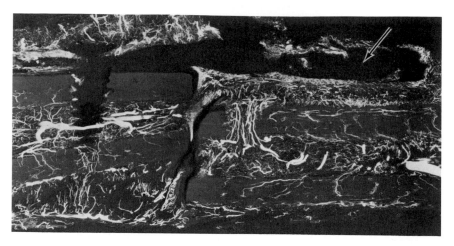

Fɪɢ. 24. Microangiogram of radius 3 weeks after transverse osteotomy and fixation by a four-hole standard plate. One end of the plate has become loosened and elevated (arrow). Blood vessels stream through the space provided by a loosened screw. Note the vascularity of cortex beneath the loose portion of the plate and the avascularity beneath the tight portion (×3.5).

in this experiment suggest that the blood supply of this area of compact bone is through-and-through where flow is concerned—in a centrifugal direction, from medulla to periosteum. This agrees with the conclusions of Brookes quoted in Section III, C above.

In view of the demonstration by the author in subsequent experiments that the type of periosteal attachment to the surface of cortex is of great significance where periosteal blood supply is concerned, it should be noted that the plate in Fig. 24 (as with all bone plates) was applied to a smooth cortical surface, where the periosteum is easy to elevate, and not to an area of heavy fascial attachment (see Section IV, F,4 below).

3. Thermal Necrosis

The avascularity of the small segment of cortex just to the right of the osteotomy in Fig. 24 (between the osteotomy and the screw hole which contains perforating blood vessels) appears to be attributable to thermal necrosis caused by the oscillating power saw (even though well cooled by saline) when the osteotomy was made. Figure 25 shows the histologic picture of this type of thermal necrosis in another 3-week experiment—one in which the plate fixation had remained secure. The osteotomized cortical surfaces have a glazed appearance. They are being attacked by osteoclasts derived from the medullary cavity. An old bone

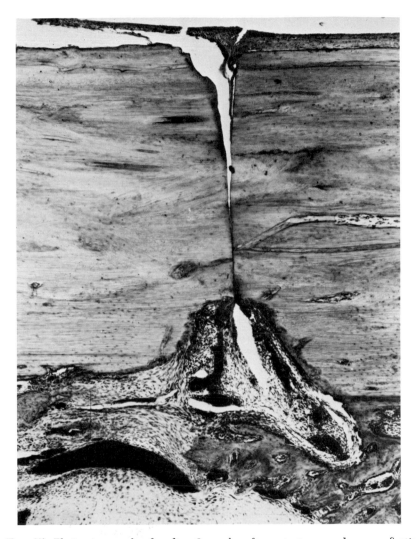

Fig. 25. Photomicrograph of radius 3 weeks after osteotomy and secure fixation by a plate (which lay along the top), showing the effects of thermal necrosis produced by an oscillating power saw (H & E, ×58.5).

canal (on the right) is being revascularized as osteoclasts enlarge it. For a measured distance of 0.8–1.5 mm from the osteotomy, the cortex is necrotic, as judged by the presence of empty lacunae. On magnification, the line of demarcation of the thermal necrosis is seen to be somewhat irregular but quite definite. This visual evidence is a reminder that, even under the best surgical conditions, thermal necrosis can be caused by an oscillating bone saw when cutting thick cortex. A dull drill, or a pin inserted by power, can produce the same effect.

4. Fibrous Nonunion—Pseudarthrosis

The microangiogram of Fig. 26 is from a 6-week osteotomy experiment in which a radius was fixed internally by a four-hole plate and screws. Two of the screws have pulled out. The left-hand bone fragment, from which the screws were extruded, has become displaced downward away from the plate and is well vascularized in contrast to the cortex beneath the tight end of the plate on the right (cf. Fig. 24, at 3 weeks). The space beneath the loosened portion of the plate has become occupied by highly vascularized tissue which is supplied by medullary arterioles that completely traverse the cortex below. The curving osteotomy gap, in the center of the illustration just to the left of the screw hole, is filled by a congested mass of vessels—not at all the orderly microangiographic pattern of fibrocartilage undergoing ossification (Fig. 19).

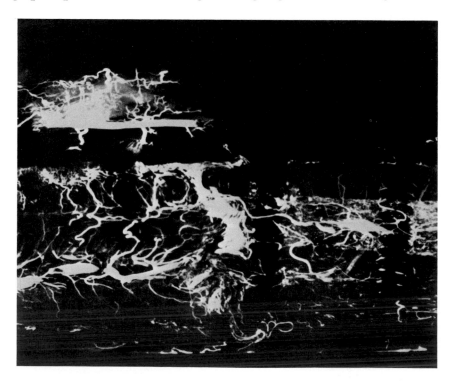

FIG. 26. Microangiogram 6 weeks after unsuccessful osteotomy and plating of a radius. One end of the plate has loosened. The disordered microvascular pattern of fibrous nonunion is demonstrated ($\times 5.1$).

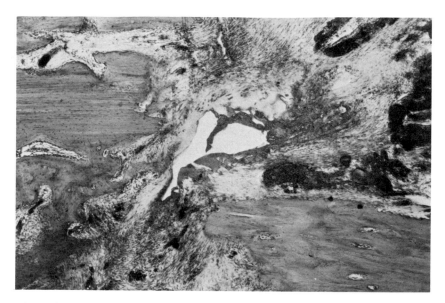

Fig. 27. Histologic enlargement from central area of vascular congestion at site of osteotomy shown in Fig. 26. Note the beginnings of a pseudarthrotic cavity (H & E, ×52.5).

Histologic enlargement of the healing area (Fig. 27) confirms the impression that there is no osseous or cartilaginous union. The increased local blood supply, observed in the microangiogram, has led to a more rapid invasion of dead bone than is usual at this stage, with the result that the smooth cortical ends, burned by the power saw, have mostly been removed. Detritus and fragments of dead bone are present in the central cavity. To its right are the engorged blood vessels which occupy the center of the microangiogram (Fig. 26). This is the early histologic picture of pseudarthrosis.

5. Effects of Wires and Bands Encircling Diaphysis

Cerclage, or the use of circumferential wires around the diaphysis of a long bone for fracture fixation, bears in some quarters (Charnley, 1957) the unjustified reputation of strangling bone from the vascular viewpoint. However, in the experimental studies of Göthman (1962a,b) on the rabbit's tibia, and in the author's extensive clinical and laboratory experience (Rhinelander, 1968; Rhinelander and Brahms, 1961; Rhinelander et al., 1967), nothing could be further from the truth when the wires are properly applied. Application is greatly facilitated by the use of appropriate surgical instruments (Rhinelander, 1958).

A 4-week canine experiment, involving a fracture of the radial shaft, serves as an example of internal fixation by an L-plate[7] and cerclage. External callus, as required for healing, grew abundantly over the six wire loops that were applied. The high-power histologic section in Fig. 28 shows the periosteal callus surrounding a wire which had secured the narrow tip of an oblique fracture fragment. There is no sign of osseous necrosis. This is the characteristic situation when wires remain tight.

The arterioles of periosteal callus run perpendicularly to the outer surface of cortex as demonstrated in Fig. 16. No significant blood vessels run longitudinally in periosteum to be pinched off by encircling wires. Furthermore, a wire, being round in cross section, makes minimal contact with the cortical surface. Problems arise only when wire loops are used erroneously or inadequately. Under such conditions wires, like screws, can produce cortical necrosis and can loosen.

The vascular effect of Parham bands (steel bands a quarter inch wide) is quite different. When they are tightened snugly around a bone, their broad surface in contact with cortex does interfere with the access of periosteal vessels (Rhinelander and Brahms, 1961). This is analogous to the blocking of periosteal vessels by a plate (see Fig. 24), but the vascular interference is more insidious because the zone of vascular blockade by a Parham band extends all around the bone while that of a plate is along one side only.

6. Types of Callus in Fracture Repair

Figure 29 summarizes by means of paired histologic sections, from the right and left radii of a dog in an 8-week osteotomy experiment (Rhinelander *et al.*, 1967), the three types of fracture repair where the formation of osseous callus is concerned. A fracture or osteotomy, when the opposed ends of cortex are not in absolute contact, heals by means of medullary bridging callus, periosteal bridging callus, and intercortical uniting callus.

Medullary bridging callus is the first to effect osseous union—as shown abundantly both in the osteotomy fixed by a six-hole screw-plate (below) and that fixed by a six-wire L-plate (above). When immobilization is adequate, medullary callus can produce osseous union without the intervention of cartilage.

Periosteal bridging callus is always interrupted at first by a zone of fibrocartilage opposite the fracture or osteotomy site. The amount of periosteal callus does not depend on the size of the surrounding hema-

---

[7] A type of sliding plate which fits into a longitudinal slot and is held in place by multiple circumferential wire loops.

toma, as has sometimes been suggested, but it depends on the degree of stabilization of the bone fragments. The bone fragments of the upper specimen in Fig. 29 had obviously been fixed less securely than those of the lower one, for they have a much larger mass of reinforcing external

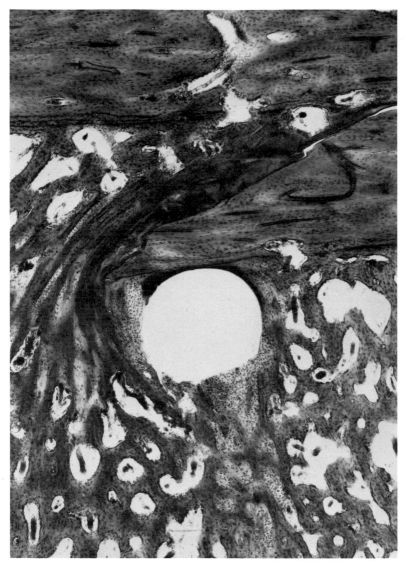

FIG. 28. Photomicrograph of periosteal callus that completely surrounded a wire loop which had securely fixed the tip of a fracture fragment for 4 weeks (H & E, ×40.5).

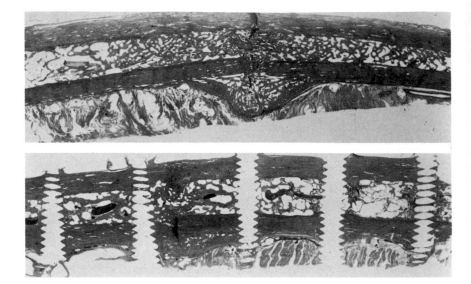

Fig. 29. Photomicrograph of paired radii 8 weeks after osteotomy and internal fixation, showing the three types of osseous callus (see text). The firmer fixation produced less external callus (H & E, ×3.5).

callus. The L-plate and wires, used above, were less rigid than the standard plate and screws, used below. With the even greater rigidity produced by compression-plate fixation (see Section IV, D), all of the required bridging callus develops within the medulla and no periosteal callus need form.

Intercortical uniting callus develops in the course of normal fracture or osteotomy healing, filling whatever gap is present between the bone ends, as demonstrated in Fig. 29. It grows in from both the medullary and periosteal surfaces, and its amount naturally depends on the size of the gap. Where there is no gap, there is, of course, no intercortical callus—as noted at the fracture cleft shown in Fig. 22. The same is observed with compression fixation.

7. Osteotomy Healing vs. Fracture Healing

The microvascular and histologic characteristics of well-advanced osteotomy healing have been examined. Fracture healing differs only in that the disrupted bone ends are irregular in outline, and the blood supply of some of the fragments, which are apt to be multiple, has generally been more compromised by the wider area of injury.

Since the final objective of fracture treatment in man is maximum restoration of total function, internal fixation may be justified when stabilization is difficult to obtain, or when other aspects such as early joint mobilization are considered particularly important. Under those conditions, the increase in stabilization achieved by the surgery must, of course, outweigh the interruption of blood supply which is perpetrated by the surgeon.

D. COMPRESSION PLATE FIXATION

1. Experiments by Other Investigators

Fixation of fractured bone fragments under longitudinal compression is advocated as producing the most perfect immobilization. What does it do to the cortical blood supply? A report by Schenk and Willenegger (1965) of the Swiss ASIF[8] group described a series of experiments on dogs' radii in which compression-plate fixation was carried out after very careful transverse osteotomy. By 6 weeks, regenerating osteons had made their way directly across the osteotomy cleft. There was no radiologically visible callus (all of the bridging callus being within the medulla, as described in Section III, C,6). The Swiss termed this development *primary healing of compact bone.*[9] It was mediated by intimate approximation, rigid fixation, and excellent vascularity of the bone fragments.

2. Experiments in the Author's Laboratory

In a series of experiments reported by Milner and Rhinelander (1968) both distal radial shafts of eight mature dogs were osteotomized by a handsaw five thousandths of an inch thick. This left viable cortex very close to the cut surfaces. The bone fragments were then fixed internally, under longitudinal compression, by the small four-hole ASIF plates and screws.

Compression of one radius of each dog was accomplished by a standard ASIF compression device (Müller *et al.*, 1970), and compression of the other radius by an experimental device designated a pin compressor. In application of either device, final fixation by the bone screws is accomplished while compression is maintained. Then the compression device is removed.

The first contact healing was observed at a 4-week osteotomy. Figure 30 demonstrates the vascular pattern. Several injected vessels traverse the osteotomy. One such vessel is shown histologically in Fig. 31—near the center of the tightly compressed but somewhat offset ends of cortex.

[8] Association for the Study of Internal Fixation (AO in German).
[9] The terms *primary healing of compact bone, primary cortical healing,* and *contact healing* are all applied to the same phenomenon.

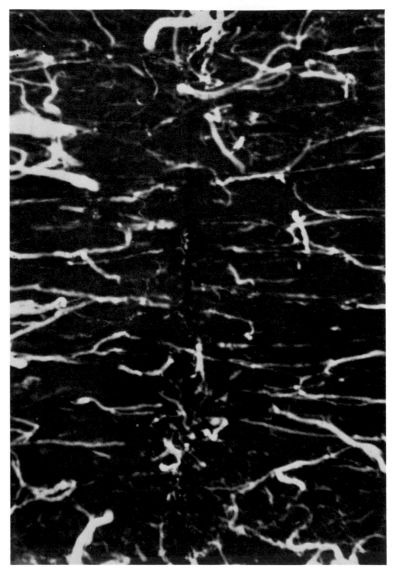

FIG. 30. Enlarged microangiogram of closely apposed cortical surfaces 4 weeks after osteotomy of radius and compression-plate fixation. Note the injected vessels crossing the osteotomy crevice ($\times$40.5).

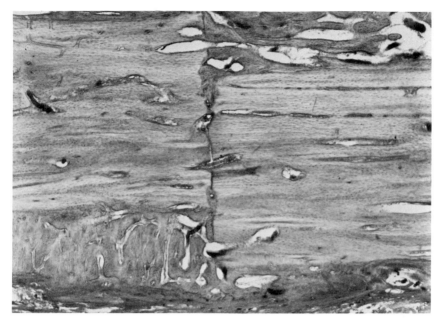

Fig. 31. Photomicrograph corresponding to Fig. 30 showing an arteriole as it crosses the center of the cortical osteotomy (H & E, ×35).

Histologic enlargement (Fig. 32) reveals that this is the central arteriole of an osteon, surrounded by a layer of osteoblasts and a sheath of new bone, both of which cross the osteotomy crevice. This regenerating osteon has evidently been progressing from left to right. Closely beneath this osteon in Fig. 32, the spearhead of another regenerating osteon, moving from right to left, is observed to have just reached the osteotomy. The osteoclastic spearheads of two other regenerating osteons are approaching the cleft, one from the right (above) and one from the left (below).

Contact healing comprises simultaneous healing and reconstruction. Its regenerating osteons are present in large numbers and converge on the osteotomy cleft from both sides; thus, the process appears to be more specifically oriented toward the site of repair than can be accounted for simply by the activities of habitual bone remodeling as suggested by Ham and Harris, Chapter 10, this volume. Furthermore, Schenk and Willenegger (1965) have clearly demonstrated, by means of tetracycline studies, that osteonic remodeling is manyfold more active in the vicinity of compressed osteotomies than it is in normal resting cortex.

A microangiogram from one of the author's 8-week experiments is shown in Fig. 33. The osteotomy site, in tight apposition, is faintly

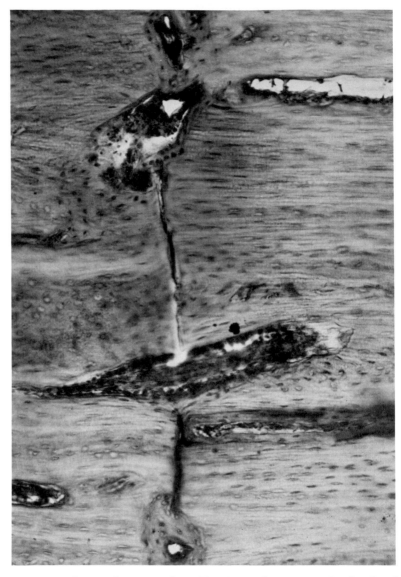

FIG. 32. Histologic enlargement from Fig. 31 to demonstrate the details of the osteon traversing the crevice. Observe also the spearheads of other regenerating osteons approaching the osteotomy cleft (H & E, ×180).

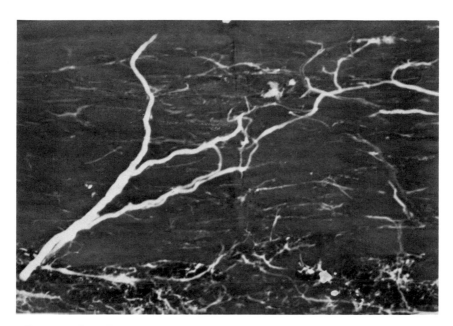

Fig. 33. Enlarged microangiogram showing cortical arterioles crossing the osteotomy crevice 8 weeks after compression-plate fixation. They supply the cortex beneath the site of the plate (×28).

visible down the center. Cortex which lay directly under the plate, above, is supplied by arterioles of medullary origin. Major medullary branches cross the osteotomy, some going to the area beneath the plate. Figure 34 presents the histology of contact healing of canine cortex at 8 weeks.

In the eight dogs with compression plating of both radii, one radius exhibited contact healing at 4 weeks, two radii showed it at 6 weeks, and all four radii at 8 weeks. Primary cortical healing, so-called, is thus easily reproducible experimentally.

3. *Value of Compression Fixation*

The two essential factors in the healing of contiguous bone fragments are blood supply and immobilization. Avascular bone fragments will not unite, and well-vascularized bone fragments will not unite when they are immobilized inadequately. Both of these factors can be compromised to a certain degree, but each must be present to an adequate extent. There are, of course, fundamental differences between bones in their ability to heal with respect to these two factors. Cancellous bone, with its richer intrinsic blood supply and looser texture, unites more rapidly than cortical bone. Ribs, although chiefly cortical in struc-

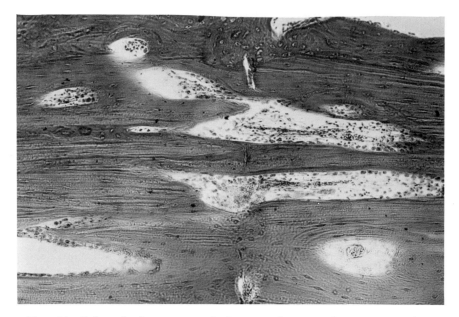

Fig. 34. Enlarged photomicrograph from another 8-week compression-fixation experiment to demonstrate the histologic patterns of advanced contact healing of cortex (H & E, ×140).

ture, heal in the presence of motion which would produce nonunion of a radius or tibia.

The major and serious problems in fracture healing in man concern fractures of the shaft of long bones. Rigid immobilization of cortical bone fragments permits the medullary circulation, which mediates the most rapid osseous healing, to regenerate most effectively. In the dog, secure plate fixation without compression leads to regeneration of medullary vessels across the osteotomy site in a week (Fig. 23). However, the standard type of four-hole plate on the radius frequently loosened in the longer experiments (Figs. 24 and 26). Although the cortex directly beneath a tight plate is initially devascularized, this is inconsequential in comparison with the improved immobilization of the bone fragments which a plate can produce. Plates and screws employed for compression fixation are stronger and stiffer than the usual plates and screws used in bone surgery. In addition to that, however, the specific virtue of compression plating is that, in effect, the strong impingement locks the bone fragments to each other, thus greatly reinforcing the support provided by a plate and screws alone.

The natural question of whether compression fixation does any damage to the compressed cortical surfaces is well answered in the negative by the extensive studies of the Swiss investigators (Perren *et al.*, 1969). The author's experiments (Milner and Rhinelander, 1968) also revealed no evidence of such damage. Acceptable compression devices are engineered to produce only a limited amount of force. Excessive force would tear the screws loose in the bone.

Contact healing, the specific type of cortical repair produced by compression fixation, is not a novel phenomenon. In Fig. 22, it was observed (although at a much later stage of healing) in a fracture treated without surgery. Along a random fracture line, however, tightly apposed surfaces of cortex are relatively rare, whether the treatment be by closed reduction or by open reduction. It is the rigid immobilization, therefore, which recommends compression fixation for the treatment of fractures where continued maintenance of a blood supply adequate to permit direct osseous union is particularly difficult to achieve.

E. INTRAMEDULLARY FIXATION WITH LOOSELY FITTING ROD

1. Blockade of Endosteal Surface

The devascularization of the full thickness of cortex observed beneath a tightly fitting plate was discussed in Section IV,C. What is the effect of blockade of the endosteal surface? This is demonstrated at 3 weeks in a fracture experiment. A closed fracture of a canine tibia was produced by a hydraulic press, which permits precise control of the force applied so that the bone fragments need not become greatly displaced. Surgery was performed immediately after the fracture, with care to avoid periosteal stripping. Internal fixation by means of a $\frac{1}{8}$-inch intramedullary rod of the Rush type was carried out. In the microangiogram, Fig. 35, the tract of the rod is included in only the right-hand two-thirds of the section because the plane of the tissue slice is somewhat oblique. The rod did not fill the medullary cavity completely. Above the rod tract, the medulla contains highly vascular osseous callus, and the adjacent cortex is well supplied by blood vessels—even though introduction of the rod must have obliterated the major medullary arteries. Below, where the rod was in direct contact with the cortex, the inner two-thirds of the cortex are avascular. To the left in the illustration, medullary vessels are observed curving around the centrally placed rod tract and supplying the cortex on both sides.

The small, detached, triangular bone fragment in the fracture line below is mostly avascular, but it is surrounded by highly vascular callus. To the right of this, where the inner two-thirds of the cortex has been

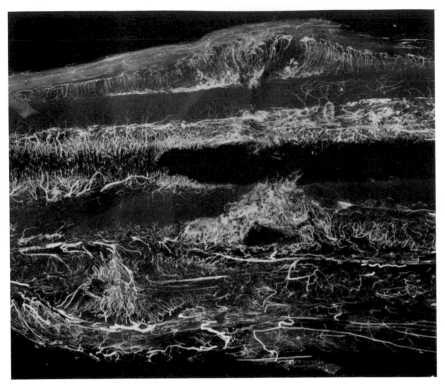

FIG. 35. Microangiogram from 3-week closed fracture of tibia fixed by a loosely
fitting medullary rod. Cortex separated from the rod tract retains its vascularity, while
cortex abutting on the rod tract (lower right) is vascularized in only its outer
third (×3.5).

devascularized, the outer third retains its blood supply via vessels of
periosteal origin. This can only be explained by a locally centripetal
arterial flow—from the periosteum inward. It suggests the proximity
of a fascial attachment carrying periosteal arterioles to the external layer
of cortex. However, in the absence of cross-sectional microangiograms,
a definite conclusion cannot be drawn (see Sections III, E,7 and IV,
F,4).

The effect of continuing blockade of a portion of the endosteal cortical
surface is demonstrated at 6 weeks in a canine osteotomy experiment.
Medullary fixation was carried out by a loosely fitting rod of the Rush
type. In the microangiogram, Fig. 36, it is observed that cortex which
was in contact with the rod (the upper cortex, to the left of the osteotomy) contains very few blood vessels, and that those are chiefly in

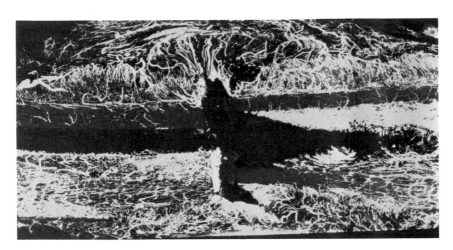

FIG. 36. Microangiogram of 6-week ulnar osteotomy fixed by a loosely fitting medullary rod. Cortex separated from the rod tract is well vascularized, especially that to the left, below. Cortex to the left, above, was in contact with the rod and is only poorly vascularized (see text) (×4.2).

the outer third. Elsewhere in this cortex there are a few additional injected arterioles which were not severed from their medullary connections, presumably because they emanated from alongside the tract of the round rod.[10] The lower left-hand cortex, which was separated from the rod, is so well vascularized that it can scarcely be distinguished from the highly vascularized medulla above it.

The corresponding histologic picture, shown enlarged in Fig. 37, is confirmatory. The lower cortex is seen to be separated from the rod tract by vascular medullary callus. It is markedly porotic, consistent with the stage of fracture healing. However, the upper cortex, next to the rod tract, is almost as dense as normal compactum over its full width. It has not been able to enter significantly into the repair process.

One of the chief vascular events following a fracture is the enormous hypertrophy of all the cortical vascular channels in the area in order to accommodate the increased blood supply required. The lower segment of cortex in Fig. 37 illustrates very well the porosity which accompanies the healing of fractures and osteotomies. As the vascular channels enlarge, bone substance must be removed, thus producing histologic porosity and radiologic demineralization.

The microangiograms from both the 3-week (Fig. 35) and 6-week

[10] A round loose-fitting medullary rod actually contacts cortex only along a narrow zone, and that zone may not correspond exactly to the tissue slice of the microangiogram—as in this illustration.

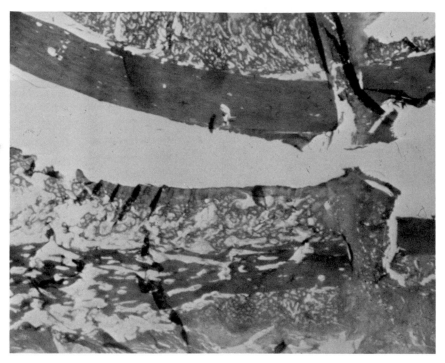

FIG. 37. Photomicrograph of cortices to left of osteotomy in Fig. 36 (somewhat distorted during histologic processing). Observe the marked porosity of the lower cortex which was highly vascularized, and the almost normal density of the upper cortex which was largely deprived of medullary blood supply by contact with the rod (H & E, ×8.5).

(Fig. 36) experiments with loosely fitting medullary rods appear to show that the periosteal circulation, in certain areas, can maintain the blood supply of an outer layer of cortex when access of medullary vessels to the endosteum is blocked by contact with the rod. However, on histologic examination (Fig. 37) it is strikingly evident that the periosteal circulation, in the same area, is not able to produce the vascular proliferation and osseous porosity which should accompany fracture healing. Subsequent experiments with tightly fitting medullary nails will further elucidate this matter.

2. Regenerative Ability of Medullary Circulation

The tremendous ability of the medullary circulation to regenerate after obliteration by an intramedullary nail is demonstrated by Fig. 38, a cross-sectional microangiogram of an ulna in a 7-week osteotomy experi-

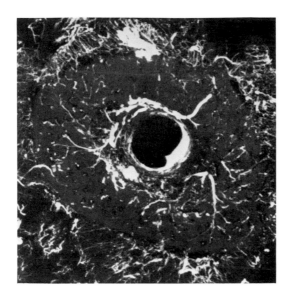

Fig. 38. Microangiogram of cross section of ulna adjacent to 7-week osteotomy fixed by a centrally placed loose-fitting medullary rod. Note the complete regeneration of the medullary blood supply (×5.7).

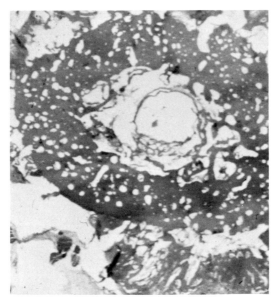

Fig. 39. Photomicrograph corresponding to Fig. 38. The porosity, indicative of enhanced blood supply, is equal in all areas of the cortex (H & E, ×5.7).

ment. The fixation rod, of which the tract lies centrally with an open area of medulla all around it, must have disrupted the medullary blood supply when it was passed. Nevertheless, all of the cortex here visualized is well vascularized by arterioles radiating from large medullary trunks. Histologically (Fig. 39) the degree of porosity is consistent with the stage of fracture repair, and it is evenly distributed all around the circumference. None of this cortex could have been deprived of blood supply for any significant period. Thus, an open space around an intramedullary fixation device permits rapid and complete regeneration of the endosteal circulation.

F. Medullary Reaming and Fixation with Nail That Fills Medulla Completely

The ultimate test of the ability of the medullary circulation to regenerate is provided by experiments in which a tightly fitting nail, completely filling the medullary cavity, is introduced. Since the canine femur was planned for these studies, a preliminary investigation of the normal vascular anatomy of that bone was first carried out.

1. Vascular Studies of Normal Canine Femur

Figure 40[11] is a microangiographic cross section of a normal canine femur at the level of entry of the nutrient artery into the medulla. The nutrient artery and two large medullary arteries are observed to be the only significant avenues of longitudinal blood supply. The cortex exhibits only a few injected vessels, and none of them is directed longitudinally. More are present posteriorly, in the region of the linea aspera, than elsewhere. This is significant in view of the sequelae to this type of medullary nailing. The corresponding histologic picture is shown in Fig. 41. Venae comites, filled with coagulated plasma, lie alongside the nutrient artery and one of the large medullary arteries. The anterior cortex, above, is traversed directly by a large emissary vein which also contains coagulated plasma. Two large nerves are in close proximity to the nutrient artery. This may be significant in view of the demonstration by Cooper *et al.* (1966) in elegant electromyographic studies that small unmyelinated nerves routinely accompany Haversian arterioles. These neurologic elements, distributed throughout the osteons of com-

---

[11] In this and in the subsequent femoral cross sections, the orientation is such that the posterior aspect of the femur (linea aspera) is at the bottom of the illustration.

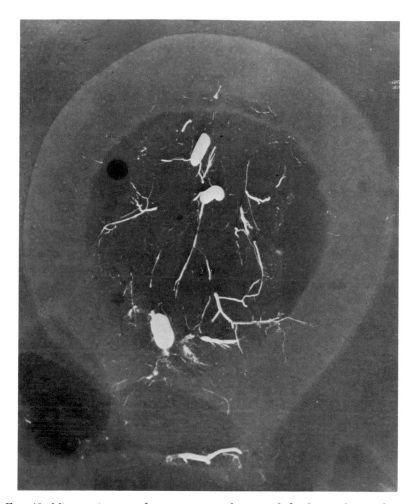

Fɪɢ. 40. Microangiogram of cross section of proximal diaphysis of normal canine femur. (The linea aspera is below, as is the case in all succeeding cross-sectional illustrations.) Observe that the principal nutrient artery and two large medullary arteries are the only major vessels conveying longitudinal blood supply at this level (×9.9).

pact bone, may well be concerned with the control of blood flow through the cortex. As discussed above, the mechanism of this control is obscure.

2. Experiments on Medullary Reaming and Nailing—Surgical Technique

Küntscher's (1967) method of medullary reaming and insertion of an oversized nail has certain clinical advantages; thus, it was adopted for

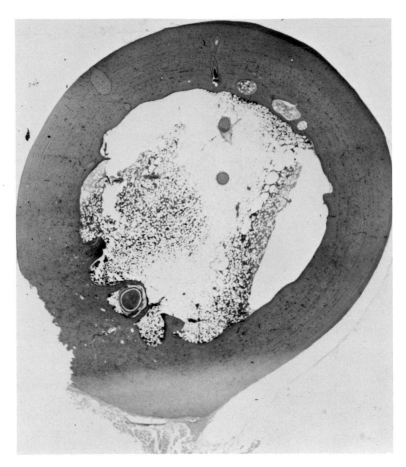

Fig. 41. Photomicrograph corresponding to Fig. 42 showing the nutrient artery just inside the medullary cavity posteriorly and the two medullary arteries anteriorly (H & E, ×9.9).

the author's experiments. However, technical difficulties were immediately encountered. In cross section, as illustrated in Fig. 42A, a Küntscher nail is hollow with three curved lobes in continuity and an opening opposite the middle lobe. The open side of the nail allows it to be slightly compressed from side to side on insertion into a medullary cavity which is slightly smaller in diameter than the overall diameter of the nail. The nail's natural expansibility then assures a tight fit with a firm grip on the endosteal surface of the bone being nailed.

All the available Küntscher nails of the appropriate diameter were too stiff in compressibility for use in dogs' femora. Besides cutting the

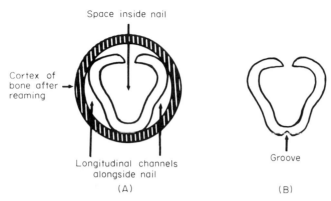

Space inside nail

Cortex of bone after reaming

Longitudinal channels alongside nail

Groove

(A)　　　　　　　　(B)

FIG. 42. Diagram of Küntscher nail in cross section. (A) Nail fitting tightly in reamed (therefore circular) portion of medullary cavity. (B) Nail with V-shaped groove as milled along its full length to enhance its compressibility. An internal expander was used inside this nail.

nails to the proper length, it was therefore also necessary to weaken them in compressibility by milling a longitudinal groove the full length of the middle lobe, as shown in Fig. 42B. The nails would then not expand spontaneously after insertion; thus, an internal expander had to be fabricated for each nail—to be activated and retained *in situ* after the nail had been inserted.

At surgery, the femora were reamed proximally and distally from the midshaft osteotomy site after thorough aspiration of the medullary contents. A small reamer, which passed freely up the medullary cavity without cutting bone, was first used to open a channel in the upper end of the femur next to the greater trochanter. As a result, the larger reamers did not cause a buildup of intramedullary pressure (see Danckwardt-Lilliström *et al.*, 1970). Since the femoral shaft is approximately round, the reamers removed endosteal bone about equally all around the circumference. Reaming was carried out until the thickness of cortex, as visualized at the osteotomy, was reduced by about half. Then a Küntscher nail, containing the internal expander, was introduced from above. Finally, the expander was tightened until the bone fragments were held securely.

3. Results of Experiments

The experiments carried out in the author's laboratory, with the use of the modified Küntscher nails in canine femora, have been described in another publication (Rhinelander, 1971b). In these experiments, tissue specimens were obtained from the midshaft osteotomy area and from the femoral shaft proximally and distally. For the limited discussion of the circulation in bone being presented herewith, the most pertinent specimens are the proximal cross sections—to be compared with the cross sections of the normal femur at the same level. The results at 4, 6, 8, and 12 weeks following surgery will be considered, with presentation of a few representative illustrations.

The microangiogram of Fig. 43 shows the vascular situation in the proximal femoral shaft at 4 weeks. The most highly vascularized tissue occupies protrusions into the medulla, corresponding to the longitudinal channels (see Fig. 42) alongside the nail; and the blood vessels in these protrusions connect with vessels in the extensive external callus. However, the cortex itself contains many more injected vessels than are ob-

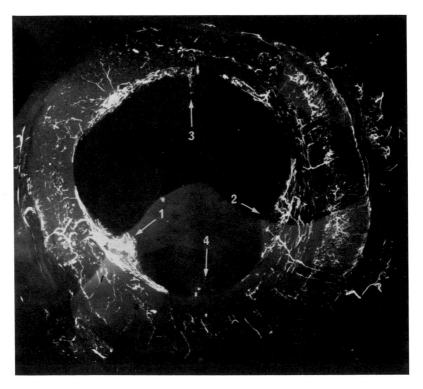

Fig. 43. Microangiogram of proximal femoral diaphysis 4 weeks after midshaft osteotomy, medullary reaming, and internal fixation with a tightly fitting Küntscher nail. (The cavity within the nail was occupied by an internal expander; see Fig. 40.) Medullary blood vessels have regenerated within the longitudinal channels (arrows 1 and 2) on the outside of the nail. Arrow 3 indicates the site of the cleft along the open side of the nail, and arrow 4 indicates the site of the milled groove (×6).

served in the normal femur (Fig. 40), and there is nothing to suggest that these vessels are derived from the periosteal circulation.

One of the medullary protrusions, containing osseous callus, is shown histologically enlarged in Fig. 44. Its small arteries are cut straight across as are also those of the subjacent cortex. This would suggest that these vessels are carrying blood in a longitudinal direction. There are many more longitudinally directed arteries within the cortex than there are in the external callus. It appears, therefore, that the suppressed medullary circulation is regenerating through the substance of cortex to revascularize the compactum in this area, and that the preserved periosteal circulation is not providing any of the new endosteal blood supply.

Examination of enlarged histologic sections shows that the inner layers of cortex adjacent to the medulla contain empty lacunae except around new blood vessels. Only a narrow external zone of the old cortex contains osteocytes. The periosteal callus blends well with the outer circumferential lamellae of cortex. Thus, the periosteal circulation has evidently maintained the viability of some external cortex, although the observed zone of viable osteocytes appears to comprise much less than a third of the original full thickness.

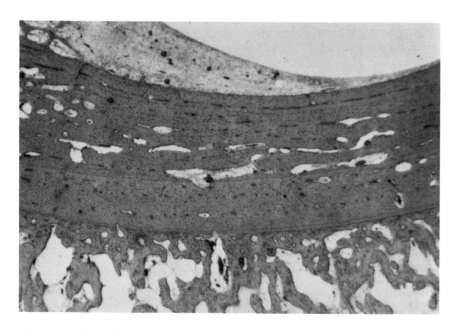

Fig. 44. Enlarged photomicrograph, corresponding to Fig. 43, showing a portion of one of the vascularized protrusions which has grown into the medulla. Observe also the cross-cut arterioles within the cortex (H & E, ×28).

By 6-weeks, the intracortical vascular channels had increased and were conveying the major longitudinal blood supply. Osteoclasts were removing necrotic cortex from the endosteal surface where the nail was in contact, as demonstrated in Fig. 45, to create space for the regenerative

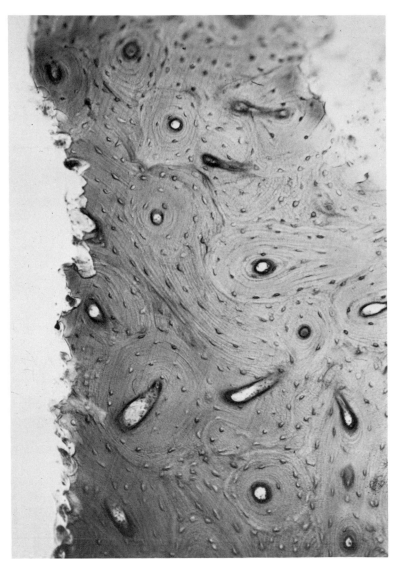

Fig. 45. Enlarged photomicrograph from 6-week experiment to demonstrate the osteoclasis of cortex along the endosteal surface and at the border of an enlarging bone canal. All of this cortex is avascular and necrotic (H & E, ×180).

and highly vascular endosteal membrane which in the longer experiments (Fig. 49) would surround the nail completely.

In the microangiogram at 8 weeks (Fig. 46) there are many vessels traversing the area between the anterior femoral cortex and the new periosteal surface outside the external callus, where two large injected arteries lie against the external surface. The principal nutrient artery is observed in its cortical canal, while a large branch, cut in cross section, occupies a protrusion into the medulla.

High histologic magnification in Fig. 47, which includes a small portion of the regenerative nutrient artery within the medulla, shows that most of the cellular lacunae of even the inner layers of cortex in this

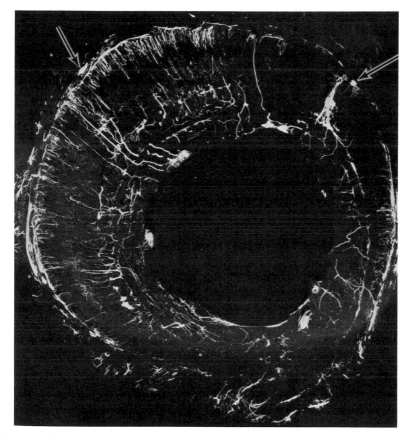

Fɪɢ. 46. Microangiogram from 8-week experiment, showing the principal nutrient artery (below, to right) and two large arteries (arrows) lying just outside the external callus. These extraosseous arteries are furnishing blood for the remodeling of the antero-lateral cortex (×6.6).

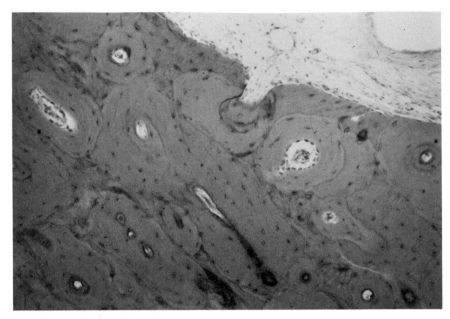

Fig. 47. High-power photomicrograph corresponding to Fig. 46 at the site of the nutrient artery (upper right-hand corner) to demonstrate that the posterior sector of the femoral cortex has remained viable, with osteocytes within most of the lacunae (H & E, ×140).

area contain osteocytes. Significantly, this is the posterior aspect of the femur, near the linea aspera.

At the anterior aspect of this femur, two large cavities within the substance of cortex are observed in the microangiogram (Fig. 46) to be well vascularized, so active repair must be in progress. The right-hand cortical cavity, and the periosteal callus above it, are shown histologically enlarged in Fig. 48. Its walls are scalloped from osteoclasis. It is evidently receiving its blood supply from the large extraosseous artery (noted in Fig. 46) which is giving off a branch inward, through the callus. New-bone formation, originating in the external callus, has crossed the old periosteal line and is invading the outer layer of old cortex.

High histologic magnification reveals that only the outermost one or two lamellae of the old cortex contain residual osteocytes. All the remainder of the anterior and lateral femoral cortices, right down to the reamed endosteal surface, contains only empty lacunae. It would appear, therefore, that the original periosteal circulation had been able to maintain the viability of only a few outer circumferential lamellae of cortex

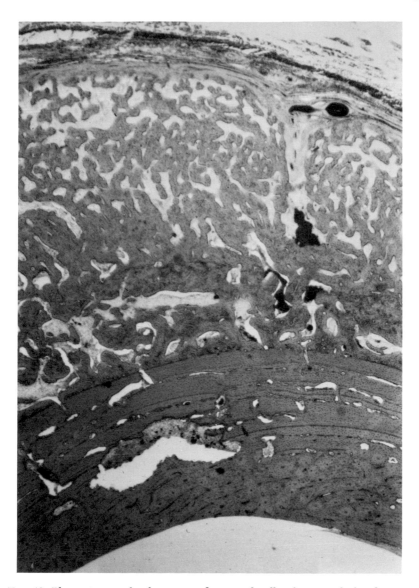

Fɪɢ. 48. Photomicrograph of cortex and external callus facing right-hand arrow of Fig. 46. The large periosteal artery is supplying blood for the remodeling of this anterior cortex, which is completely necrotic except for one or two of the outer circumferential lamellae (H & E, ×22).

(see Fig. 3) after the medullary blood supply was obliterated. Brookes (1964) mentioned a report of areas of cortex where only the most external lamellae appeared to be nourished, through diffusion, by periosteal vessels.

From the 8-week experiment, two important observations are to be made concerning the normal blood supply of the mature dog's femoral diaphysis:

(1) The vascularity of the posterior cortex, in the region of the linea aspera, is only slightly suppressed by medullary reaming, and it comes back rapidly via regeneration of intracortical blood vessels. This is consistent with the further statement by Brookes that accessory nutrient arterioles may be found along the linea aspera. These evidently supply the posterior cortex directly, in anastomosis with arterioles of medullary origin (cf. Fig. 6 regarding the ulna).

(2) The vascularity of the anterior and lateral femoral cortices is almost completely suppressed by medullary reaming. Only a minute external layer of cortex remains viable, evidently having been nourished by periosteal blood vessels. The anterior and lateral femoral cortices, therefore, are in effect supplied exclusively by the medullary arterial circulation. However, after the medullary blood supply has been completely and persistently obliterated, new arteries derived from the surrounding soft tissues are able, belatedly, to penetrate the external callus and furnish blood for the processes of cortical repair. This is not the reversal of the normal centrifugal flow of blood through cortex which Brookes described, for these extraosseous arteries are large new vessels.

There are, thus, highly significant differences in the patterns of normal blood supply, and of reparative blood supply, to different areas circumferentially around the shaft of the femur.

At 12 weeks, the most striking feature of the microangiogram (Fig. 49) is the thick and highly vascularized endosteal membrane which surrounds the entire nail tract. It must have been formed through osteoclastic removal of cortex next to the tight nail, such as was demonstrated in Fig. 45. Arterioles radiate from this endosteal membrane to the cortex all around the circumference of the femur. This was not observed at the earlier time intervals. Scattered longitudinal arterioles persist within the external callus, but they are now not as large as the intracortical arteries observed posteriorly. These, in a group, point right up at the observer when viewed in stereo; thus, unquestionably, they are short segments of major longitudinal trunks.

The cortex everywhere contains fine and irregular vessels, suggesting that revascularization has become more complete than it was at 8 weeks.

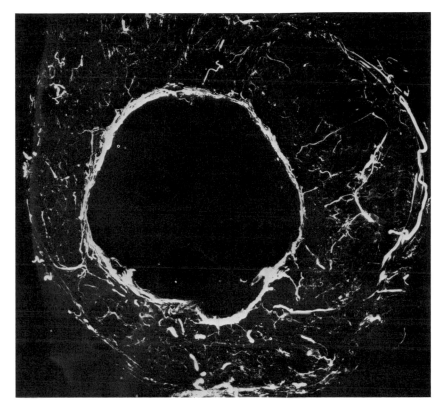

FIG. 49. Microangiogram from 12-week experiment demonstrating a regenerative, highly vascular endosteal membrane completely surrounding the nail tract. Note also, in the posterior cortex, the short segments of arteries which traverse the full thickness of this 1-mm tissue slice as observed stereoscopically. They are, therefore, directed longitudinally in the femur (×6.6).

Many endosteal vessels radiate out into the external callus, consistent with the finding in the fracture experiments (Figs. 13, 14, and 21) that the periosteal callus comes to be supplied by the medullary circulation.

The histologic section of the entire circumference of the femur (Fig. 50) reveals that all of its cortex is osteoporotic, which would indicate supernormal vascularization. The osteoporosis is somewhat greater in the vicinity of the linea aspera, where the major longitudinal intracortical arteries are located. Observe the thick endosteal membrane and its multitudinous small blood vessels. Many of these are cross-cut, as shown on enlargement (Fig. 51), which would indicate that they also are directed longitudinally.

Figure 51 also includes the group of intracortical arteries observed

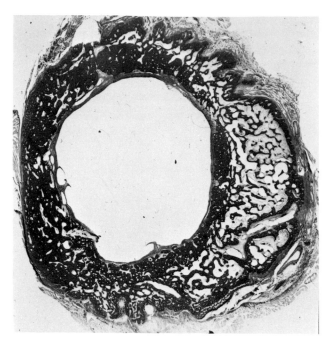

FIG. 50. Photomicrograph corresponding to Fig. 49 showing the increased porosis of all the residual femoral cortex, indicative of advancing revascularization and remodeling (H & E, ×5.2).

in the microangiogram (Fig. 49) posteriorly near the linea aspera. These, as judged by their size, must be conveying the chief longitudinal blood supply to the area of bone repair at the osteotomy site more distally.

In the anterior and lateral cortices, as observed in the overall histologic section (Fig. 50), the repair processes have also advanced as more of the normal medullary blood supply has been restored via the new endosteal membrane. The old external cortex often blends with the surrounding callus, and the external circumferential lamellae have generally been replaced by osteonic new bone. Detailed histologic study reveals, however, that a zone of cortex, directly surrounding the endosteal membrane, remains necrotic and is being replaced. There are still areas where even the external cortical lamellae contain empty lacunae.

The 12-week experiment thus shows progression of the differing revascularization and repair processes of the anterior and posterior femoral cortices. During the progression, the differences have become less marked as the endosteal circulation has continued to proliferate. The most striking features are (1) the advanced regeneration of the medullary

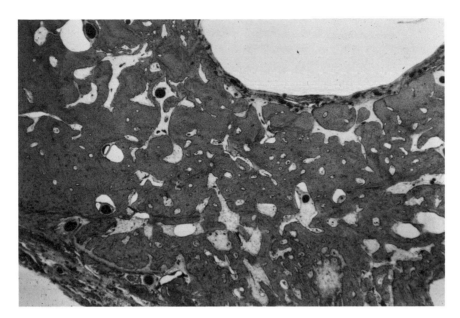

FIG. 51. Enlarged photomicrograph of posterior femoral cortex of Fig. 50, to demonstrate the major intracortical arteries carrying the longitudinal blood supply. Observe also the great number of arterioles in the endosteal membrane (H & E, ×14).

circulation via large intracortical arteries, and (2) the concomitant regression of the new, temporary extraosseous arterial supply to portions of the devitalized cortex which the proliferating endosteal circulation had previously been unable to reach.

4. Critique of Observations on Cortical Blood Supply following Medullary Reaming and Tight Nailing

From the experiments on medullary reaming and internal fixation of canine femora by a tightly fitting nail, it is evident that the normal blood supply of the femoral shaft is different anteriorly and laterally from what it is posteriorly. This is in keeping with the well-known variability of certain aspects of cortical blood supply in different long bones and in different portions of the same bone. The author's experiments demonstrate these differences for the central region of the diaphysis of canine femora, as represented diagrammatically in Fig. 52. Particular aspects of the observations made on these femora are worthy of further analysis.

In all portions of the femoral diaphysis, the medullary circulation,

Anterior

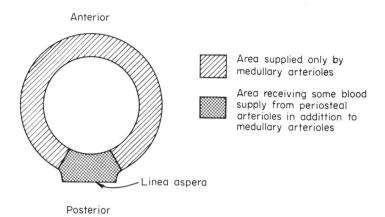

Area supplied only by
medullary arterioles

Area receiving some blood
supply from periosteal
arterioles in addittion to
medullary arterioles

Linea aspera

Posterior

Fig. 52. Drawing from cross section of canine femoral shaft to demonstrate the experimentally observed difference in arterial supply to the anterior and lateral, and to the posterior, portions of the cortex. The indicated limitations of these areas are only approximate, and at their junctions there are undoubtedly an overlap and blending of the two types of afferent blood supply.

derived from the principal nutrient artery, is the primary supplier of cortex. Posteriorly, however, this blood supply is supplemented by periosteal arterioles which reach the diaphysis along the linea aspera. These arterioles have their counterparts along the fascial attachments to other long bones. Since all such arterioles originate in the soft tissues surrounding a long bone, they are generally classified as belonging to the periosteal circulation. This classification leads to much confusion.

As discussed in Section III, C above, the great majority of the vascular connections at the periosteal surface are venules and capillaries, and the normal flow of blood through cortex is centrifugal. Therefore, it would appear to the author helpful to avoid the terms periosteal circulation and periosteal vascular system, which include the few periosteal arterioles, and to use the term efferent vascular system to encompass the predominating efferents at the periosteal surface plus the specific veins which drain the medulla. Likewise, it would appear more meaningful to group together, into their overall nutrient function, the periosteal arterioles (already sometimes called accessory nutrients), the medullary arteries (derived from the principal nutrient), and the metaphyseal arteries, and to describe them all as comprising the afferent vascular system of a long bone.

Further reason for classifying the periosteal arterioles with the metaphyseal arteries is that they are clearly the same type of vessel. Their differences are solely related to the different areas of the long bone where they enter. Both are multiple and approach the bone through soft-tissue planes. Both arborize upon entering the bone, and finally anastomose with terminal branches of medullary arteries to assist in the blood supply of the compactum. Such an anastomosis, in longitudinal section, was illustrated in Fig. 6 from the author's investigation of the blood supply of the normal ulna.

The foregoing basic classification on functional grounds (afferent and efferent) of the blood vessels participating in the circulation of a long bone, rather than on anatomic grounds (medullary and periosteal), helps to clarify some of the conflicting results reported by other investigators in suppressive vascular experiments as described by Brookes (1964). And it elucidates the author's experimental observation that only the outermost lamellae of the cortex (and in some areas, no cortex at all) remain viable around the anterior and lateral aspects of the femoral diaphysis after medullary reaming and tight nailing. This observation is in conflict with the usual description of the blood supply of a long bone, namely, that the inner two-thirds of the cortex are supplied by the medullary circulation and the outer one third, by the periosteal circulation. The discrepancy is explained in simplest terms when one ignores the periosteal circulation as such, and describes the anterior and lateral cortices of the femur as areas where the entire afferent blood supply comes from arterioles of medullary origin.

In consequence of the differing types of afferent blood supply between the posterior, and the anterior and lateral, femoral cortices, the local processes of repair would also be expected to differ. This was, indeed, observed experimentally. Following medullary reaming and tight nailing, the posterior cortex at the linea aspera (which had been only incompletely devascularized, being supplied normally in part by accessory nutrient arterioles) was able rapidly to become fully revascularized via the preserved accessory nutrients plus the regenerative endosteal arteries emanating from the remnants of the medullary afferent system. On the other hand, the anterior and lateral cortices (which had been almost completely devascularized) were very slowly revascularized and remodeled. Transitory aid was provided by new extraosseous arteries that gave off branches which passed inwardly through the external callus. These supplied localized areas of the necrotic cortex until the endosteal afferent circulation, derived from the medullary, could regenerate and once more take over completely. Thus, as osseous repair advanced toward completion, the twofold nutrient supply (mostly medullary, in small part periosteal) became again the sole source of blood for all areas of cortex.

V. Vascularization of Cancellous Chip Grafts and Transplants

A. BACKGROUND

The primary objective of bone grafting, in the author's estimation, is to accomplish complete incorporation of living graft material into host bone as rapidly as possible without regard to the provision of immediate stabilization by the graft itself. Stabilization of the grafted bone, when lacking, is of course essential, but extensive clinical experience has demonstrated (Rhinelander, 1971a) that stabilization is provided more effectively by suitable metallic support than by any type of bone graft. Furthermore, massive cortical bone grafts, used to bridge defects in human long bones, have been found still to be avascular in the center when they fractured and were regrafted several years after the original application. On the other hand, grafts composed of small particles (cancellous chips and thin cortical slivers) have been observed to be rapidly incorporated and remodeled to become as strong as the neighboring host bone. For example, a 6-inch defect in the femoral shaft of a World War II casualty was bridged by autogenous bone grafts consisting entirely of thin slivers and chips, introduced in three surgical stages. Several years later, in a fall, this man sustained a supracondylar fracture of the same femur. The extensively grafted femoral shaft remained intact.

The difficulty in finding a sufficient amount of suitable autogenous graft material in one individual, for bridging a large bone defect, led the author to set up a research project to examine other types of grafts of small particle size. The experimental work in Trueta's laboratory, as reported by Stringa (1957), suggested that the most sensitive indicator of the take of a bone graft was its vascularization. The author's studies were begun with an examination of cancellous bone chips of various types—homogenous and heterogenous implants in comparison with autogenous grafts.

B. EXPERIMENTAL METHODS

Two recipient sites were used in canine experiments (Rhinelander, 1967; Rhinelander *et al.*, 1971): an *incomplete* defect $\frac{1}{2}$ inch in diameter, made in the proximal tibial metaphysis by means of a hand-turned plug cutter, and a *complete* defect consisting of a 1-cm discontinuity in the proximal ulnar diaphysis, made by a saline-cooled double-bladed power-driven bone saw. A Teflon spacer was placed in the complete defect for 3 or 4 weeks before the bone grafting in order to create an environment which resembled an established clinical nonunion.

All cancellous chips were of approximately match-head size and were packed firmly into the recipient sites. The autogenous chips were obtained freshly from the ilium or the proximal tibia. The homogenous chips were harvested from dogs' ilia and were stored at —4°F before implantation. The heterogenous chips consisted of commercially processed calf bone.

C. Incomplete Bone Defects

1. Autogenous Cancellous Chips

Autogenous cancellous chips became vascularized very rapidly, as shown at 1 week in the microangiogram of Fig. 53. Blood vessels have already invaded the entire grafted area. Histologically, new-bone formation was observed in contact with the dead chips everywhere. At 3 weeks (Fig. 54) and thereafter, the intensity of the vascularization was found to be decreasing progressively as the formation of new-bone was advancing to fill the spaces between the grafts. Less local blood supply

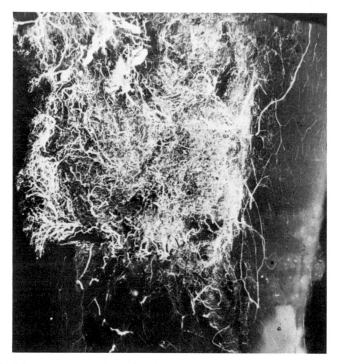

FIG. 53. Microangiogram 1 week after insertion of fresh autogenous cancellous chip grafts into incomplete defect in canine tibial metaphysis, showing vigorous permeation of the entire graft recipient site by injected blood vessels (×6.7).

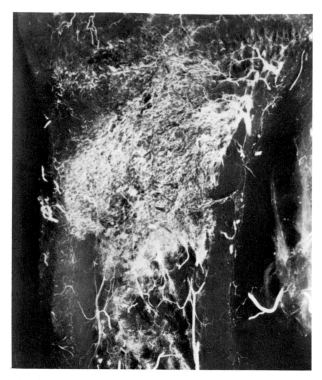

Fig. 54. Microangiogram 3 weeks after insertion of fresh autogenous cancellous chips into incomplete bone defect, showing decrease in the vascularity as compared to the 1-week observation (×5.7).

was then required than had been brought in by the initial wave of granulation tissue. By 12 weeks (Fig. 55), the microvascular pattern of the graft site approached that of the surrounding host cancellous bone.

2. Homogenous Cancellous Chips

Homogenous cancellous chips at 1 week in Fig. 56 appear to have fallen out of the recipient site, but on scrutiny of this microangiogram it is evident that some have been vascularized along a narrow zone at the periphery, in contact with host bone. Examination of the histologic sections reveals grafts throughout the whole area, but granulation tissue and new-bone formation peripherally only. By 3 weeks in Fig. 57 most of the graft site has been vascularized. Thereafter, the vascularization decreased, as it had with the autogeneous chips, but the repair process continued to lag in comparison.

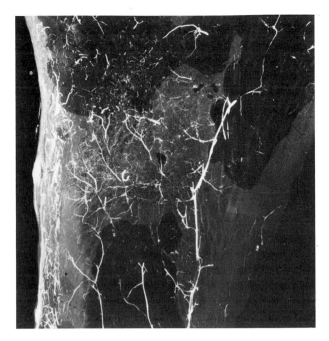

FIG. 55. Microangiogram 12 weeks after insertion of fresh autogenous cancellous chips into incomplete bone defect, showing regression of the vascular pattern to nearly the normal for the surrounding cancellous bone (×4.75).

3. Heterogenous Cancellous Chips

Heterogenous cancellous chips were frequently extruded into the overlying soft tissues. In the best experiment, fine blood vessels pervaded the recipient site at 4 weeks. However, the vascularization was never as intense as had been observed with the autogenous chips. Avascular pockets containing grafts continued to be present even up to 12 weeks. Histologically, the new-bone was not as adherent to the heterogenous graft spicules as it had been to the autogenous and homogenous spicules. Furthermore, there were scattered areas of round-cell infiltration indicative of a local inflammatory reaction.

D. COMPLETE LONG BONE DEFECTS

The ultimate test of the efficacy of a bone graft material is its ability to be incorporated completely into a discontinuity in the shaft of a long bone. Only the experiments with autogenous cancellous chips have so far been completed in the author's laboratory. Within 1 week, as

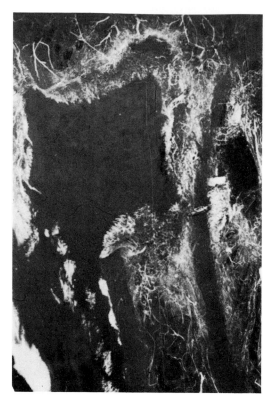

Fig. 56. Microangiogram 1 week after insertion of frozen homogenous cancellous chip grafts into incomplete bone defect, showing injected blood vessels in only a narrow zone around the periphery of the graft site (×4.75).

demonstrated in Fig. 58, these were vascularized as rapidly as they were when introduced into an incomplete defect (Fig. 53). Equally rapid incorporation of the grafts also took place histologically, and by 12 weeks the recipient site was a solid mass of mature cancellous bone with a shell of new cortex covering the external surface. Regeneration of a new medullary cavity to complete the remodeling would be expected to follow, but experiments covering this phase have not yet been carried out.

E. CONCLUSIONS REGARDING VASCULARIZATION OF CANCELLOUS
   CHIP GRAFTS

The rapidity with which highly vascular granulation tissue pervades a mass of fresh autogenous cancellous chips is remarkable. In the dog,

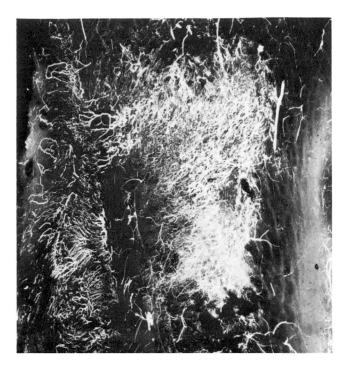

Fig. 57. Microangiogram 3 weeks after insertion of frozen homogenous cancellous chips into incomplete bone defect, showing vascularization of almost the entire graft site and spread of increased vascularity into the adjacent metaphysis (×5.7).

a ½-inch trephine hole in cancellous bone and a 1-cm discontinuity in cortical bone were completely and intensely vascularized within 1 week after the grafts had been introduced. Control experiments, in which the same bone defects were created but were left to become filled only by blood, showed vascularization very much more slowly, as the hematoma organized and new-bone grew in from the periphery. In the homograft experiments, the defects also became fully vascularized more rapidly then they did in the controls. (The heterografts used in this study had apparently not been adequately processed. They gave generally poor but variable results and will not be discussed further.)

It is thus evident that autogenous and homogenous cancellous chips, packed closely within the hematoma in a prepared bone defect, act as a three-dimensional scaffold over which capillaries can progress with enhanced ability. Fresh autogenous chips appear to act as more than just a scaffold. They evidently possess some factor, not possessed by homografts, which induces especially rapid capillary invasion and new-bone production.

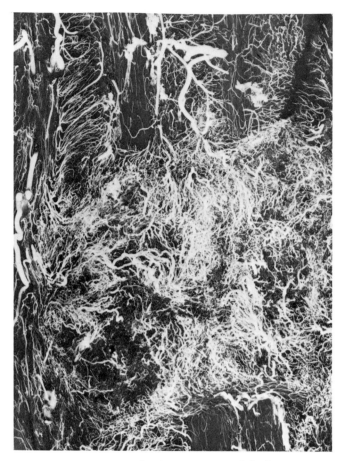

Fig. 58. Microangiogram 1 week after insertion of fresh autogenous cancellous chips into a discontinuity in a canine ulnar diaphysis, showing invasion of the entire recipient site by active blood vessels (×5.7).

These experiments also confirm the author's impression that vascularization, as judged by microangiography and correlated histology, is the most sensitive indicator of the complete incorporation by the host of a bone graft or implant.

VI. Summary of Circulation in a Mature Long Bone

All of the vessels concerned in the blood supply of bone are conveniently described as either *afferent* or *efferent*, depending upon whether they enter the bone bearing nourishment or leave it bearing waste products. Within the substance of bone, the two systems possess, respectively, their distributing and collecting branches which come together in the capillaries. Having this functional concept in mind, the fundamental aspects of the circulation in mature long bones, based upon the author's experimental observations in the dog and supplemented by some observations of other investigators, may be summarized as follows.

A. The Afferent Vascular System

The three primary components of the afferent vascular system bringing blood to every portion of a long bone may be grouped together as the total nutrient supply. These components are (1) the principal nutrient artery, (2) the metaphyseal arteries, and (3) the periosteal arterioles (see Fig. 59).

(1) The principal nutrient artery (which may be dual) penetrates the diaphyseal cortex without giving off collaterals and divides into ascending and descending medullary arteries. The latter subdivide into

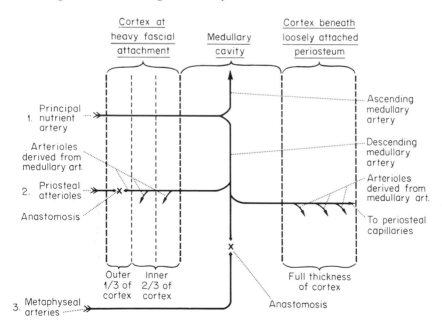

Fig. 59. Diagrammatic representation of author's concept of the afferent vascular system of a mature long bone and its distribution. 1, 2, and 3 constitute the total nutrient supply. Arrows indicate direction of blood flow.

arterioles which are distributed to all areas of the endosteal surface and furnish the major arterial supply to all diaphyseal cortex.

(2) The metaphyseal arteries enter each metaphysis and arborize to provide the blood supply of the constituent cancellous bone. They are also in important anastomoses with terminal branches of the ascending and descending medullary arteries—with the effect that they can rapidly divert a major amount of blood to the medullary circulation and thereby can maintain the nourishment of diaphyseal cortex when the primary branches of the principal nutrient artery have been disrupted by a fracture.

(3) The periosteal arterioles (sometimes termed accessory nutrient arterioles) enter diaphyseal cortex along heavy fascial attachments (such as along the linea aspera of the femur and the ridge for the interosseous membrane of the ulna) and aid in the supply of compact bone close to where they enter, but not elsewhere. They anastomose locally, within the outer third or quarter of cortex, with arterioles derived from the medullary arteries. When the medullary circulation is obliterated by insertion of an intramedullary nail in fracture fixation, the periosteal arterioles appear able to maintain the viability of the compactum in their immediate vicinity but not more widely.

B. The Efferent Vascular System

The components of the efferent vascular system of a long bone are (1) the large emissary veins and vena comitans of the principal nutrient artery, (2) the cortical venous channels, and (3) the periosteal capillaries (see Fig. 2).

(1) The emissary veins and nutrient vena comitans arise from the central venous sinus of the medulla and are concerned chiefly with drainage from the hematopoietic elements of the marrow. Minute vascular channels in the diaphyseal compactum, close to the endosteal surface, have been observed returning postcapillary blood back to the medullary cavity (Brånemark, 1959). However, the drainage from the greater proportion of the cortex is via venous channels which reach the periosteal surface.

(2) The cortical venous channels, which drain most of the compactum, are numerous and ill defined. They empty into the venous system of the surrounding soft tissues via interfascicular venules. The normal flow of blood through the full thickness of diaphyseal cortex is functionally centrifugal—from medulla to periosteum.

(3) The periosteal capillaries are distributed throughout the apparently smooth surfaces which predominate over diaphyseal cortex.

These are the surfaces where the periosteum is only loosely attached beneath the bellies of muscles and where punctate bleeding occurs when the periosteum is stripped from living bone. Such periosteal capillaries are in continuity with the capillaries of the external layers of cortex and are terminations of the medulla-derived circulation which nourishes these layers. They are thus final participants in the centrifugal flow of cortical blood.

C. The So-called Periosteal Circulation

The commonly used term, periosteal circulation, is confusing (and in the author's opinion should be avoided) because it includes types of vessels of diametrically opposed function: arterioles, venules, and capillaries. The arterioles are a lesser component—supplying blood to the compactum only in the immediate vicinity of the fascial attachments through which they reach the cortex. The venules and the capillaries are predominant components—engaged in the final stages of the centrifugal flow of blood through most of the diaphyseal compactum.

Regardless of their anatomic location, the components of the circulation in bone are classified most clearly in terms of whether they belong to the afferent or to the efferent vascular system.

D. The Effects of Fracture

Both temporal and anatomic factors affect the blood supply of healing compact bone.

(1) In the early repair of fractures, an extraosseous arterial supply, derived from the surrounding soft tissues, furnishes the blood for external callus formation. However, periosteal callus is always traversed by a zone of fibrocartilage; it does not provide the first osseous union unless the fracture be extremely comminuted with multiple small bone fragments, in which case all the blood reaching these fragments must come from the arterioles of the surrounding muscles. Under these conditions, osseous union is greatly delayed.

(2) In the later repair and remodeling of the major fragments of the diaphysis following fracture, the medullary circulation provides all the blood supply. When the two major fragments of cortex are in contact with each other at the fracture site, the medullary vessels in each fragment meet and supply the area of initial osseous union. After 5 weeks in the dog, medulla-derived arterioles penetrate the full thickness of cortex to furnish the chief blood supply even to the external callus.

The flow of blood through cortex must then be very definitely centrifugal—as it is through normal cortex.

(3) When the medullary arteries in a segment of mature canine femur are totally disrupted by reaming and the introduction of a tightly fitting intramedullary nail, by far the greater proportion of diaphyseal cortex, being supplied only by medullary arteries, becomes necrotic. The one or two most external of the circumferential lamellae can remain nourished—presumably by means of a reversal of the usual centrifugal direction of flow through the periosteal capillaries. Penetration of a possibly reversed periosteal blood supply more deeply than the few external lamellae was not observed in the author's experiments. Even the most external lamellae in some areas contained only empty cellular lacunae.

(4) Following the disruption of the medullary circulation by the passage of a nail, the normal periosteal arterioles (accessory nutrients) are able to maintain the viability of cortex in the limited areas where they enter, but they are not able to proliferate in the manner required for repair of an adjacent fracture (see Section IV, E,1 above). For an intermediate period during the repair, new extraosseous arteries can aid in the revascularization of cortex which has been totally devitalized by passage of a tight medullary nail; but a few weeks later, regenerative arteries of the medullary system are again supplying all areas of cortical healing and remodeling. The regenerative powers of the medullary circulation are enormous, leading even to the formation, when necessary for carrying blood to a distance, of new arteries directed longitudinally through compact bone.[12]

E. The Effect on Bone Grafts

A bone graft picks up whatever blood supply is available along its borders in the recipient site. At first, this is always at the capillary level. There is some evidence that the old bone canals in a cortical graft may become revascularized, but complete permeation of an entire massive graft by nutrient-bearing bone canals and canaliculi is an extremely slow process. In man, it requires several years.

Cancellous bone, being structurally a latticework, is much more readily permeated by capillaries than is compact bone. A cancellous graft in

---

[12] It should be emphasized that the above descriptions take into account the observed differences in afferent vascular supply to various areas circumferentially around the diaphysis of the mature canine femur. Danckwardt-Lillieström (1969, Danckwardt-Lillieström *et al.*, 1970) reported a major contribution to cortical repair by the "periosteal vascular system" without reference to circumferential distribution of the vessels.

the form of small chips packed closely together is more rapidly vascularized than is a cancellous block or slab.

Autogenous grafts are vascularized more rapidly than are homogenous transplants, and this is especially striking with cancellous chip grafts. In the dog, a 1-cm discontinuity in the ulnar diaphysis, packed with autogenous cancellous chips, is intensely vascularized throughout within 1 week.

F. Outline of Normal and Reparative Blood Supply

Figure 59 indicates diagrammatically the basic features of the author's present concept of the normal arterial supply of a mature long bone. It is based on the microangiographic findings obtained with a normal canine ulna after physiologic vascular stimulation (Fig. 6) and with a series of canine femora after medullary reaming and nailing (Fig. 52). The difference in distribution of arterial blood to different areas of diaphyseal cortex, with respect to the type of periosteal attachment to the surface in the area, is emphasized.

The left-hand portion of the diagram represents the relatively small area (or areas) where a strong fascial attachment is present, transmitting periosteal arterioles to assist in the supply of the outer third of cortex and to anastomose with arterioles of medullary origin.

The right-hand portion of the diagram represents the predominant areas beneath muscles where the periosteum is only loosely attached and is not able normally to convey blood vessels for supply of the compactum. (Under abnormal conditions, the efferent periosteal capillaries in these areas do appear able to reverse their direction of flow and maintain the vitality of a few outer circumferential cortical lamellae.)

The arterial supply of diaphyseal cortex appears, thus, to be derived overwhelmingly from the medulla, and the flow of blood through cortex (taking account also of the efferent system) appears to be in effect entirely centrifugal from medulla to periosteum.

Because the so-called periosteal circulation of a normal long bone contains both arterioles and venules, this designation is confusing in a description of osseous blood supply. The term *afferent vascular system* clearly covers the three components of the total nutrient supply (Fig. 59), and the term *efferent vascular system* covers all veins, venules, and capillaries which drain the various areas of a long bone regardless of their anatomic locations.

When a fractured long bone is undergoing repair, an important early contribution of blood (for external callus formation) comes from the arterial system of the surrounding muscles which have been torn by the injury. This is an entirely new avenue of blood supply, and it should not be classified with the nutrient supply of the uninjured bone. The term periosteal circulation, as frequently applied to this new source of blood, is confusing here also because of the protean implications of the word periosteal in vascular anatomy. A better designation of the source of early additional blood for healing bone would appear to be the extraosseous circulation.

In the later stages of fracture repair, the arterial supply reverts entirely to the intraosseous vessels of the normal afferent system.

Acknowledgments

The experimental work carried out in the author's laboratory was supported by United States Health Service Research Grant No. AM 2579.

Many of the illustrations have been published previously by the author. Figures 4, 5, 8–14 are reproduced from Rhinelander and Baragry (1962). Figure 24 is reproduced from Rhinelander (1965). Figures 17–19, 21, and 22 are reproduced from Rhinelander *et al.* (1968). Figures 6, 15, 16, 20, 23, 25, 28, and 38 are reproduced from Rhinelander (1968). Figures 31 and 33 are reproduced from Milner and Rhinelander (1968). All of the other figures have not previously been published or have their sources indicated in the legend.

References

Barclay, A. E. (1951). "Micro-Angiography and Other Radiological Techniques Employed in Biological Research." Blackwell, Oxford.

Bellman, S. (1953). *Acta Radiol., Suppl.* **102.**

Brånemark, P.-I. (1959). *Scand. J. Clin. Lab. Invest.* **2,** Suppl. 38.

Brookes, M. (1960). *J. Anat.* **94,** 552–561.

Brookes, M. (1964). *In* "Modern Trends in Orthopaedics" (J. M. P. Clark, ed.), Vol. 4, Chapter 6, pp. 91–125. Butterworths, London.

Brookes, M. (1971). "The Blood Supply of Bone." Butterworths, London. (Published after this chapter went to press.)

Brookes, M., and Harrison, R. G. (1957). *J. Anat.* **91,** 61.

Brookes, M., Elkin, A. C., Harrison, R. G., and Heald, C. B. (1961). *Lancet* **1,** 1078–1081.

Charnley, J. (1957). "The Closed Treatment of Common Fractures," pp. 18–20. Livingstone, Edinburgh.

Cooper, R. R., Milgram, J. W., and Robinson, R. A. (1966). *J. Bone Joint Surg., Amer. Vol.* **48,** 1239–1271.

Danckwardt-Lillieström, G. (1969). *Acta Orthop. Scand., Suppl.* **128.**

Danckwardt-Lillieström, G., Lorenzi, G. L., and Olerud, S. (1970). *Acta Orthop. Scand., Suppl.* **134.**

de Marneffe, R. (1951). "Recherches Morphologiques et Expérimentales sur la Vascularisation Osseuse." Editions Acta Medica Belgica, Bruxelles.

Güthmann, L. (1900). *Acta Chir. Scand.* **120,** 201–210.

Göthman, L. (1961). *Acta Chir. Scand., Suppl.* **284.**
Göthman, L. (1962a). *Acta Clin. Scand.* **123,** 1–8.
Göthman, L. (1962b). *Acta Chir. Scand.* **123,** 1–11.
Ham, A. W. (1969). "Histology," 6th ed., Fig. 18–41, p. 427. Lippincott, Philadelphia, Pennsylvania.
Hulth, A., and Olerud, S. (1960). *Acta Chir. Scand.* **120,** 220–226.
Johnson, R. W. (1927). *J. Bone Joint Surg.* **9,** 153–184.
Kane, W. J. (1968). *J. Bone Joint Surg., Amer. Vol.* **50,** 801–811.
Küntscher, G. (1967). "Practice of Intramedullary Nailing." Thomas, Springfield, Illinois.
Leriche, R., and Policard, A. (1926). "Les problémes de la physiologie normale et pathologique de l'os." Masson, Paris.
Milner, J. C., and Rhinelander, F. W. (1968). *Surg. Forum* **19,** 453–456.
Müller, M. E., Allgöwer, M., and Willenegger, H. (1970). "Manual of Internal Fixation," Chapter II, pp. 19–41. Springer-Verlag, Berlin and New York.
Perren, S. M., *et al.* (1969). *Acta Orthop. Scand., Suppl.* **125.**
Rhinelander, F. W. (1958). *J. Bone Joint Surg., Amer. Vol.* **40,** 365–374.
Rhinelander, F. W. (1965). *Clin. Orthop. Related Res.* **40,** 12–16.
Rhinelander, F. W. (1967). *Proc. Int. Congr. S.I.C.O.T., 10th, 1966* pp. 636–637.
Rhinelander, F. W. (1968). *J. Bone Joint Surg., Amer. Vol.* **50,** 784–800.
Rhinelander, F. W. (1971a). "The Use of Iliac Bone in Bone Defects. Orthopaedics in World War II—Zone of the Interior." Office of Surgeon General, Department of the Army, Washington, D.C. (in press).
Rhinelander, F. W. (1971b). Vascular Effects of Intramedullary Fixation. (To be published).
Rhinelander, F. W., and Baragry, R. A. (1962). *J. Bone Joint Surg., Amer. Vol.* **44,** 1273–1298.
Rhinelander, F. W., and Brahms, M. A. (1961). *J. Bone Joint Surg., Amer. Vol.* **43,** 599–600.
Rhinelander, F. W., Gracilla, R. V., Phillips, R. S., and Steel, W. M. (1967). *J. Bone Joint Surg., Amer. Vol.* **49,** 1006–1007. (A.A.O.S. Sound-Slide Lecture, No. 134.)
Rhinelander, F. W. Phillips, R. S., Steel, W. M., and Beer, J. C. (1968). *J. Bone Joint Surg., Amer. Vol.* **50,** 643–662.
Rhinelander, F. W., Felber, D. W., Gracilla, R. V., Phillips, R. S., and Steel, W. M. (1971). The Vascularization of Cancellous Chip Bone Grafts—An Experimental Study. (To be published).
Schenk, R., and Willenegger, H. (1965). *Calcif. Tissues 1964, Proc. Eur. Symp. 2nd, 1964* pp. 125–133 Université de Liège, Liège, Belgium.
Shim, S. S. (1968). *J. Bone Joint Surg., Amer. Vol.* **50,** 812–824.
Stringa, G. (1957). *J. Bone Joint Surg., Brit. Vol.* **39,** 395–420.
Trueta, J. (1964). *In* "Bone Biodynamics" (H. M. Frost, ed.), Chapter 15, pp. 245–258. Little, Brown, Boston, Massachusetts.
Trueta, J., Barclay, A. E., Daniel, P. M., Franklin, J. J., and Pritchard, M. M. L. (1947). "Studies of the Renal Circulation." Blackwell, Oxford.
Wray, J. B., and Lynch, C. J. (1959). *J. Bone Joint Surg., Amer. Vol.* **41,** 1143–1148.
Wray, J. B., and Spencer, M. P. (1960). *Surg. Forum* **11,** 444–445.

CHAPTER 2

Phosphatase and Calcification

G. H. BOURNE

I. Historical

Although the phosphatase activity of bone had been discussed as early as 1907 (Suzuki *et al.*, 1907) not much attention was paid to it until the early 1920's when R. Robison, studying the dephosphorylation of hexosemonophosphate by various enzymes, noted that when the soluble calcium and barium salts of this ester were used in his experiments, he obtained a precipitate of calcium and barium phosphate.

This suggested to him that the calcium phosphate of bone might be precipitated *in vivo* in the same way. He therefore placed fresh bones of young rats in solutions of barium hexosemonophosphate and in a few hours found a precipitate of barium phosphate on the bone. Further work (Robison, 1923) showed that bone contains a phosphatase, active not only against hexosemonophosphate but also against a number of other phosphoric esters, e.g., hexosediphosphate, glycerophosphates, and nucleotides (Kay and Robison, 1924). It was also shown that this enzyme was not present in cartilage which was not ossifying but that at the stage of ossification which is represented by hypertrophy of the cells the enzyme appeared. According to Robison, cartilage which never ossifies never shows any phosphatase. The enzyme was found to be present in greatest activity in the ossifying cartilage, bones and teeth of young animals. Bone, in fact, was found to contain very much more phosphatase than any other organ in the body—twice as much as kidney and twenty times as much as liver. It is of interest that Kay (1926) found that in the embryonic animal there was very little phosphatase activity in the kidney but a good deal in the developing bones. Rossi *et al.* (1951a,b,c) have found histochemically, however, a good deal of alkaline phosphatase in the human kidney from the period when it begins to differentiate onward. Phosphatase has been found to be associated not only with ossifying cartilage but also with regions of membranous ossification. Robison conclusion (1932) was that "it was considered legitimate to conclude that the production of the enzyme is a part of those cellular activities which result in the formation of bone." It is of interest that Robison recorded the fact that rachitic bones actually contain more phosphatase than normal.

Robison and his co-workers carried out a good deal of *in vitro* calcification experiments, comparing bones from normal animals with those suffering from rickets. They soaked rib junctions or entire heads of bones of rachitic rats for 8–24 hours in $M/10$ solutions of calcium hexosemonophosphate or calcium glycerophosphate at 37°C. Some bones were split longitudinally. After incubation the bones were washed and fixed and finally stained by treatment with silver nitrate and exposure to light. Robison found that whereas in the bones of a rachitic animal there was a broad metaphysis of uncalcified hypertrophic cartilage, when this bone was incubated with phosphoric ester calcification occurred in large areas of hypertrophic cartilage in the metaphysis which would be calcified *in vivo* if the animal had been placed on a normal diet. This indicated that phosphatase was present in these rachitic bones, and it seemed as though lack of phosphoric ester was a factor in the failure of calcification. It may be of interest in this connection that

Zetterstrøm and Ljunggren (1951) have shown that vitamin D_2 activates alkaline phosphatase at pH 9.7.

An additional series of experiments designed to show further the association between phosphatase and calcification was initiated by Fell and Robison (1929). Fell had previously shown (1925, 1928; Strangeways and Fell, 1926) that if fragments from the end of the limbs of an 8-day chick embryo were explanted *in vitro,* one of two things was likely to happen: If cartilage was already present in the explanted portion it tended to differentiate into a diaphyseal portion with hypertrophied cells and an epiphyseal portion with small cells and, in some cases, bone was deposited in the diaphyseal portion; if, however, a piece of limb bud which contained only undifferentiated mesenchyme was explanted, eventually cartilage was formed from it. However, this cartilage was of the small-celled type and calcification scarcely ever occurred. Fell and Robison found that if cartilage was present in the explant, even if it was the small-celled variety and could be shown by chemical estimation of the control limb rudiments of the other side to contain no phosphatase, it developed the enzyme after a period of incubation. In the second type of explant, i.e., containing undifferentiated mesenchyme, the small-celled cartilage which formed but did not calcify did not develop phosphatase. Robison (1932) believed that the phosphatase was synthesized by osteoblasts and by the hypertrophied cartilage cells.

Similarly, explants of Meckel's cartilage which contained a nonossifying portion which did not calcify *in vitro* did not develop phosphatase while the neighboring palatoquadrate did both.

These experiments (now over forty years old) of Robison and his colleagues appeared to establish an intimate relationship between ossification and phosphatase and Robison adduced the following scheme to explain the role of phosphatase in ossification.

SCHEME OF CALCIFICATION

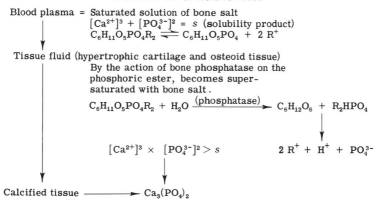

Blood plasma = Saturated solution of bone salt

$$[Ca^{2+}]^3 + [PO_4^{3-}]^2 = s \text{ (solubility product)}$$

$$C_6H_{11}O_5PO_4R_2 \rightleftharpoons C_6H_{11}O_5PO_4 + 2\ R^+$$

Tissue fluid (hypertrophic cartilage and osteoid tissue)

By the action of bone phosphatase on the phosphoric ester, becomes supersaturated with bone salt.

$$C_6H_{11}O_5PO_4R_2 + H_2O \xrightarrow{\text{(phosphatase)}} C_6H_{12}O_6 + R_2HPO_4$$

$$2\ R^+ + H^+ + PO_4^{3-}$$

$$[Ca^{2+}]^3 \times [PO_4^{3-}]^2 > s$$

Calcified tissue $\longrightarrow Ca_3(PO_4)_2$

Robison explained that for simplification he assumed that bone salt was tricalcium phosphate and the ester, hexosemonophosphate, but that the scheme would apply equally well if a more complex bone salt such as carbonato-apatite were precipitated or any other phosphoric ester which could be split by the phosphatase were available.

Martland and Robison (1927) subsequently showed that bone phosphatase would synthesize phosphoric esters from glycerol, glycol, mannitol, glucose, and fructose in the presence of inorganic phosphate. Robison's theory of calcification suggests therefore that the bone phosphatase can synthesize phosphoric esters and then later, by dephosphorylating them at specific sites, secure local concentrations of phosphate which in the presence of calcium would precipitate as bone salt. Robison felt, however, that there was probably a second factor in addition to phosphatase involved in the actual precipitation of the bone salt, but he did not actually establish the nature of such a factor.

II. Identity of Bone Phosphatase and Comparison with Soft Tissue Phosphatase

An enzyme (or enzymes) which hydrolyzes glycerophosphate and other monoesters of phosphoric acid at an alkaline pH is widespread throughout the body. Some soft tissues, e.g., the kidney, contain considerable quantities of it. Such alkaline phosphatase is also normally found in serum.

Whether the soft tissue phosphatases are the same as bone phosphatase is not certain. Various substances inhibit the activity of phosphatases derived from different tissues to a different extent. For example, Bodansky (1937) showed that the activity of bone and kidney phosphatase was retarded by bile acids and that intestinal phosphatase (as might be expected) was not. That there is a similarity between kidney and bone phosphatase is also suggested by the work of King and Hall (1930), who showed in the hen that the phosphatase activity of both these organs was reduced by feeding irradiated ergosterol. On the other hand, a similarity between kidney and intestinal phosphatases was shown by Page and Reside (1930) who found that irradiated ergosterol fed to dogs produced a reduction in the activity of both types of phosphatase. Cloetens (1939) found that the inhibition by CN– takes place in such a way that the presence of two alkaline phosphatases is indicated and Monche *et al.* (1947) claimed that the inhibition produced by the methyl ester of the two tautomeric forms of HCN differed with purified phosphatases derived from a variety of different tissues. There is also evidence that metals such as magnesium, manganese, cobalt, and zinc produce activating effects in phosphatase extracts of different tissues (see Kay, 1930; Massart and Vandendriessche, 1944). Although these results give no clear-cut answer to the identity of various phosphatases it seems reasonable to suggest that the phosphatases of various organs like many of their constituent proteins have a certain degree of specificity (see review by Roche, 1950). The present author has studied histochemically the distribution of the phosphorolytic activity of soft tissues toward a number of phosphate esters (Bourne, 1954a,b,c). These include riboflavin-5-phosphate, pyridoxal phosphate, various sugar phosphates, naphthohydroquinone phosphate, hexesterol, stibestrol and estrone phosphates, two chalcone phosphates and glycerophosphate.

In most organs the pattern of activity was similar to glycerophosphate in the case of the sugar phosphates and the naphthohydroquinone phosphates. But even in the case of the former there were in some organs, e.g., the adrenal cortex, differences between the reaction with glycerophosphate and with sugar phosphates. With the latter, for example, there was much greater nuclear activity. The two vitamin phosphates, the estrogen phosphates, and the chalcone phosphates were all dephosphorylated in a pattern which was in most cases quite different from that of the conventional alkaline phosphatase preparation. The conclusion derived from this work and which is indeed supported by a considerable amount of biochemical work which has gone before is that the body contains a spectrum of phosphatases with overlapping substrate preferences. The various substrates used above have not been applied yet to the study of the dephosphorylating activity of bone, but it seems reasonably certain that there are a number of nonspecific phosphatases present in this tissue. It is of interest to record that Huggins (1931, 1933) found that pieces of urinary and gall bladder epithelium which contain appreciable amounts of glycerophosphatase, when transplanted into the sheath of the rectus muscle, produced bone. If phosphatase plays any part in the formation of bone, therefore, one might well ask why it does not form bone in all parts of the body where it occurs. Huggins and Sammet (1933) found that the artificially produced areas of bone formation were rich in phosphatase. Although bone does not normally form in soft tissues we must remember that occasionally ectopic bone does sometimes occur. For example, Keith (1928) has described the formation of such bone in laparotomy scars, in the choroid coat of the eye, in the breast, the thyroid gland, the aorta, and in the uterus. Kohno (1925) has found ectopic bone in the adrenal. Phosphatase has been found histochemically in all these sites although in some, e.g., the adrenal cortex, it is restricted to the walls of the sinusoids (at least in rats). Huggins and Sammet pointed out that probably the reason why urinary epithelium, for example, does not normally produce bone is that it needs a different type of connective tissue from that usually in contact with it. So perhaps some fibroblasts can be stimulated to form bone in the presence of phosphatase and some cannot. Presumably most of the former are present in association with the various bones which constitute the skeleton, but, in addition, they may occur elsewhere, e.g., rectus muscle sheath. If this is so then the occasional migration of these fibroblasts into regions where phosphatase is present (perhaps only in the capillary vessels which in all organs and tissues appear to be rich in this enzyme) may be the reason for the occurrence of ectopic bones in unusual sites. That different races of fibroblasts do exist in the body has been shown by various authors (see Weiss, 1934).

III. Histological Distribution of Phosphatase in Mature and Developing Bone

A. METHODS

The experiments of Robison and his colleagues in which the ability of bone phosphatase to precipitate calcium phosphate from solutions of calcium salts of hexosemonophosphate and its subsequent demonstration with silver nitrate served to adumbrate the histochemical method for the localization of phosphatase activity in bone and soft tissues which was devised by Gomori (1939) and Takamatsu (1939). Kabat and Furth (1941) and Gomori (1943) subsequently described the localization of the enzyme in fetal bones, and a description of the application of the technique to adult bone was given by the present author (Bourne, 1943a). Most of the latter author's preparations were made on rather thick nondecalcified sections of femur, humerus, and parietal bone and of costochondral junctions of rat and guinea pig.

Kabat and Furth (1941) studied the distribution of phosphatase in the developing bones of human fetuses after decalcification with diammonium citrate.

Lorch, in 1947, produced a method of decalcifying adult mammalian bones with sodium citrate-HCl buffer at pH 4.5, subsequently regenerating the phosphatase with barbitone and then demonstrating it in wax sections of the bone obtained in the usual way. Similar techniques were also introduced by Morse and Greep (1948) and by Zorzoli (1948).

B. MATURE BONE

In mature bone the phosphatase reaction appeared to be restricted to the periosteum (osteoblasts, capillaries, and some fibers) and end-

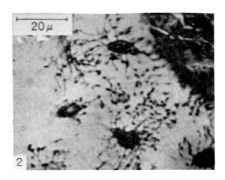

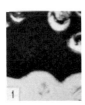

Fig. 1. Wave of phosphatase activity in cartilage matrix prior to ossification in association with damaged rat femur.

Fig. 2. Phosphatase-positive osteocytes in bone. Note positive processes and also positively staining fibers extending from endosteum: taken from the compact bone of rat's rib near the marrow cavity. (Lorch 1947, 1949c. By courtesy of the author and the *Quarterly Journal of Microscopical Science.*)

osteum (including that of the Haversian canals) and to the more super-ficially placed osteocytes (see Bourne, 1942; Lorch, 1947; see also Figs. 1 and 2). These results were confirmed by those of Mäjno and Rouiller (1951) and by other authors, e.g., Morse and Greep (1951). The latter authors found that at edges of bones where bone was actually being formed, not only were the bone-enclosed osteoblasts (including their nuclei, cytoplasm and canaliculi) positive but the matrix was positive too. They also noted a positive reaction in the osteoclasts, confirmed by Mäjno and Rouiller (1951).

Mäjno and Rouiller (1951) showed that osteoblasts have considerable phosphatase activity and that as bone substance encloses them they show less activity and as they become more deeply embedded, and thus older, they become more and more enzymically inactive until finally they become negative. However, they have not lost their ability to syn-thesize phosphatase because in onkosis (which the authors describe as a special form of osteocytic necrobiosis) they show signs of intense phosphatase activity again (see Fig. 3).

C. Bones of Embryos and Newborn Animals

A number of studies have been made on the distribution of alkaline phosphatase in embryonic bone; these include those of Horowitz (1942), Gomori (1943), Zorzoli (1948), Lorch (1949a,b), Bevelander and John-son (1950), Pritchard (1952), Rossi and co-workers (1951a,b,c), and Borghese (1952, 1953) (see Figs. 4 and 5). The findings of these authors are substantially in agreement with each other, but individual reference will be made to some of the results.

Gomori (1943) studied the embryos of mouse, rat, guinea pig, rabbit, dog, pig, chicken, and man and found that the first signs of phosphatase activity in developing bone was in the perichondrium of the vertebrae and the ribs. Zorzoli (1948) also found in mouse embryos that the first signs of ossification occurred in the "connective tissues surrounding the cartilage in a localized region which was destined to become a centre of ossification." Similar findings were described by Borghese (1953) in the mouse embryo and by Lorch (1949a) in *Scyliorhinus canicula* (an elasmobranch) and (1949b) in the trout embryo.

Subsequently, according to Gomori, the perichondrium of practically all cartilage that will later ossify showed the presence of the enzyme. Later still, the cartilage (usually about 20–50 μ across) near the positive portions of the perichondrium gave an intense positive reaction in the cell nuclei and in the matrix. It was in the region of localization of the first reaction within the cartilage that, according to Gomori, the first signs of calcification appeared. The first granules of bone salt were always found at the centers of the phosphatase-positive areas. Borghese (1953) described and figured similar results; see also Zorzoli (1948) and Lorch (1949a,b). In the development of membrane bones Gomori recorded the development of phosphatase activity in strands of connective tissue which later became bone. Within these strands calcium salts, at first granular, and later coalescing, were deposited. Bevelander and

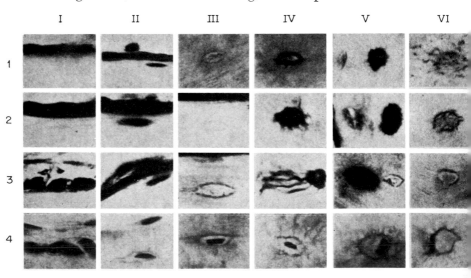

FIG. 3

Johnson (1950) showed in the development of membrane bones in heads of embryo pigs that phosphatase was present in the embryonic mesenchyme in osteoblasts, osteocytes, and in the young spicule of the fibrous matrix prior to calcification. With the progression of mineralization the activity of the enzyme became greatly reduced in the matrix although it persisted in the cells. They noted also that glycogen was present in the periosteal fibroblasts and in osteoblasts and osteocytes. Also, muco-

---

Fig. 3. The human osteocyte cycle in relation to alkaline phosphatase. The scheme illustrated in this figure is a resumé of the evolution of the human osteocyte from the osteoblastic stage to that of necrobiosis (onkosis, see text). The distinction between the six stages is based on the morphological aspect of the cell and its alkaline phosphatase reaction. In each of the vertical columns the first three photographs represent the result of applying the Gomori technique to bone tissue decalcified by the Lorch method. The bottom figure in each column shows an osteocyte in the same stage as those above it but stained with hematoxylin and eosin.

I. Osteoblasts.
    (1) Resting. Three osteoblasts can just be distinguished.
    (2) Active. Showing intense phosphatase activity. Individual osteoblasts cannot be distinguished; black and white line represents a layer of osteoid.
    (3) In Paget's disease. Phosphatase is present in both nucleus and cytoplasm.
    (4) Appearance of osteoblasts with hematoxylin and eosin (bone is below them and marrow above).
II. Young osteocytes.
    (1) (2) (3) Young osteocytes are phosphatase positive.
    (4) Stained hematoxylin and eosin.
III. Adult osteocytes.
    (1) (2) (3) Show loss of phosphatase activity by older osteocytes.
    (4) Appearance with hematoxylin and eosin.
IV. Beginning of necrobiosis. Reappearance of alkaline phosphatase.
    (1) Only slight morphological change in the osteocyte.
    (2) (3) More advanced stages. There is enlargement of the lacunar space in which the osteocyte lies and beginning of phosphatase reaction in the canaliculi.
    (4) Morphological changes and enlargement of the lacuna can be seen in hematoxylin and eosin preparation.
V. Established necrobiosis.
    (1) (2) (3) The phosphatase activity is now as intense as it was in the osteoblasts.
    (4) The hematoxylin and eosin preparation shows considerable enlargement of the lacunar space.
VI. End of necrobiosis.
    (1) At this stage the osteocyte has undergone lysis and phosphatase has disappeared except in the small amounts in the canaliculi.
    (2) (3) Empty lacunae.
    (4) The remains of the nucleus can be seen in the left of the lacuna.
(Reproduced by permission of Dr. Mäjno and Dr. Rouiller and *Virchow's Archiv. für pathologische Anatomie und Phyoiologie und für klinische Medizin.*)

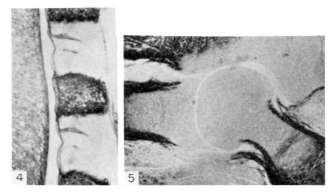

Fig. 4. From 17-day mouse fetus. Sagital section of the vertebral column, showing phosphatase in the hypertrophic cartilage at the stage of onset of ossification.

Fig. 5. From a 17-day mouse fetus. In the right-hand bottom corner is the humerus and the radius; the ulna is to the left. Phosphatase can be seen in hypertrophic cartilage and in the perichondrium. (Figures 9 and 10 are from Borghese (1953), by permission of the author and the *Zeitschrift fur Anatomie und Entwicklungsgeschichte*.)

polysaccharide was present in the periosteal fibers and fibroblasts and later in the bone matrix. It appeared to increase in amount as mineralization of the bone progressed (Figs. 6 and 7). Pritchard (1952) studied the first development of phosphatase in the embryo rat (see Chapter 2, Volume I of this treatise) for some details of his results).

Siffert (1951) also made a study of phosphatase in the bones of growing rabbits and newborn human beings. In general his results agree with those already described but there were some differences and simul-

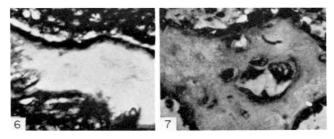

Fig. 6. Phosphatase in membrane bone of embryo pig head. Regions negative for phosphatase are those which have become calcified.

Fig. 7. Phosphatase in section of membrane bone of embryo pig head (decalcified and enzyme reactivated). Note positive osteoblasts lining the bone trabeculae and some positive osteocytes. (Figures 11 and 12 are from Bevelander and Johnson (1950), by permission of the authors and the Wistar Institute of Anatomy and Biology.)

taneously with his phosphatase studies he examined his sections for the presence of free phosphate and chondroitin sulfate (the latter by metachromatic staining with toluidine blue). Siffert also classified cartilage cells approaching zones of ossification into three groups but separated the aligned cells from the hypertrophied cells. In the undifferentiated cells (in agreement with all other authors) he found phosphatase only in the nuclei. He found a complete absence of phosphatase from cytoplasm and matrix and like many other authors found considerable metachromatic staining material in the matrix.

In the next zone (that of aligned cartilage cells) the nuclei of the cells and the matrix were positive; no phosphatase was present in the matrix, but it still stained metachromatically. In the region of hypertrophied cells, at the inner zone of which provisional calcification is beginning, phosphatase was found at first to be intensely active in the cells and matrix and then present in the matrix but not in the cells; the metachromatic substance was still present in the matrix. The simultaneous presence of metachromasia and alkaline phosphatase activity is claimed by Siffert to be in contradistinction to the findings of Sylvén (1947) who suggested that chondroitin sulfate disappeared from cartilage matrix before phosphatase made its appearance and that the removal of the former permitted an alkaline milieu to develop which was favorable to alkaline phosphatase activity.

Siffert (1951), in this study of endochondral ossification, pointed out that alkaline phosphatase, phosphates, and chondroitin sulfate were present in relatively large concentrations in remnants of cartilage present in the metaphysis. He said that these remnants appeared to become calcified without further apparent morphological change almost; as he put it, "as if the remaining constituents were reorganized to form bone matrix." The metachromatic staining ability of these remnants disappeared as calcification took place. During this process they became surrounded by osteoid in which both matrix and cells showed considerable alkaline phosphatase reaction. That free phosphates and phosphatase were found in cartilage cells and fibrocallus in the absence of demonstrable calcium phosphate suggests, ccording to Siffert, that the enzyme may be basically concerned with cellular functions associated with the elaboration of matrix. It is of interest that Follis (1949) found that costochondral cartilage and periosteum contained not only alkaline and acid phosphatases but also an enzyme which attacks depolymerized yeast nucleic acid at neutrality.

Lorch found that in the ribs of a newborn kitten the cartilage at a distance from the costochondral junction was negative. Nearer to the junction the nuclei of the chondrocytes began to give a positive reaction—those of the periphery more strongly than those of the center—but no reaction was given by the matrix or by the perichondrium. In the region of alignment of the cartilage cells the perichondrium became strongly positive, the inner layer being much more intense than the outer layer. A reaction was also present in the nuclei and cytoplasm of the chondrocytes.

At the junction itself the hypertrophic cartilage cells gave no reaction, and only a slight one was given by the matrix.

In long bones of the kitten the endosteum and bone marrow of the epiphysis were positive but the matrix negative. In the diaphysis the matrix was uniformly negative, but the linings of the Haversian canals stood out as black (positive) areas. In the older bone the osteocytes were negative but nearer the epiphysis some cells (including their processes) were obviously positive. In the epiphyseal plate the small-celled cartilage gave no reaction, but in the hypertrophic regions the nuclei of the cells and the matrix did show signs of enzymic activity.

The cells of the articular cartilage also had positive nuclei and their capsules also contained phosphatase—a similar reaction was given in the epiphyseal plate at the region of transition between the small-celled and the hypertrophic cartilage. Morse and Greep (1951) found no evidence of enzymic activity in the outer regions of articular cartilage; they speculated on the possibility of the enzyme being present in the outer region but not being demonstrable. In membrane bone it is of interest that the periosteum on the outer side was positive, but in that on the inner side no evidence of enzymic activity could be seen. The endosteum lining the marrow spaces was uniformly positive.

It is of interest that, besides Lorch, other authors have shown that in the three characteristic zones of cartilage approaching a region of ossification (e.g., at costochondral junctions and at epiphyseal junctions) there are three characteristic zones of phosphate distribution which correspond with these. Morse and Greep (1951) for instance, classified these zones as (1) proliferative zone, (2) hypertrophic zone, and (3) zone of provisional calcification (compare with zones listed by Siffert, 1951). In the first of these zones where the cartilage cells are small and unorientated they found phosphatase only in the nuclei of the cells. In the second zone where the cells are aligned and hypertrophied the cells become progressively richer in enzymic activity as the junction was approached. The increase in activity began first in the nuclei, then in the cytoplasm, and finally in the matrix. The third zone, Morse and Greep found to be relatively free of phosphatase. Similar results have been recorded by Zorzoli (1948) and Borghese (1952, 1953) in the mouse, by Greep et al. (1048) in the rat, by Zorzoli and Mandel (1953)

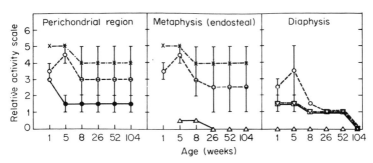

Fig. 8. ATPase activity of mouse bone cells at different age: (●———●) osteo-chondrogenic cells, (○- - -○) osteoblasts, (×-··-×) osteoclasts, (○--○) osteo-blasts, (△———△) osteocytes, (×-··-×) osteoclasts, (□———□) fibrous peristeum, (▽-▽) pre-osteoblasts, (○--○) osteoblasts (periosteal and endosteal), and (△———△) osteocytes. (From Tonna and Severson, 1971.)

in the guinea pig, and by Follis (1949) in man and dog. Tonna and Severson (1971) studied the distribution of ATPase in developing and aging bones of mice and found that osteoclasts had strong activity and that the next most active cells were osteoblasts, osteochondrogenic cells, and osteocytes, in that order. The activity of these cells reached its peak 5 weeks after birth, but the activity then decreased progressively with age except in articular cartilage cells (see Fig. 8).

D. Tumors

The localization of the enzyme in osteogenic sarcomas was described by Gomori (1943). He examined four tumors and found them all to be positive for phosphatase and that the reaction was present both in the cells and in the "fibrillar-intercellular substance." In those tumors which showed areas of sclerosis the sclerotic areas were found to be enzymically much less active. In an osteoblastic metastasis of the breast, Gomori found the tumor cells to be negative but the stroma to show a strong positive reaction. He also showed that in two giant cell tumors and two fibrosarcomas of bone which showed no signs of bone cell formation there was no phosphatase.

E. Developing Bones of Fish

Lorch has examined the distribution of phosphatase in the developing bones of cartilaginous (elasmobranchs) and bony fishes.

The representative of the elasmobranchs used (Lorch, 1949a) was *Scyliorhinus canicula* (Fig. 9A and B). This is of particular interest because the skeleton of this animal, as of other elasmobranch fishes, is composed of calcified cartilage not of bone. In these animals, according to Lorch, calcification always starts at the periphery of a piece of cartilage and is usually remote from and not associated with the cartilage cells. The granules of calcium which are first formed later coalesce and form a series of crystalline plates. The relation of phosphatase to this process had previously aroused the interest of other authors. For ex-

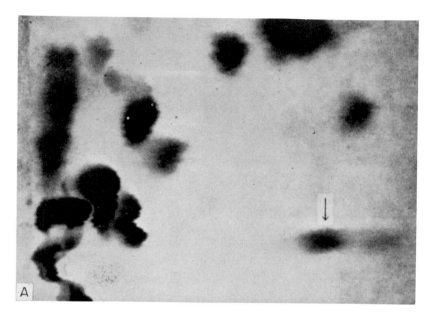

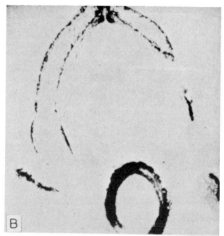
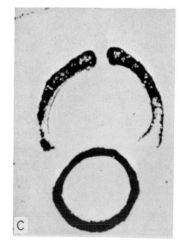

Fig. 9

ample, as long ago as 1931, Bodansky, Bakwin, and Bakwin had shown that alkaline phosphatase was present in the elasmobranch skeleton and Roche and Bullinger (1939) had shown that it was present in both cartilaginous and bony fishes and that it was similar to the bone phosphatase of mammals. Furthermore, these authors found by biochemical means that the enzyme was present in the calcifying portions of cartilage and not in those parts which did not calcify. They also found the enzyme to be present in association with the calcification of scales and teeth. Some important points from Lorch's work can be obtained from the following quotation from her paper:

> Phosphatase is absent from the cartilages of the young embryos and appears first in the chondrocyte nuclei and in the perichondrium. At a stage just prior to calcification the enzyme is also detected in the cartilage matrix. The maximum extracellular phosphatase activity occurs during the first stage of calcification. The phosphatase positive zone then retreats in front of the wave of calcification.

It seems reasonable to claim from these results that phosphatase is concerned with calcification here, as it is in ossification in mammals and (Pritchard, 1950) in frogs and lizards. One important point noted by Lorch was that calcification was found only to occur where *extracellular* phosphatase was present. Also, there was a lag from the time of first appearance of phosphatase to the first signs of calcification. In the cyclostomate fishes, of which the lamprey is a characteristic representative, the skeleton is cartilaginous and never calcifies, although the nuclei of the peripheral chondrocytes gave a positive reaction phosphatase was never found in the matrix. Lorch concluded that in the case of the

---

Fig. 9A. Two-dimensional chromatogram of an acid hydrolyzate of rachitic rat cartilage sprayed with ninhydrin. (Similar results have been obtained by the authors with trichloroacetic acid-extracted material and embryonic chick cartilage.) The arrow indicates the presence of a previously undescribed compound. If the hydrolyzate is treated with phosphatase this spot disappears. It appears to be a galactose amine phosphatase ester and is discussed in section V. (By permission of Dr. DiStefano, Dr. Neuman, and Dr. Rouser, and the *Archives of Biochemistry and Biophysics.*)

Fig. 9B. Phosphatase in a transverse section through the vertebral column of a 75-mm *Scyliorhinus* embryo (decalcified and reactivated specimen). The positive ring at the bottom of the photograph is the notochordal sheath. Note phosphatase is absent from the interior of the neural plates (enclosing the spinal cord) which has become calcified but is still present at the outer edges. This should be compared with

Fig. 9C. Phosphatase in a transverse section through the vertebral column of a 58-mm *Scyliorhinus* embryo. Calcification of the neural plates is just beginning and phosphatase can be seen extending through most of the thickness of the portion enclosing the spinal cord. (B and C are from Lorch, 1949b), by permission of the author and the *Quarterly Journal of Microscopical Science.*)

elasmobranch fishes the only interpretation of the function of phosphatase was that it is concerned directly with calcification and not much with the formation of an organic matrix (see Fig. 9B and C).

In a later paper on the development of the skull of the trout, Lorch (1949b) found that in the early stages of development as in mammals alkaline phosphatase was present in most cells although confined mostly to the nuclei. In mesenchyme and cartilage which was to form bone the activity of the enzyme increased in the nuclei and later spread to the cytoplasm of the cells and to the matrix, while in cartilage which was not to ossify, and in undifferentiated mesenchyme, enzymic activity decreased. Bone was found never to form in the absence of extracellular phosphatase. This is in keeping with the findings in mammalian bone, and in general the relationship of alkaline phosphatase to the processes of ossification observed by Lorch follows in all important respects that were seen by her and by other authors in mammalian skeletal development.

F. Calcification in Other Animals

The possibility that alkaline phosphatase may be concerned with the deposition of calcium salts in other animals has been investigated histochemically by Bourne (1943a) and Wagge (1951).

Manigault, in 1939 and 1941, had shown biochemically that there was a direct correlation in mollusks between liver, mantle and blood phosphatase in the snail, *Helix pomatia,* and calcium precipitation in the shell. The present author investigated histochemically the distribution of alkaline phosphatase in the mantle edge of two representatives of the Mollusca. In these animals the mantle is an organ which is responsible for the production of the shell, and the mantle edge is believed to be the most active portion in this respect. It is by constant deposition of calcium salts from this part of the mantle that the shell grows in size. The two genera of mollusks used for this study were a bivalve mussel, *Mytilus,* and a gastropod, *Callistoma.*

In both these species the mantle edge gave a very strong positive phosphatase reaction, and there was also a good deal of preformed phosphate present which appeared to be in the form of granules of shell substance. Whether phosphatase plays a direct part in the formation of these granules is not known for certain. If it does one would expect, on the precipitation theory, the shell of mollusks to contain appreciable quantities of phosphate, but Pelseneer (1906) stated that in most mollusks only about 1–2.5% of the shell is calcium phosphate. On the other hand, Plate (1922) claimed that the calcium of the mollusk shell is secreted first as the phosphate and that it later changes to the carbonate. Wagge (1951) studied the distribution of alkaline phosphatase in the repair of the damaged shell of the snail, *Helix aspersa.* She found that amoebocytes played an important part in the repair of such damage by transporting calcium carbonate and proteins from other parts of the shell or from the digestive gland (which stores calcium) to the damaged area. After injury the mantle became applied to the area and exuded a fluid containing many amoebocytes over it. The amoebocytes secreted at first a protein membrane which rapidly became calcified. Wagge found that abundant alkaline phosphatase was present during shell repair, both in the injured area and in the calcium-storing cells of the digestive gland. Small amoebocytes were massed around these cells and their nuclei were strongly phosphatase positive; a good deal of extracellular phosphatase was also present. It is of interest that the larger amoebocytes which carry a large quantity of calcium both within their nuclei and within the cytoplasm did not appear to contain phosphatase. The enzyme was also found to be present in the small amoebocytes and extracellularly in the region where the shell was being regenerated.

The present author has also studied (Bourne, 1943a) the phosphatase activity of the shell-secreting membrane of the lobster (*Homarus*). However, the animal was not in a state in which active shell secretion was occurring, and phosphatase was found to be present only in the nuclei of the cells of the membrane and not in the cytoplasm. Further investigations on the relationship between phosphatase and calcification have been carried out by the present author on the oviduct of the fowl.

It is of interest that in the laying hen the alkaline phosphatase activity of the serum is increased by 30% during the period of shell formation. The egg shell appears to be secreted by the uterus, which showed more phosphatase activity than other parts of the reproductive tract. Conrad and Scott (1938) stated that shell deposition begins the moment the egg reaches the uterus. There was some variation in the amount and distribution of phosphatase in this region according to the physiological state in relation to egg laying. In a hen which was killed 36 hours after having laid a well-shelled egg, the walls of the blood vessels in the uterus gave a strong reaction (mainly in the interna), and there was a slight diffuse reaction in the epithelium which was most intense at the brush border. In a hen that had a soft-shelled egg in the uterus and other smaller ones in the upper part of the oviduct the epithelium of the uterus was definitely more positive than any of the other uterine tissues. This reaction was diffuse and was particularly intense at the cuticular borders. The nuclei were also positive. Below the epithelium the cells of tubular glands showed positive nuclei and the outermost portion of the distal regions of the cells contained numerous granules of positive material. It appears therefore that phosphatase may play some part in the secretion of the egg shell in the hen; but when one considers the rapid and spectacular way in which this shell is laid down it is surprising, if phosphatase does play a part, that its activity in the uterus is not very much greater.

The consideration of the calcificatory activities of other animals has shown in general that in these animals, even where, not calcium phosphate but calcium carbonate is being laid down, phosphatase seems to be associated with the process. If the enzyme therefore plays a part in these processes it seems unlikely that it is responsible for the direct precipitation of calcium salt on the lines suggested originally by Robison for bone. However, this problem will be discussed later in the chapter.

For biochemical studies on the association of phosphatase with calcificatory processes in a variety of animals, see the review of Roche (1950).

IV. Phosphatase and Bone Repair

The association of phosphatase with normal bone formation has been demonstrated in the preceding sections, and it remains now to be shown that phosphatase is also associated with the processes of bone repair.

It has been shown (Bourne, 1943a,b, 1948) that phosphatase is involved in the process of healing of 1 mm holes bored in the femur, and in the skulls of guinea pigs, with a dentist's drill. Within 24 hours intense activity was shown by the periosteum surrounding the injured area. This reaction mainly resulted from the strong reaction of the osteoblasts and the capillaries in the osteogenetic layer. The fibrous layer, as has been shown by other authors in ordinary endochondral ossification, gave very little reaction. The osteoblasts showed a diffuse reaction in the cytoplasm and in the nucleus, of about the same intensity. In some preparations a small amount of cartilage had been formed near the hole by the periosteum by the end of one week, and osteoblasts near such regions gave a very intense reaction. It was noticed that where hypertrophied cartilage cells, which were surrounded by only small quantities of matrix, occurred, they often showed intense enzymic activity. In some cases when such cells were surrounded by abundant matrix which had itself given a positive phosphatase reaction, the cell appeared to contain very little of the enzyme. A site of strong activity was seen to occur at the boundary of the cell capsule and the matrix. The impression given by these observations was that the cartilage cell had charged itself with phosphatase presumably by synthesis and then as it elaborated and excreted the cartilage matrix it excreted the phosphatase with it. Similar observations have been made by some of the other authors mentioned earlier. Some specimens of cartilage were found, however, in which the cartilage cells, embedded in a matrix containing phosphatase, themselves demonstrated a high enzymic activity. In some preparations, and rather more noticeable in animals receiving a little less than the normal amount of vitamin C, "fibroblasts" were seen which were outlined by a black border indicating phosphatase activity. The presence of phosphatase at this site probably resulted from either the synthesis of the enzyme by that region of the cell membrane or by its absorption there from the phosphatase-containing medium in which the cell was bathed. Other "fibroblasts" were found with one process stretched out until it had become an elongated thread which gave a positive phosphatase reaction. This suggested the spinning of a fiber made of phosphatase-impregnated protein.

Masses of phosphatase-active fibers were also seen bunched together to form trabeculae (Fig. 10), and in many cases these appeared to be aggregated around phosphatase-active capillaries. All fibers in the repair tissue of many of these holes gave a positive reaction for phosphatase (Fig. 11). It should be noted that although in some cases bone regenerated in these holes in association with the production of small quantities of cartilage, in most cases regeneration was obtained by the process of intramembranous ossification.

Theoretically, therefore, there should be little difference between the changes seen in the repair of these small holes in a bone such as the femur and in a membrane bone such as the parietal. In practice this is so, the main difference being that repair is a very much slower process in the parietal. The present author has studied the phosphatase reaction in healing parietal bones at various periods after the injury. Twenty-four hours after 1 mm holes were bored in the parietals, an accumulation of cells with phosphatase-positive nuclei was found in the injured area

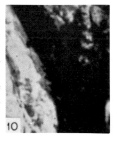

Fig. 10. Phosphatase-positive osteoid trabecula in second stage of repair in damaged *rat* femur.

Fig. 11. Mass of phosphatase-positive fibers in first stage of repair of damaged rat femur.

and in the periosteum and endosteum near the region of the injury. These cells were similar to those found by Fell and Danielli (1943) in injuries to the skin and described by them as polymorphs. Those polymorphs present in the preparations now being described had come probably from the blood vessels in the periosteum, although some may have come also from the blood vessels within the bone itself. It is of interest that it was only when they were relatively close to the area of injury that they gave a strong phosphatase reaction, farther away from the hole it was slight or moderate. It appeared that something was diffusing from the injured area which was inducing phosphatase synthesis or phosphatase absorption by polymorphs when they had migrated close enough to the injured area to come under its influence. Botterell and King (1935) claimed weak phosphatase activity in a fracture callus by the fourth day and strong activity by the eighth day, but Mäjno and Rouiller (1951) claimed that phosphatase-rich cells were present in the periosteum of a fracture callus within 48 hours and that they persisted until the end of the repair processes. In addition to the polymorphs a second type of cell was present at the site of injury after 24 hours. In this type there was a strong positive reaction in both cytoplasm and nucleus and many possessed elongated processes which were rich in enzymic activity. These cells appeared identical with those which could be seen in healing holes in the femur and with those described by Fell and Danielli (1943) in healing skin wounds. It seems fairly certain that they were fibroblasts. Toward the central part of the hole phosphatase-positive cells of a similar appearance seemed to be joining up to form phosphatase-positive capillaries. From many of these cells greatly elongated phosphatase-positive processes could be seen which at their distal ends were of the same size and appearance as the few fibers present in the hole by this time. These cells appeared similar to those found in the healing holes of the femur. At 3 days after injury many phosphatase-positive fibers were seen, but quite a number were also present (probably the more mature fibers) which gave no signs of enzymic activity. Positive osteogenetic fibers could be seen both in the injured area and also in the cellular layers of the nearby periosteum. Most of the nuclei of the periosteal cells gave a positive phosphatase reaction.

After a week of healing two massive concentrations of phosphatase appeared in the repair tissue, one on either side of the hole, and there were histological signs that in these regions formation of osteoid trabeculae was beginning and associated with them were a number of strongly positive and typical osteoblasts.

After 2 weeks phosphatase-positive osteogenetic fibers were still forming, but a lot of negative fibers could also be seen. The greatest concentration of enzymic activity was where the trabeculae were forming and enlarging. None of the enzyme-positive polymorphs could be seen at this stage.

The injured area was invaded during the early period not only by polymorphs and fibroblasts but also by masses of histiocytes. These appeared to flock to the injured area along the blood vessels and along the fibrous layer of the periosteum. Trypan blue preparations showed enormous numbers of them aggregated in the injured area by 24 hours. Phosphatase reactions made on such trypan blue preparations showed, however, that none of the cells containing this dye possessed any phosphatase activity. From these results it is possible to list the apparent cycle of events in such an injury and the association of phosphatase with them.

Following the injury, the hemorrhage, and the clotting of the blood, there was an invasion of the clot by polymorphs (phosphatase positive), histiocytes (phosphatase negative), and fibroblasts (phosphatase positive, at first in the nuclei and around the cell membrane). The fibroblasts then appeared to spin a series of phosphatase-impregnated fibers through the area of injury (see Fig. 12). This continued for some days and then after a period, presumably at maturation of these fibers, the latter lost their enzymic activity. This is in keeping with the findings of Fell and Danielli who found that the first-formed fibers in healing skin wounds were phosphatase positive and that as they matured they lost this activity.

The loss of phosphatase activity by these fibers represents the end of the first stage of repair of bone injury, and it seems to follow essentially the same pattern as in skin. In skin, repair was effected by this time; in bone, however, a second cycle of phosphatase activity soon began and it appeared to be initiated in, and by, obvious osteoblasts. Where these cells were aggregated a great deal of extracellular phosphatase appeared on or among the osteogenetic fibers, and in these regions bony trabeculae began to form. Apparently fresh phosphatase-containing fibers were laid down (see Bourne, 1943a,b) which already contained bone

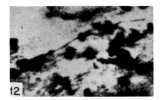

Fig. 12. Repair tissue in healing hole in rat parietal. Note fibroblast-like cell in which both cytoplasm and nucleus give a very strong phosphatase reaction. An elongated phosphatase positive process. (fiber ?) can be seen extending a considerable distance from the cell.

salt: The two processes of production of a phosphatase-impregnated fiber and deposition of bone salt seemed to occur simultaneously. The simultaneous production of matrix and bone salt has also been observed by Urist and McLean (1941). Following the formation of bone, phosphatase activity was again lost from the bone cells and from the matrix. This is in keeping with the results of other authors (see, particularly, Mäjno and Rouiller, 1951). McKelvie and Mann (1948) have suggested that there are two types of osteoblasts, both of which contain alkaline phosphatase. One group, in their opinion, includes the osteocytes of mature bone and the other comprises "matrix cells" which are concerned with matrix formation and which undergo a process of morphological disintegration and physiological death. Both types of cell eventually lose their phosphatase.

Pritchard has made a study of fracture repair in rat, lizard, and frog as representative of three groups of vertebrates. He found very little phosphatase activity associated with the healing of fractures in a frog. He suggested that a reason for this might be that the enzyme in the Amphibia was excessively thermolabile and had been largely destroyed by heat during the process of embedding. However, he suggests that the enzyme may, in fact, be lacking in repair processes in the frog's skeleton and that this might be the explanation for the virtual absence of calcification in the cartilage which forms in association with a healing fracture in this animal. It is of interest too that the author found a deficiency of the enzyme in the normal epiphyseal cartilage of the frog.

In the rat and lizard the relationship of phosphatase to the healing process was more or less the same. The enzyme was found to appear in the region of the fracture as soon as signs of proliferation by medullary and periosteal cells became evident. The reaction was found to be in the proliferating cells, in their nuclear membranes and nucleoli, and also in the intercellular fibers. Some osteoblasts showed a concentration of phosphatase in the Golgi region. In the periosteum it was found that the cells of both layers gave a positive reaction. In general, a reaction was found in the callus in osteoblasts, in the external zone of proliferating cells, and in a patchy manner in cartilage (some cells positive, others with positive capsules, matrix positive in parts). In the frog what small amount of activity appeared to be present was mainly in the nuclei of the osteoblasts and in the nuclei of certain cartilage cells.

The presence of phosphatase in osteoblasts has been confirmed by all authors who have described the relationship of the phosphatase to ossification. Pritchard has described the development of nuclear phosphatase in fibroblast-like cells as an indication that they are or are about to change into preosteoblasts. This became more intense as the osteoblasts became differentiated and the reaction sometimes spread diffusely into the cytoplasm or in some cases into the Golgi apparatus. It is of interest that Cappelin (1948) claimed that phosphatase in fact changes the distribution of the nucleic acids in the fibroblasts of the periosteum, which are undergoing evolution to osteoblasts. The coincidental development of cytoplasmic basophilia and alkaline phosphatase in the developing osteoblast is also recorded by Pritchard, but he did not suggest a causal relationship. It is of interest that he also found glycogen in preosteoblasts but not in the fully differentiated osteoblast.

Mäjno and Rouiller (1951) have studied and figured the life cycle of the human osteoblast in relation to alkaline phosphatase in some detail. They showed the osteoblast to possess potential enzymic activity even in the resting stage and demonstrated that there was an increase of enzymic reaction with the onset of activity both in osteogenesis and in bone resorption such as that found in Paget's disease. Once the osteoblast became incorporated into the bone substance and turned into an osteocyte phosphatase activity was retained for a time, but it became progressively less and less until the cells appeared completely negative. Whether this resulted from loss of the enzyme or from the enzyme's becoming inactive cannot be said, but under certain conditions, e.g., in necrobiosis or onkosis, enzymic activity returned to the osteocyte, apparently developing mainly in the cytoplasm at first. During this stage the processes of the osteocyte in the canaliculi gave a positive reaction. As the onkotic activities developed both nucleus and cytoplasm of the osteocyte showed considerable enzymic activity which eventually became as intense as that found in osteoblasts. With this increase of activity the cell enlarged considerably. Finally, there was a disappearance of the enzyme and a lysis of the cell.

In the ordinary process of bone resorption, Mäjno and Rouiller also found phosphatase played a part because they found that osteoclasts in human beings and in rabbits were very rich in the enzyme, which they thought might be concerned with the synthesis of phosphoric esters, although the significance of this in bone resorption is not obvious. The authors also claimed that osteoclasts have a positive tropism for bone salts. While phosphatase-positive osteoclasts have not been observed by the present author, it is of interest that intense enzymic activity was found extracellularly in bone chips undergoing resorption in the repair tissue in the holes bored in guinea pig bones.

The evident association of phosphatase with ossification and calcificatory processes have led to some experiments in which the enzyme was used to stimulate ossification. Blum (1944) found that if experimental fractures were treated with a mixture of phosphatase and calcium glycerophosphate with or without alginate gel to hold the mixture in position the fractures healed more rapidly. However, Slessor and Wyburn (1948) injected alkaline phosphatase solutions into leg muscles of rabbits and implanted pellets of the enzyme and substrate into muscle but obtained no sign of bone formation or calcification. The present author (Bourne, 1944) has attempted to stimulate bone formation in drill holes in the femur and the parietal of rabbits by packing the hole with crude alkaline phosphatase powder obtained by the method described by Cameron (1930) and by covering such holes with pieces of fresh or alcohol fixed gall and urinary bladder: There was no evidence of increased bone formation. Also, no signs of bone formation or of calcification were obtained when similar pieces of these bladders or of phosphatase powder or of filter paper impregnated with phosphatase were implanted in the sheath of the rectus muscle. It seems from these results that ossification and calcification are processes which are carefully timed *in vivo* and require a balanced reaction between the right types of cells and soft tissues and the initiating factor, whatever this may be.

V. Significance of Phosphatase in Bone Formation

Despite the widespread distribution of alkaline phosphatase in the soft tissues of the body, the intimate asociation of the enzyme with ossification indicates that it plays some special role in this proces. What can this role be? Robison's original view that phosphatase liberated phosphate ions until their concentration exceeded the limits of solubility and they were precipitated in association with calcium is an attractive hypothesis, but their is no evidence that precipitation of bone salt actually occurs, and according to Neuman and Neuman (1953) there is in fact evidence against this occurring. X-ray crystallographic analysis of bone salt shows that it is crystalline and that the crystal structure is compatible with that of a hydroxyapatite. Neuman and Neuman pointed out that the simplest structural unit of such apatite would contain eighteen ions and be such that "a solid phase of apatite could not possibly form spontaneously by precipitation. It can only form by crystallisation, either by a step-wise addition of ions to a nucleation centre or by a similar process involving the hydrolysis of secondary calcium phosphate." They went on to point out that they failed to see how a highly orientated crystal structure can be formed by precipitation.

In a personal communication, Neuman and Neuman (1958) has stressed that the normal serum values of ionic calcium and phosphate are very much below their precipitation points and that if a local factor such as phosphatase were to cause such precipitation it would have to increase the local concentration of phosphate by 300%.

Another argument against the precipitation theory was advanced quite early and was in fact anticipated by Robison and his colleagues; this was that suitable phosphate esters were not present in bone. However, Robison and Martland (1927; see Robison, 1932), as has already been mentioned, showed that bone phosphatase was able to synthesize phosphate esters from glycerol, glycol, and some sugars. That this ability may not have resulted from the phosphatase but from the simultaneous presence of a phosphorylase was indicated by Gutman and Gutman (1941). It is also possible that the phosphatase might act as a transphosphorylase as they have also suggested. In the process of glycolysis one or more phosphate esters could be formed which would serve as substrates for the action of phosphatase. In particular, glucose-1-phosphate was suggested. The association of glycogen with osteogenic processes has been well established, e.g., Glock (1940), Gutman and Yu (1950), and Marks and Shorr (1952). Also, Pritchard (1952) showed that both chondrocytes in the early stages of hypertrophy prior to ossification, and osteoblasts, contain considerable stores of glycogen.

Roche (1950) published a scheme of ossification in which phosphatase took part and which incorporated the conception of the provision of a phosphate ester from glycogen.

Roche pointed out that plasma contained only traces (0.1–0.2 mg) of esterified phosphorus per 100 ml and that since virtually no phosphate ester could be found in cartilage and bone its production from glycogen must be an integral part of the ossification processes.

Dallemagne (1947, 1948, 1950, 1951) has claimed that when PO_4^{3-} ions are released by the action of phosphatase during the period of polymerization of matrix to form ossein there are not sufficient calcium ions brought in by the blood to secure precipitation of all of the phosphate ions. Some, therefore, become temporarily attached to the preosseous organic substance. Later, they are freed to combine with calcium to form more bone salt. As evidence of this, Dallemagne cited the fact that first-formed bone has a calcium to phosphorus ratio of 1.29, which later rises to 2.20.

In support of the agency of phosphatase in causing precipitation of bone salt are the results of Lorch on calcification in the cartilaginous fish, *Scyliorhinus*. In such an animal she could not find any demonstrable change in matrix or cells prior to calcification other than that of phosphatase distribution, although this is not to say that some changes did not occur at a submicroscopic level. Crystalline bone salt, however, appears to be deposited straight into the cartilage matrix. Lorch could not see that phosphatase can have any role in this instance except that of causing precipitation of bone salt.

That such precipitation can in fact lead to the formation of crystalline calcium phosphate is suggested by work on soft tissues using Gomori's histochemical technique. It is known that in this technique precipitation of calcium phosphate takes place by liberation of phosphate ions from the substrate (in most cases glycerophosphate). The resultant precipitate, which is subsequently made visible by the cobalt chloride and ammonium sulfide technique, appears to be amorphous. In preparations of small intestine a deposit of calcium phosphate can be detected by these means in a matter of seconds after incubation, and by 1 minute quite a heavy deposition of the phosphate can be seen in the brush border of the epithelial cells after visualization with cobalt chloride and ammonium sulfide. However, if incubation is continued for some hours the calcium phosphate appears to have disappeared from this region which now gives a negative reaction. Although the cobalt chloride–ammonium sulfide reaction is negative in this case, if the sections after incubation are examined under phase contrast illumination or are treated with silver nitrate and exposed to light, a considerable amount of calcium phosphate is seen still to be present. It can also be shown that this difference is due to a change of the calcium phosphate from the amorphous to the crystalline condition. It is also of interest that the cobalt–ammonium sulfide technique appears to stain recently deposited bone salt but will not stain older bone. On the other hand, silver nitrate will stain mature crystalline bone salt. Can we assume therefore that bone salt is in fact originally deposited in an amorphous condition and changes subsequently to the crystalline form? On the other hand, Carlsen *et al.* (1953) have shown that the calcium phosphate precipitated in a test tube in the Gomori incubation medium used for the histochemical localization of alkaline phosphatase gives the X-ray diffraction pattern of apatite. Thus, although the precipitation theory does not bar the possibility of crystalline bone salt being formed in this way, the strictures of Neuman and his colleagues based on the ionic concentration of Ca^{2+} and PO_4^{3-} in normal serum still apply.

The presence of glycogen in pre-osteoblasts and prehypertrophic chondrocytes may not necessarily be connected with the synthesis of phosphoric esters directly concerned with the formation of bone salt. Many cells accumulate glycogen before entering into a phase of rapid multiplication and/or synthesis or differentiation (the cells of the basal layers of the skin are one example) and it may be that the accumulation of glycogen in bone-forming cells is associated with the secretion of mucopolysaccharides or protein which forms part of the osteoid substance or, as Pritchard has suggested, with differentiation of these cells (see also Follis, 1949; Borghese, 1952). In other words, the glycogen may simply be acting as an energy source and its phosphorolytic breakdown may simply be part of this process.

Despite the earlier claims which denied the existence of phosphate-donating esters in cartilage, work by Albaum *et al.* (1952) has confirmed the presence of adenosine triphosphate (ATP) in preosseous cartilage. As they pointed out, the presence of glycogen and some of the enzymes necessary for its breakdown have already been demonstrated but the presence of ATP had not. They quoted the work of Cartier (1950) who found that calcification of the cartilage of the bones of embryonic sheep was enhanced if ATP was added to the medium. Albaum and his colleagues found that preosseous cartilage contained ATP at the level of brain, kidney, and liver; however, they were not able to say whether it was contained primarily in the matrix or in the cells. The presence of ATP, however, does not mean necessarily that it provides the phosphate actually used in the formation of bone salt; it is more likely to be concerned in the energy exchanges associated with the oxidation of the glycogen.

The apatite crystals of bone (about 350–400 Å long and broad, and about 25–50 Å thick) have been shown by various authors (see Robinson and Watson, 1952, 1955) to be associated with the collagen of bone and to be distributed between the characteristic bands which can be seen in collagen fibers under the electron microscope, the longitudinal axis being parallel to the long axis of the fibers. Neuman and Neuman stated: "The organic phase of osteoid or endochondral cartilage may bind either calcium or phosphate ions in the proper space relationships of the apatite lattice." DiStefano *et al.* (1953) have searched for specific chemical groups in the matrix which, acting as a template, would bind either calcium or phosphorus. Chondroitin sulfate is usually associated with collagen, and calcium ions are known to form complexes with it, but Boyd and Neuman (1951) have shown that such complexes have a high dissociation and that this would reduce the value of the chondroitin sulfate as a template. However, DiStefano and his colleagues discovered in calcifiable cartilage a phosphate ester associated with a matrix substance insoluble in trichloracetic acid. The presence of this, they state, "correlates well with the ability of the cartilage preparation to calcify *in vitro*." The evidence at present available indicates that this ester is a "five- or six-membered heterocyclic compound with ester phosphate and amine groups present but carbonyl groups absent." There is some evidence that it is a galactose derivative possibly 2-amino galactose-6-phosphate (see Fig. 9A). The authors found that if fresh cartilage is given an overnight incubation in saline (which destroys its calcifiability) the amount of this ester is reduced to negligible amounts. They suggested that the ester may form part of the proposed template which is thought to aid the crystallization of bone salt. If this compound is in fact able to function partly or completely as a template for the crystallization of bone salt the role of phosphatase becomes somewhat obscure. The compound is in fact actually attacked by phosphatase, an activity which would certainly destroy its value as a template. This suggests however that Gutman's suggestion of a trans-phosphorylase activity for the enzyme concerned perhaps in the reaction chains associated with the synthesis of such an ester is a more likely field of activity than that of the liberation of phosphate.

In the template theory of bone salt crystal formation in which a phosphate ester forms part of the template the phosphate moiety is already present, and its position controls the point of deposition of the calcium ions which come down little by little in steplike fashion to build up characteristic crystals. In this theory there is no need at all for phosphatase to split off the phosphate in order to secure *precipitation* of the calcium ions. Dallemagne's theory of the binding of phosphate to the matrix fits in well with the template theory—the only point at issue is that he conceives of a subsequent release of the phosphate to *precipitate* the calcium ions, but by the template theory no such release is necessary.

The template theory of calcification may help to explain the deposition of crystalline bone salt in the cartilage of *Scyliorhinus* as described by Lorch. Although some sort of template, probably protein, but not necessarily containing phosphate, is probably concerned with laying down of the shell in mollusks and the shell in birds' eggs it is difficult to see where phosphatase is involved in this process.

Although chondroitin sulfate has been said to be not suitable as a template, recent work suggests that it may play an important part in calcification. Toluidine blue combines with chondroitin sulfate to form a metachromatic staining substance, and Sobel and Burger (1954) have shown that when toluidine blue is present in a calcifying medium the degree of inactivation is a function of the concentration of the dye. This suggests that chondroitin sulfate is responsible in some way for the deposition of bone substance. In addition, Sobel (1956) obtained a complex of chondroitin sulfate and collagen which, when placed in a test tube in solutions employed for *in vitro* calcification, produced 20% ash against control collagen giving only 0.1% ash. Here then, is a preparation which catalyzes deposition of bone salt without the mediation of an enzyme at all.

Where again does phosphatase come in?

Neuman *et al.* (1951) have obtained some results that suggest another possible function for the enzyme. They found that traces of ester phosphates are strongly adsorbed by the bone mineral. The phosphate added onto the crystal and the organic part of the molecule inhibited further crystal growth. Phosphatase, therefore, by hydrolyzing the ester phosphates would permit crystallization to occur on a template which would not otherwise take place in the presence of the latter type of compound.

One other complicating factor, they stated, is that if the template itself contains phosphate esters then the phosphatase is capable of destroying it but does not do so. However, Neuman has shown that in *in vitro* calcification at unphysiological concentrations of the ester the enzyme can be kept busy preferentially hydrolyzing other phosphate esters during the supposed formation of the template; in theory once this is formed and the first bone crystals deposited on it, the template is then protected from attacks by the enzyme. One cannot, of course, say that this is what happens *in vivo*.

It is of interest that bone contains a relatively large amount of citrate and that this has an inhibitory effect on alkaline phosphatase (Baccari and Quagliarello, 1950).

Bones contain a surprising amount of citrate (see Table I). The earlier work was carried out by Dickens (1940, 1941) who demonstrated that compared with other tissues, bone contains substantially more citrate. For example, 70% of the total citric acid in the whole body of the mouse is present in the skeleton. The amount of citrate gradually decreases in old bones (e.g., in medioval and prehistoric bone).

If citrate is added to a solution containing Ca^{2+} ions, it complexes with the calcium and pulls it out of solution. This could be significant in calcium metabolism from many points of view. For example, citrate can facilitate the solution of bone salt even under conditions of high pH.

Dixon and Perkins (1956) believed that calcium bound to citrate represents the major part of the ultrafilterable, nondissociated fraction of serum calcium.

It is possible that the incorporation of citrate into bone could make bone salt more soluble. Dixon and Perkins said about this:

> Evidence of the precise stage at which citrate is involved in the deposition of bone salt is lacking, since citrate cannot readily be demonstrated histologically. It is also difficult to prove that citrate plays any part in causing local dissolution of bone salt. Assuming, however, that resorption takes place without appreciable change of pH, the equilibria governing the stability of precipitated bone salt must be affected by the presence of a substance such as citrate which will remove calcium in the form of a soluble relatively nondissociated compound.

TABLE I

CITRATE CONCENTRATION OF BONES OF VARIOUS SPECIES

Species	Dry, fat-free (%)	Reference[v]
Man (adult)[a]		
Collar bone	1.88	Thunberg, 1948
Femur	1.62	Thunberg, 1948
Rib	1.75	Thunberg, 1948
Vertebra	0.89	Thunberg, 1948
Iliac crest[b]	1.19	Zipkin et al., 1960
Rib[b]	1.08	Zipkin et al., 1960
Vertebra[b]	0.97	Zipkin et al., 1960
Iliac crest[c]	1.13	Zipkin et al., 1960
Rib[c]	0.92	Zipkin et al., 1960
Vertebra[c]	0.68	Zipkin et al., 1960
Iliac crest[d]	1.03	Zipkin et al., 1960
Rib[d]	0.94	Zipkin et al., 1960
Vertebra[d]	0.68	Zipkin et al., 1960
Iliac Crest[e]	0.92	Zipkin et al., 1960
Rib[e]	0.80	Zipkin et al., 1960
Vertebra[e]	0.68	Zipkin et al., 1960
Femur[f]	1.25	Leaver et al., 1963
Femur[g]	0.82	Leaver et al., 1963
Man (Fetus)[a]		
Femur[h]	0.98	Gedalia et al., 1967
Femur[i]	0.94	Gedalia et al., 1967
Femur[j]	0.81	Gedalia et al., 1967
Femur[k]	0.86	Gedalia et al., 1967
Mandible[h]	0.92	Gedalia et al., 1967
Mandible[i]	0.96	Gedalia et al., 1967
Mandible[j]	0.78	Gedalia et al., 1967
Mandible[k]	0.88	Gedalia et al., 1967
Bovine[a]		
Foreleg[l]	0.27	Dickens, 1941
Foreleg, red marrow[l]	0.04	Dickens, 1941
Metatarsal[m]	0.81	Zipkin et al., 1964
Metatarsal[n]	0.69	Zipkin et al., 1964
Metatarsal[o]	0.62	Zipkin et al., 1964
Metatarsal[p]	0.62	Zipkin et al., 1964
Tibia[q]	0.82	Leaver et al., 1963
Kitten[a]		
Bone[r]	0.37	Dickens, 1941
Cartilage[s]	0.03	Dickens, 1941
Normal[t]	0.64	Dickens, 1941
Rachitic[t]	0.35	Dickens, 1941
Puppy[a]		
Normal[t]	1.31	Dickens, 1941
PTH[u]	1.66	Dickens, 1941

However, another function of phosphatase is possible, and that is that it is concerned with the production and maturation of the protein matrix on which the bone salts are received. There are some findings which might be interpreted as providing evidence in favor of this. Fell and Danielli (1943) and Danielli *et al.* (1943) showed that the first-formed fibers in repair of skin wounds always contained phosphatase. Danielli (1951) has suggested that as this phosphatase disappears when the scar contracts, that is, at the time of maturation of the collagen fibers, the enzyme is concerned with the maturation of these fibers. The present author (Bourne, 1943b, 1948) has shown that the first-formed fibers in bone regeneration are also impregnated with phosphatase and that in fact if the fiber is formed at all it also contains the enzyme. Dietary experiments in which animals were deprived of vitamin C (see Chapter 6, this volume) showed that such deficiency could inhibit the production of fibers, but any which formed contained, as far as could be estimated by their histochemical reactions, a normal quota of enzymic activity. In this connection it should be remembered that Bloom and Bloom (1940) maintained that the property of calcifiability was conferred upon osseous tissue as it was deposited and that the actual process of deposi-

---

[a] Whole bone used.

[b] From individuals drinking water containing 1.0 ppm F.

[c] From individuals drinking water containing 1.0 ppm F.

[d] From individuals drinking water containing 2.5 ppm F.

[e] From individuals drinking water containing 4.0 ppm F.

[f] Midshaft from 77-year-old subject.

[g] Midshaft from 12-year-old subject.

[h] Taken at 5 months *in utero* from mothers drinking water containing 0.1 ppm F.

[i] Taken from mothers at 5 months *in utero* drinking water containing 1 ppm F.

[j] Taken at 9 months *in utero* from mothers drinking water containing 0.1 ppm F.

[k] Taken at 9 months *in utero* from mothers drinking water containing 1 ppm F.

[l] Method may have allowed for only partial extraction of citrate from the bone.

[m] Animals received 12 ppm F in ration for 7 years.

[n] Animals received 27 ppm F in ration for 7 years.

[o] Animals received 49 ppm F in ration for 7 years.

[p] Animals received 93 ppm F in ration for 7 years.

[q] Not specified, so presumably whole tibia.

[r] Legs and ribs including marrow.

[s] From ribs and leg joints.

[t] Bones, not specified.

[u] Parathyroid hormone administered.

[v] For references see Zipken, 1970.

tion of calcium salts was simply a matter of these salts being deposited
into the osteoid when it had reached the appropriate stage of acceptabil-
ity. Bradfield (1946) has also shown that a very active alkaline phos-
phatse is always present in the silk-spinning glands of insects. That
the enzyme is associated with protein synthesis may also be suggested
from its frequent presence in nucleoli which are important centers, if
the available evidence is interpreted correctly, of protein synthesis.
Caspersson (1947), for example, has claimed that an increase in cytoplasmic basophilia associated with an increase in nucleolar size is a
diagnostic feature of cells engaged in active protein synthesis. At the
time of matrix formation in bone there is also a great increase in the
alkaline phosphatase activity of the osteoblast (see Cappellin, 1948) and
of cytoplasmic basophilia. McKelvie and Mann (1948) have found accumulations of alkaline phosphatase in periosteal fibrosarcomata in
which bone was never formed and in polyostotic fibrous dysplasia in
which there is a great overproduction of fibrous tissue which is rich
in alkaline phosphatase activity (but see contrary results of Gomori,
1943). Also, Siffert (1951) has pointed out that the frequent association
of alkaline phosphatase with the matrix in both cartilaginous and fibrocallus would indicate an association with the elaboration of cartilage
and bone matrix rather than with their calcification. Furthermore, the
presence of phosphatase in the uterus of the hen and the mantle of
mollusks (Bourne, 1943a; Wagge, 1951; Bevelander, 1952), the shell
of which contains no significant amount of phosphates (Pelseneer, 1906;
Turek, 1933), also suggests some connection with the formation of the
protein matrix on which the calcium salts of the hen egg and the mollusk
shell are deposited rather than with the deposition of these salts. In
further support of this thesis is the work of Moog (1944), Rossi *et
al.* (1951a,b,c), and Engel and Furuta (1942) who showed the widespread diffusion of phosphatase in embryonic soft tissues during the
process of growth and differentiation, and that of Jeener (1947) who
showed that alkaline phosphatase was associated with cell proliferations
in organs stimulated by sex hormones.

A suggestion, purely speculatory, regarding the role of phosphatase
in fiber formation has been made by Neuman and Neuman (1958). They
pointed out that collagen fibrils can be dissolved in acetic acid and that
following removal of the acid the small units so formed may recombine to
form characteristic collagen fibrils. In this case it is necessary to ask why
these small units do not combine within the cell itself. He suggested
that they are synthesized and secreted as phosphate esters and that
as they pass to the cell surface the phosphate is hydrolyzed off by
extracellular phosphatase and the units then combine to form fibrils.

A. Mechanism of Calcification

According to Schiffman *et al.* (1970), some organic matrices possess the ability of heterogeneous nucleation, that is, the ability to precipitate calcium and phosphate ions. These matrices include bone collagen, enamel protein, and the elastin of the aorta. They pointed out that the collagen of most vertebrates contains three specific amino acids; these are four hydroxyproline, three hydroxyproline, and five hydroxylsine. Sobel and Burger (1954) showed that if a bone is decalcified in ethylenediaminetetraacetic acid then treated with calcium chloride and sodium hydrogen phosphate and finally placed in calcifying fluid, it will recalcify. This mineralization appears as complete as in normal bone. Sobel believed that the first two processes (following decalcification) result in the formation of nuclei for initiatory crystallization processes and that the calcifying fluid then deposits calcium phosphate on the nuclei. Glimcher (1959) indicated that crystals of bone salt appear to be deposited on collagen in regions where the most polar side chains are concentrated.

In 1958, Neuman and Neuman found that if they added bone mineral to blood serum, the former pulled calcium and phosphate out of solution and formed additional bone mineral. Strates and Neuman (1958) then discovered that decalcified bone tendon and reconstituted collagen could do the same thing. Schiffman and his colleagues (1970) then pointed out that Glimcher (1959; see Schiffman *et al.*, 1970) had produced a variety of collagen fibrils by reconstituting disaggregated collagen units. These collagen fibers varied from each other only in the way the collagen molecules were stacked, and when they were placed in supersaturated solutions of Ca and PO_4, only the fibrils which had an arrangement of collagen molecules identical with "native" collagen caused precipitation of mineral salts. Schiffler and his colleagues indicated that this result suggested: "the mechanism of nucleation involved a specific stereochemical configuration which resulted from a particular state of aggregation of collagen macromolecules." It is of interest that Glimcher and Krane (1962) found that if collagen fibers are incubated with solutions containing phosphate ions, a considerable number of the latter were bound to the collagen (150 moles of PO_4 per mole of collagen). Twenty percent of these moles could not be dialyzed out again. In this connection, the observations of Krane and his colleagues (1965), in which they found that connective tissue contains kinases that can act on ATP to transfer phosphate to gelatin, are significant. These results suggest that a phosphorylated matrix (and those above) may act as nucleators for the deposition of bone salt; but Miller and Martin (1968) pointed out that there is very little phosphate associated with bone collagen, and Schiff-man *et al.* (1970) pointed out that mineralization has not yet been shown to be dependent upon the phosphorylation of the matrix.

Various authors have suggested that the ε-amino groups of collagen play a part in the bonding of mineral salts to the matrix (Solomons and Irving, 1958; Cartier and Lanzetta, 1961; Wuthier *et al.*, 1964), but some of the results are conflicting and others can be explained in other ways. However, the weight of evidence suggests that they may play some part.

Eanes and Posner (1970) have summarized the evidence that bone mineral is first deposited and that it subsequently reorganizes to form apatite. In 1955, Robinson and Watson, studying calcification in the rib bone of the human infant, described a haze in the tissue immediately in front of the advancing area of calcification. Fitton Jackson and Randall (1956) found that the new matrix produced by periosteal bone growth was opaque to electrons which again suggested an amorphous type of calcification. Molnar (1959) found the same thing in the parietal bones of young mice, and Hancox and Boothroyd (1965, 1966) found in the skull bones of the embryonic fowl that the "pre-osseous matrix" contained a "cloudy granular material" which they believed represented deposits of bone mineral. Harper and Posner (1966) and Termine and Posner (1967) showed from X-ray diffraction studies that these areas probably were in fact due to amorphous bone salt.

Studies by Bourne (1943b) and others in the demonstration of phosphatases have also provided results which suggest that the first-formed salts of calcium phosphate are amorphous in nature. In the technique for the histochemical demonstration of phosphatases calcium phosphate salt is deposited on those areas where phosphatase is located. This calcium phosphate is visualized for observation under the microscope by treating the section first with cobalt chloride and then with ammonium sulfide. The black product produced demonstrates the localization of phosphatase. If sections are incubated for a long period of time, however, before being put through the visualization process, they do not react with the reagents used for this purpose—in other words, areas which appeared positive with short incubations become negative on long incubations. This is shown especially by the brush borders of intestinal cells. Presumably, this results from a reorganization of the calcium phosphate precipitate. Crystals of apatite also do not react with the cobalt chloride ammonium sulfide reagents, so presumably in these *in vitro* experiments, the calcium phosphate first comes down in the amorphous form and then changes to apatite. We seem here to have a test tube model of what happens in bone formation.

Eanes and Posner (1970) have pointed out that "synthetic amorphous calcium phosphates are not stable in aqueous media . . . if they are kept in contact with their preparative solution, these materials will incongruently hydrolyze into crystalline apatite." (See Fig. 13.)

This discussion has suggested that bone becomes mineralized by some noncellular process such as nucleation, but evidence has been presented earlier in this chapter which indicated that there is not a period in the production of normal bone when pure matrix is formed and mineral salts then deposited on it. The author's studies have demonstrated that in the formation of bone trabeculae, if a trabecula (osteoid) forms at all, it will be calcified when it is formed. This suggests that the cells may themselves play as important a role in the mineralization of collagen as they do in the formation of collagen units (See Fig. 14).

Eanes and Posner (1970) gave a number of reasons why cells may be concerned directly with calcification. The first reason is that cells are usually closely associated with areas of calcification, and they made the point that if calcium and phosphate have to pass through and be mobilized by the cells, then the serum concentrations of these two ions are not important in the mineralization process. They quoted Pautored (1966) who demonstrated intracellular deposits of apatite in the baleen of whales, and they quoted Greenwald *et al.* (1964) who showed that mitochondria can take up calcium and phosphorus even from very low concentrations of these salts and can form granules of calcium phosphate. Bernard and Pease (1967) have produced evidence that "the initial

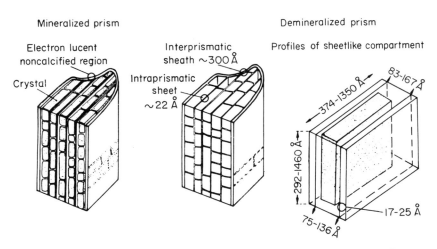

Fig. 13. The comparative ultrastructure and organization of five calcified tissues. A diagram summarizing the inorganic crystal–organic matrix relationship (from Travis, 1970).

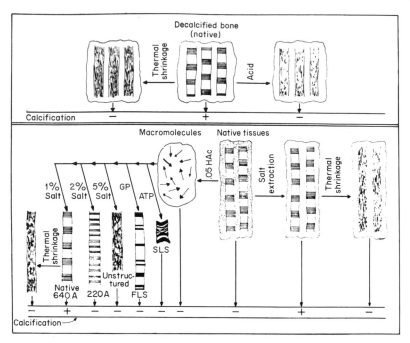

FIG. 14. Diagrammatic illustrations of specificity of macromolecular aggregation state of native-type collagen fibrils in calcification and possible role of ground substance in inhibiting and controlling it (from Glimcher, 1959).

calcification locus appears to be a cellular derived globule, apparently originating from an osteoblastic Golgi vesicle." Eanes and Posner went on to say that one cannot depend upon extracellular mechanisms to produce the degree of supersaturation that would be needed *in vivo* to secure the precipitation of amorphous bone salt. They proposed a cellular model for calcification assuming that "amorphous calcium phosphate is a product of direct cellular activity." Through the ion pumping activities of the cell, the local concentration of calcium and phosphate can be raised to the supersaturation level and at this level there can be a spontaneous precipitation of calcium phosphate. They pointed out that at this time there is no evidence to show whether this supersaturation occurs in the cell cytoplasm with the production of amorphous granules of bone salt which are then secreted and later reorient themselves molecularly into apatite, or whether the calcium and phosphorus are pumped by the cell across the cell membrane to form local extracellular supersaturation. Eanes and Posner quoted the work of Taves (1965) who, as a result of his studies, indicated the possibility of the formation of a calcium phosphoprotein complex by the Golgi apparatus which was excreted from the cell. This would correspond very well with the results of Bourne, mentioned above, that the matrix when it is formed is already calcified. According to Jones, when this complex is outside the cell, the phosphatase also located extracellularly liberates the phosphate so it is free to combine with calcium and thus appear as amorphous calcium phosphate on the protein matrix—this salt then is the origin of the ions which form apatite. Eanes and Posner concluded their theory by stating:

> In this model, the primary factor responsible for limiting the formation of apatite crystals to those areas that normally calcify, is not alkaline phosphatase, or a pyrophosphatase, but a cellularly derived amorphous calcium phosphate. Thus in this proposal, the cell ultimately governs the entire calcification process.

(See Fig. 15.)

VI. Summary

The facts regarding the distribution of phosphatase in bone are summarized as follows.

In mature bone, the endosteum and the periosteum are phosphatase positive and in the latter nearly all of this reaction is localized in the inner layer of the membrane. The superficial osteocytes are positive and so is recently deposited bone matrix. Older osteocytes and bone matrix are negative.

In developing embryos condensations of mesenchyme destined to form membrane bone show phosphatase activity, those destined to form cartilage do not. Phosphatase does not appear in cartilage until just prior to ossification; in cartilage which never ossifies phosphatase is never found.

When cartilage ossifies the first phosphatase appears in the perichondrium near the regions where ossification of the matrix will first appear. The cartilage cells show signs of enzymic activity when they begin to hypertrophy; phosphatase appears at first in the nuclei and then spreads to the cytoplasm and the matrix. Once the matrix shows activity the cytoplasmic reaction decreases. Calcification appears to occur only in the presence of *extracellular* phosphatase. Periosteal osteoblasts appear to go through a cycle of phosphatase activity in growing bone. Originally possessing considerable phosphatase activity, they retain this activity when they eventually become surrounded by bone matrix and become young osteocytes; as they become older osteocytes they lose their phosphatase but under certain circumstances, particularly in break-

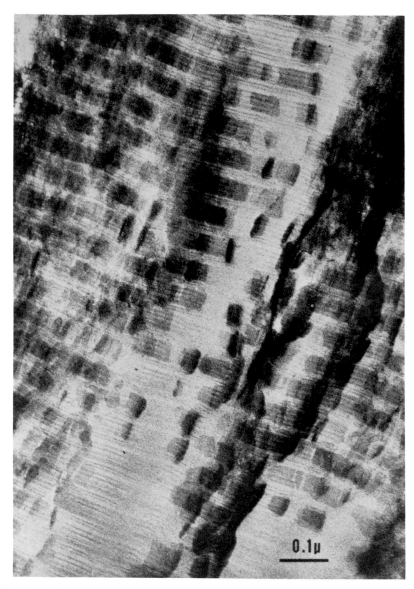

Fig. 15. Electron micrograph of a thin section of rat tail tendon calcified after implantation into the peritoneal cavity of a rat. The platelike crystals are arranged to correspond with the periodicity of the collagen bonds (from Mergenhagen *et al.*, 1960).

wn of bone, they may show signs of renewed activity. Osteoclasts so contain some phosphatase (see Hancox, Chapter 3, Volume I of is treatise).

In the regeneration of bone and of skin wounds after injury, large numbers of phosphatase-positive polymorphs migrate into the injured area within 24 hours. They are accompanied and followed by phosphatase-positive fibroblasts which appear to produce a mass of phosphatase-positive fibers. There is then a loss of phosphatase activity in the fibers. In the skin wounds this signals the virtual completion of the repair process; in bone injuries this is followed by a second cycle of phosphatase production associated with the production of calcified osteoid.

In addition to the association of phosphatase with bone formation, the enzyme is also present when the shell of mollusks and hens' eggs are being laid down.

The views regarding the significance of phosphatase in bone formation are: (1) it is associated with production of phosphate ions which secure the precipitation of calcium as bone salt; (2) it is associated with the formation of the organic matrix of bone; (3) it is concerned with the formation of a phosphate ester which acts as a template or part of a template for the catalytic crystallization of bone salt; and (4) it keeps the surface of bone crystals free of ester phosphate, thus permitting continued growth of the crystals.

References

Albaum, H. G., Hirshfeld, A., and Sobel, A. E. (1952). *Proc. Soc. Exp. Biol. Med.* **79**, 238.

Baccari, V., and Quagliarello, E. (1950). *Boll. Soc. Ital. Biol. Sper.* **26**, 596.

Bernard, G. W., and Pease, D. C. (1967). *Abstr. 49th Meet. Int. Ass. Dent. Res.* p. 72.

Bevelander, G. (1952). *Biol. Bull.* **102**, 9.

Bevelander, G., and Johnson, P. L. (1950). *Anat. Rec.* **108**, 1.

Bloom, W., and Bloom, M. A. (1940). *Anat. Rec.* **78**, 497.

Blum, G. (1944). *Lancet* **2**, 75.

Bodansky, A. (1937). *J. Biol. Chem.* **118**, 341.

Bodansky, A., Bakwin, R. M., and Bakwin, H. (1931). *J. Biol. Chem.* **94**, 551.

Borghese, E. (1952). *Boll. Soc. Ital. Biol. Sper.* **28**, 801.

Borghese, E. (1953). *Z. Anat. Entwicklungsgesch.* **116**, 610.

Botterell, E. H., and King, E. J. (1935). *Lancet* **2**, 1267.

Bourne, G. H. (1942). *J. Physiol. (London)* **101**, 327.

Bourne, G. H. (1943a). *Quart. J. Exp. Physiol.* **32**, 1.

Bourne, G. H. (1943b). *J. Physiol. (London)* **102**, 319.

Bourne, G. H. (1944). Unpublished results.

Bourne, G. H. (1948). *J. Anat.* **82**, 81.

Bourne, G. H. (1949). *Brit. J. Nutr.* 3, xi.

Bourne, G. H. (1954a). *Quart. J. Microsc. Sci.* 95, 359.

Bourne, G. H. (1954b). *J. Physiol.* (*London*) 124, 409.

Bourne, G. H. (1954c). *Acta Anat.* 22, 289.

Boyd, E. W., and Neuman, W. F. (1951). *J. Biol. Chem.* 193, 245.

Bradfield, R. G. (1946). *Nature* (*London*) 157, 876.

Cameron, G. R. (1930). *J. Pathol. Bacteriol.* 23, 939.

Cappellin, M. (1948). *Boll. Soc. Ital. Biol. Sper.* 24, 1228.

Carlsen, F., Jensen, E., and Johansen, G. (1953). *C. R. Trav. Lab. Carlsberg Ser. Physiol.* 29, 1.

Cartier, P. (1950). *C. R. Soc. Biol.* 144, 331.

Cartier, P., and Lanzetta, A. (1961). *Bull. Soc. Clin. Biol.* 43, 981.

Caspersson, T. (1947). *Symp. Soc. Exp. Biol.* 1, 127.

Cloetens, R. (1939). *Enzymologia* 6, 46.

Conrad, R. M., and Scott, H. M. (1938). *Physiol. Rev.* 18, 481.

Dallemagne, M. J. (1947). *Acta Physiother. Rheumatol. Belg.* 3, 77.

Dallemagne, M. J. (1948). *Nature* (*London*) 161, 115.

Dallemagne, M. J. (1950). *Annu. Rev. Physiol.* 12, 101.

Dallemagne, M. J. (1951). *J. Physiol.* (*Paris*) 43, 425.

Danielli, J. F. (1951). *Nature* (*London*) 168, 464.

Danielli, J. F., Fell, H. B., and Kodicek, E. (1943). *Brit. J. Exp. Pathol.* 24, 196.

Dickens, F. (1940). *Chem. Ind.* (*London*) 59, 135.

Dickens, F. (1941). *Biochem. J.* 35, 1011.

DiStefano, V., Neuman, W. F., and Rauser, G. (1953). *Arch. Biochem. Biophys.* 47, 218.

Dixon, T. F., and Perkins, H. R. (1956). *In* "The Biochemistry and Physiology of Bone" (G. H. Bourne, ed.). Academic, New York.

Eanes, E. D., and Posner, A. S. (1970). *In* "Biological Calcification" (H. Schraer ed.), p. 1. Appleton, New York.

Engel, M. B., and Furuta, W. (1942). *Proc. Soc. Exp. Biol. Med.* 50, 5.

Fell, H. B. (1925). *J. Morphol. Physiol.* 40, 417.

Fell, H. B. (1928). *Arch. Exp. Zellforsch. Besonders Gewebezuecht.* 7, 390.

Fell, H. B., and Danielli, J. F. (1943). *Brit. J. Exp. Pathol.* 24, 196.

Fell, H. B., and Robison, R. (1929). *Biochem. J.* 23, 767.

Fitton Jackson, S., and Randall, J. T. (1956). *Bone Struc. Metab., Ciba Found. Symp., 1955* p. 47.

Follis, R. H., Jr. (1949). *Bull. Johns Hopkins Hosp.* 85, 368.

Follis, R. H., Jr. (1950). *Bull. Johns Hopkins Hosp.* 87, 181.

Glimcher, M. J. (1959). *Rev. Mod. Phys.* 31, 359.

Glimcher, M. J., and Krane, S. M. M. (1962). "Radioisotopes and Bone," p. 393. Blackwell, Oxford.

Glock, G. E. (1940). *J. Physiol.* (*London*) 93, 1.

Gomori, G. (1939). *Proc. Soc. Exp. Biol. Med.* 42, 23.

Gomori, G. (1943). *Amer. J. Pathol.* 19, 197.

Greenwald, J. W., Rossi, C. S., and Lehningen, A. L. (1964). *J. Cell Biol.* 23, 21.

Greep, R. O., Fischer, C. J., and Morse, A. (1948). *J. Amer. Dent. Ass.* 36, 427.

Gutman, A. B., and Gutman, E. B. (1941). *Proc. Soc. Exp. Biol. Med.* 48, 687.

Gutman, A. B., and Yu, T. F. *Conf. Metab. Interrelations, Trans.* 2, 167.

CHAPTER 3

Elaboration of Enamel and Dentin Matrix Glycoproteins

ALFRED WEINSTOCK

I. Introduction

The mineralized matrices of enamel, dentin, and bone contain carbohydrates in addition to the main organic constituent, protein. These carbohydrates are believed to be linked to protein, and as such they constitute the matrix glycoproteins and proteoglycans (mucopolysaccharides).

Dentin and bone matrices, both produced by mesodermally derived cells, possess many similarities in structure and chemical composition. The principal organic component is collagen. In both tissues the collagen fibers are tightly packed and intimately associated with mineral deposits; together they form the structural framework of each tissue and provide mechanical rigidity. Although calcified tissue collagen has many features in common with soft tissue collagen, there is evidence that chemical and structural differences may exist (Veis *et al.*, 1969; Volpin and Veis, 1971; Miller, 1972).

Enamel matrix, on the other hand, is an ectodermal product and differs from the other two both structurally and chemically; most notable is the fact that it lacks collagen. In view of the close relationship and spatial orientation of the large apatite crystals of enamel relative to the enamel matrix subunits, it is likely that these subunits serve a function in the epitaxis and orientation of the mineral crystals.

In this chapter, the elaboration of the matrix glycoproteins of enamel and dentin will be examined with emphasis placed on intracellular sites of synthesis, pathway of migration, and mode of secretion of these substances by the respective cellular elements. Much of the available information was obtained by means of light and electron microscope radioautography and the findings interpreted in light of current biochemical data.

II. Background

It has become increasingly evident that most animal cell secretions are composed of glycoprotein (Eylar, 1965; Spiro, 1969), a class of substances occurring almost universally in vertebrates as well as invertebrates. Glycoproteins are composed of carbohydrate and protein which are held together by firm convalent bonds. While the complete structure of very few of the glycoproteins in nature has been established, progress has been made toward establishing the structure and composition of the carbohydrate moieties of several of these substances. Relatively few types of simple sugars seem to occur in the carbohydrate side chains, and only six are commonly found: D-galactose, D-mannose, L-fucose, D-glucosamine, D-galactosamine, and D-neuraminic acid (sialic acid). A few glycoproteins, including those of enamel and bone, contain D-glucose. When uronic acid sugars, like glucuronic acid, or sulfate ester sugars are present as carbohydrate constituents, the carbohydrate moiety of this type of glycoprotein (proteoglycan) is referred to as a glycosaminoglycan. Figure 1 illustrates the biosynthetic pathways whereby some sugar residues may become incorporated into glycoproteins.

Protein synthesis occurs on ribonucleoprotein particles in association with messenger RNA. This synthetic process is regulated according to information coded on DNA. Many radioautographic studies utilizing a variety of secretory cell types have shown that labeled amino acids are synthesized into polypeptides in the ribosome-laden rough endoplas-

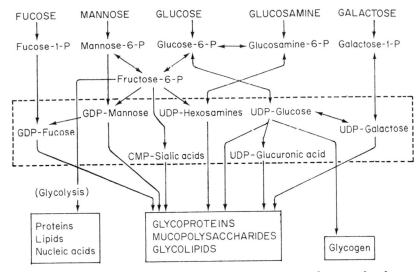

FIG. 1. A schematic chart showing the biosynthetic pathways whereby some sugars may become incorporated into glycoproteins.

mic reticulum (rER), the cytoplasmic component that appears basophilic in routinely stained histological tissue sections (see review by Leblond, 1965). Accordingly, the rER is referred to as the *site of protein synthesis*.

Recently, attention has been drawn to the question of the intracellular site of synthesis of the carbohydrate moiety of glycoproteins, for it appears that a synthetic pathway unique from that of proteins exists. Peterson and Leblond (1964) and Neutra and Leblond (1966a,b) were the first to present evidence suggesting that polysaccharide precursors such as glucose and galactose were incorporated into high molecular weight compounds in the Golgi region of a variety of cell types. Indeed, by means of electron microscope radioautography, they showed that the Golgi apparatus of colonic goblet cells was the site of incorporation of glucose-³H into mucus glycoprotein. Evidence also suggests that sulfation of glycosaminoglycans may occur in the Golgi region (Godman and Lane, 1964; Fewer et al., 1964). Finally, cytochemical work with the periodic acid–silver methenamine technique (Rambourg and Leblond, 1967) has clearly pointed to the presence of carbohydrate, probably in the form of glycoprotein, in the Golgi apparatus of a variety of cell types.

Since it was known that the organic matrices of mineralizing tissues were composed in part of glycoproteins, we chose to investigate the synthesis and sequence of events leading to the secretion of some of these glycoproteins. The continuously erupting rat incisor was selected to serve as a model for some of these studies inasmuch as it contains two different types of mineralized tissues situated adjacent to one another, namely, enamel and dentin. The organic matrices of both of these tissues are elaborated simultaneously at the growing end of the tooth (Fig. 2a); thus, we were able to observe the ameloblasts and odontoblasts in stages of active matrix secretion, as will presently be discussed. Insofar as more is known about the elaboration of enamel matrix glycoprotein, this will be reviewed initially in some detail; the synthesis and secretion of dentin matrix glycoprotein will then be considered.

III. Enamel Matrix

A. Presence of Glycoproteins in the Organic Matrix of Enamel

The organic matrix of enamel in embryonic teeth constitutes approximately 20% of the total enamel (Deakins, 1942; Weinmann *et al.*, 1942; Eastoe, 1960; Burgess and Maclaren, 1965). After mineralization is completed in the adult, the matrix content is reduced to about 0.5% (Losee and Hess, 1949; Stack, 1954; Battistone and Burnett, 1956; Burnett and Zenewitz, 1958).

Enamel matrix consists essentially of protein, the amino acid composition of which is distinctly different from that of collagen (Eastoe, 1960, 1963; Piez, 1961; Glimcher *et al.*, 1961, 1964a). Mature bovine enamel matrix is believed to be composed of low molecular weight peptides with smaller amounts of high molecular weight proteins (Glimcher and Levine, 1966). Carbohydrates constitute 1.5–2% of the organic matrix in mature human and bovine enamel (Egyedi and Stack, 1956; see also Pincus, 1949; Stack, 1954) and 1% in embryonic bovine enamel (Seyer and Glimcher, 1969). These carbohydrate components have been shown to exist in the form of glycoprotein (Stack, 1954; Egyedi and Stack, 1956; Burgess *et al.*, 1960; Clark *et al.*, 1965; Glimcher and Levine, 1966; Seyer and Glimcher, 1969) and glycosaminoglycan (Clark *et al.*, 1965). Analysis of the individual sugar residues in mature human and bovine enamel matrix has demonstrated the presence of galactose, glucose, and mannose as principal components, with smaller amounts of fucose, xylose, and rhamnose (Burgess *et al.*, 1960).

Two glycoprotein-containing fractions have been isolated from mature bovine matrix; one consisting of material with a molecular weight higher than 30,000 and the other lower than 30,000 (Glimcher and Levine, 1966). Thin-layer chromatography revealed the presence of glucose, galactose, mannose, and fucose in the former, and galactose as the only hexose in the latter. Glucosamine and galactosamine are constituents of both fractions, a finding that is consistent with studies on human enamel in which hexosamine-containing glycoproteins are found (Clark et al., 1965).

Finally, embryonic bovine enamel matrix, which is similar to rat enamel matrix in amino acid composition (Levine and Glimcher, 1965), can be separated into two main fractions according to solubility. One is soluble in acid and the other soluble at neutral pH (Glimcher *et al.*, 1964a). Both fractions contain galactosamine. The acid-soluble fraction, believed to come from the rod sheaths (Glimcher *et al.*, 1964b) contains only galactose as neutral hexose. The fraction soluble at neutral pH, believed to represent the rods themselves, contains about 75% of its hexoses as galactose, the rest consisting of mannose with some glucose (Seyer and Glimcher, 1969).

B. Ameloblasts and the Elaboration of Enamel Matrix

It is well known that the enamel matrix of the rat incisor is elaborated by ameloblasts at a time when these cells are very tall; at this stage they are referred to as *secretory ameloblasts*.[1] While numerous studies have been done on the structure of these cells in the incisor teeth of rat (Fearnhead, 1960, 1961a,b; Reith, 1960, 1961; Watson, 1960; Kallenbach et al., 1963; Warshawsky, 1968; Jessen, 1968a; A. Weinstock, 1970b; Moe, 1971) and mouse (Nylen and Scott, 1960; Garant and Nalbandian, 1968), their mode of secretion was poorly understood until recently (A. Weinstock and Leblond, 1971).

1. Cytology

The secretory ameloblasts are arranged in a single layer on the labial surface of the rat incisor tooth (Fig. 2a). They are tall columnar cells in which the organelles are found in specific locations. Mitochondria are grouped below the nucleus at the base of the cell (Fig. 2b). Above the nucleus, a tubular-shaped Golgi apparatus is visible as a double-

[1] Between the region of enamel matrix secretion and the incisal tip of the tooth the ameloblasts become smaller and acquire different morphological features. They are thought to be involved in processes other than matrix secretion (Wassermann, 1944; Marsland, 1952; Reith, 1963, 1970; Reith and Coty, 1967; Kallenbach, 1970); nevertheless, recent evidence indicates that they also have a secretory function (A. Weinstock, 1970a; 1972). According to general usage, the term *secretory amelo-blasts* will be restricted in this chapter to those cells that elaborate the enamel matrix (see also Bélanger, 1955).

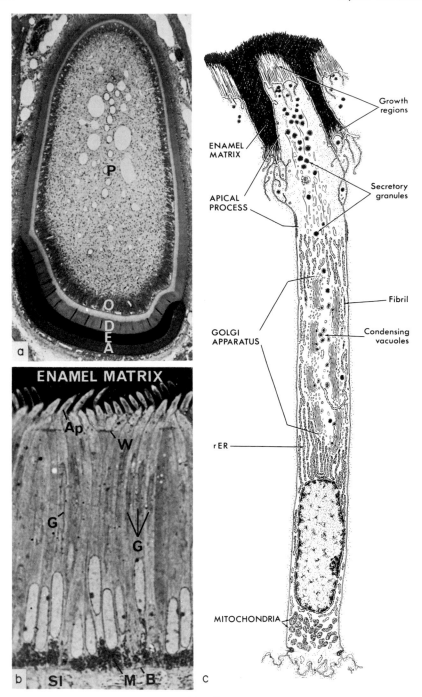

FIG. 2.

stranded structure running longitudinally along the cell axis. On all sides of the Golgi, cisternae of rough endoplasmic reticulum are abundant (Fig. 2c). Above the level of the apical terminal web is a cytoplasmic extension called the *apical (Tomes') process* (Fig. 2b). The distal portion of this process is embedded in enamel matrix; within its central core toluidine blue–positive material can be seen which, in the electron microscope, corresponds to groups of secretory granules (Figs. 2c and 3).

Electron microscopy has shown that the Golgi appears as a double array of stacks of saccules, one on either side of the cell axis. Each array consists of successive stacks aligned end-to-end in a linear fashion. In three dimensions, the Golgi resembles a hollow cylinder enclosing a central cytoplasmic core (Kallenbach *et al.*, 1963). Within each stack, those saccules situated medially, that is, facing the central cytoplasmic core, are referred to as *inner saccules*, whereas those located laterally— facing the surrounding rough endoplasmic reticulum and plasma membrane—are referred to as *outer saccules*. The inner Golgi saccules give rise to strings of condensing vacuoles which, after breaking up into "free"

Fig. 2. (a) A rat maxillary incisor tooth as seen in a 1-μ thick transverse section through the region of enamel matrix secretion (within the proximal one-third of the tooth). Toluidine blue stain; Epon. ×51. The enamel organ is located on the labial surface of the incisor (lowermost part of figure). From the base up, the lettering points to the layer of secretory ameloblasts (A), the enamel matrix (E) intensely stained by toluidine blue, the dentin (D) separated from the layer of odontoblasts (O) by the lightly staining predentin, and finally the pulp (P). (From A. Weinstock and Leblond, 1971.) (b). Secretory ameloblasts as they appear in a 1-μ thick transverse section through the region of enamel matrix secretion in a rat maxillary incisor. Toluidine blue stain; Epon. ×850. The ameloblasts from the base up show a faintly visible basal web (B), the groups of mitochondria intensely stained with toluidine blue (M), the elongated nucleus, the supranuclear cytoplasm with the Golgi apparatus appearing as a double-stranded structure (G), the terminal web (W) and the apical (Tomes') process (Ap) which is partially embedded in the enamel matrix. The toluidine blue–stained content of the processes represents secretory granules [cf. (2c)]. Since the apical processes of ameloblasts in a given row interdigitate with those in other rows, the cut-off portions of several rows of processes are visible. (SI, stratum intermedium). (From A. Weinstock and Leblond, 1971.) (c) A diagrammatic representation of the structure of a secretory ameloblast from the region of enamel matrix secretion in a rat maxillary incisor. Mitochondria are usually grouped between basal web and nucleus. The supranuclear region contains an elongated tubular-shaped Golgi apparatus which is surrounded on all sides by rER. Within the central core of cytoplasm demarcated by the Golgi saccules are condensing vacuoles and a few secretory granules. The apical process extends apically from the terminal web and its distal portion is embedded in the enamel matrix. Secretory granules abound within its central core. The "growth regions" represent the most recently deposited matrix, as described in the text. (From A. Weinstock and Leblond, 1971.)

condensing vacuoles, gather for a short time within the core of cytoplasm surrounded by the stacks of saccules (A. Weinstock and Leblond, 1971). These condensing vacuoles then evolve into secretory granules which rapidly migrate from the Golgi apparatus to the apical process wherein

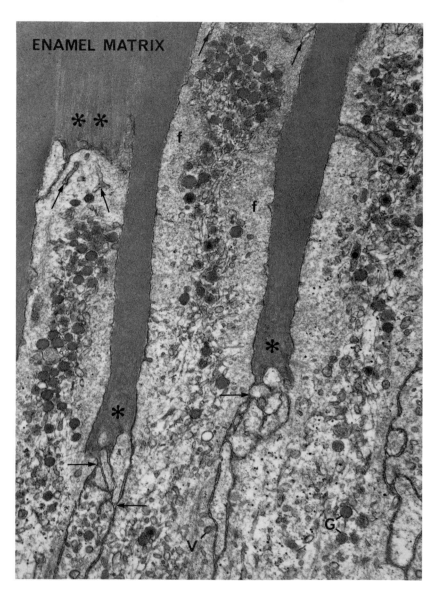

Fig. 3.

they accumulate (Fig. 3) prior to discharging their content (A. Weinstock and Leblond, 1971).

2. Histochemical Detection of Glycoprotein

Histochemical investigations using phosphotungstic acid (Pease, 1966; Marinozzi, 1967, 1968) acidified according to Rambourg (1967, 1969) for the detection of glycoprotein have demonstrated the presence of glycoprotein in ameloblasts as well as in the enamel matrix itself (A. Weinstock and Leblond, 1971). Briefly, when thin sections of glycol methacrylate-embedded ameloblasts are treated with phosphotungstic acid at low pH, the content of the Golgi saccules takes up the stain. While the outermost saccules in a stack exhibit little or no reactive content, a gradient of increasing staining intensity is observed from the next saccule to the innermost one (Fig. 4a). The innermost saccules usually display a relatively large amount of stained material, which is of a density and texture similar to that observed in the nearby condensing vacuoles and secretory granules. Indeed, these secretory granules stain like the readily identified secretory granules of the apical processes (Fig. 4b). Finally, the enamel matrix takes up the stain, mainly in the parallel, linear subunits (Fig. 4b). Judging from their size, these delicate structures represented the long tubular subunits previously described in the enamel matrix (Jessen, 1968b; Warshawsky, 1971). Hence, these subunits appear to contain glycoprotein material. They presumably con-

---

FIG. 3. Apical (Tomes) processes and associated enamel matrix. ✕10,000. The proximal portion of each process (lower one-third of micrograph) contains scattered secretory granules (G) as well as smooth membranous elements admixed with fragments of rER, microtubules, bristle-coated vesicles (V), and a few glycogen granules. The distal portion of each apical process (upper two-thirds of micrograph) is embedded within enamel matrix. Each process is limited by a plasma membrane which is closely applied to the matrix. At the distal end, the plasma membrane is thrown into folds that invaginate inward (see arrows at the tip of each process). Invaginations are infrequent along the lateral aspects of a process. Secretory granules abound within the central core of the processes in association with microtubules and smooth membranous elements. The core of cytoplasm containing the secretory granules is usually ensheathed by a feltwork of fine filaments (f) which extends to the plasma membrane. The junction between the proximal and distal regions is indicated by the tips of the enamel prongs. There the cell membrane is thrown into elaborate infoldings (e.g., arrows, lower left). Although the enamel matrix appears relatively homogeneous at this magnification, it shows an arrangement of parallel lines in two regions: (1) the matrix abutting the distal end of each process (**, upper left), and (2) at the proximal ends of the prongs of matrix (*) projecting between the processes. These are the two regions where the nearby plasma membrane shows numerous infoldings (arrows). (From A. Weinstock and Leblond, 1971.)

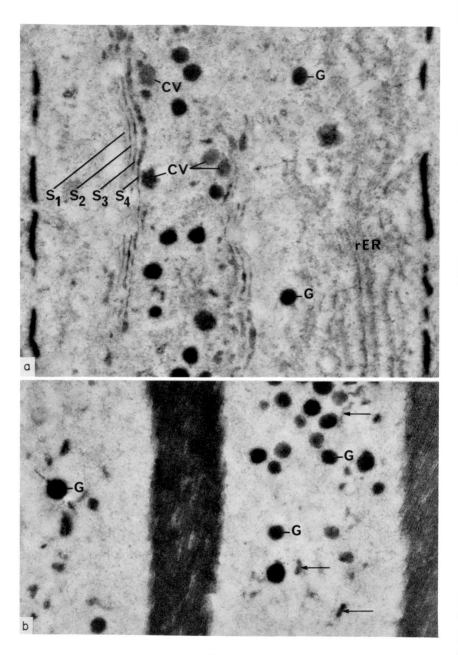

Fig. 4.

tained galactose since this sugar was identified biochemically in all the glycoprotein fractions of enamel described above.

3. Radioautography

Extensive radioautographic investigations using labeled amino acids have shown that ameloblasts are able to rapidly synthesize proteins which ultimately become incorporated into new enamel matrix (Bélanger, 1956; Karpishka *et al.*, 1959; Hwang *et al.*, 1962, 1963; Young and Greulich, 1963; Greulich and Slavkin, 1965; Warshawsky, 1966). Radioautographic studies at the ultrastructural level have demonstrated that the rough endoplasmic reticulum is the initial site over which silver grains appear very soon after injection of a labeled amino acid. Accordingly, the rough endoplasmic reticulum of ameloblasts, as in other protein-secreting cells, is the site of protein synthesis (Warshawsky, 1966; Frank, 1970a). Newly labeled protein is then transported from the rER compartment to the Golgi apparatus. In this regard, morphological evidence has been found that may explain the way in which the intracellular transport of material takes place between the rough endoplasmic reticulum and the Golgi. Briefly, membranous buds are seen on ribosome-free regions of rER cisternae adjacent to the Golgi apparatus (A. Weinstock, 1970b; A. Weinstock and Leblond, 1971). These fuzz-coated buds are often attached by long stems, suggesting *extrusion* of membrane rather than fusion and, therefore, the buds are believed to give rise to small vesicles (ca. 400–700 Å in diameter) referred to as *intermediate vesicles* (A. Weinstock and Leblond, 1971). Furthermore, fuzz-coated buds which often lack stems are present on outer Golgi saccules (A. Weinstock

---

Fig. 4. Electron micrographs of secretory ameloblasts embedded in glycol methacrylate and "stained" with phosphotungstic acid at low pH for the detection of glycoprotein. ×36,000. (a) Golgi region. On either side, the discontinuous vertical stained line represents cell coat material present in the intercellular space between adjacent ameloblasts. The Golgi apparatus appears as a double array of stained saccules which demarcate a core of cytoplasm containing stained condensing vacuoles (CV) and secretory granules (G). A staining intensity gradient exists among Golgi saccules in a given stack. The outermost saccule (S_1) contains little or no stained material, whereas the other saccules show increasing amounts (S_2–S_4). The density and texture of the stained material within S_4 is similar to that seen within the condensing vacuoles. Secretory granules stain more intensely than the vacuoles. (From A. Weinstock and Leblond, 1971.) (b) Portions of two apical processes and their surrounding enamel matrix. The processes are unstained, except for the secretory granules (G) and structures which may correspond to smooth tubular elements (arrows). The staining of the enamel matrix may be assigned to linear subunit components running parallel to one another. (From A. Weinstock and Leblond, 1971.)

and Leblond, 1971), suggesting *fusion* of vesicles with these saccules. In short, we believe that the intermediate vesicles transfer newly synthesized protein from the rough endoplasmic reticulum to the outer saccules of the Golgi apparatus.

Since galactose had been found biochemically in all of the enamel matrix glycoprotein fractions in which its presence was analyzed, galactose-^{3}H was deemed a useful precursor for studying the biosynthesis of enamel glycoprotein. Thus, light microscope radioautographs of ameloblasts obtained minutes after injection of galactose-^{3}H (A. Weinstock, 1967; A. Weinstock and Leblond, 1971) showed silver grains localized in discrete columns over the supranuclear region corresponding to the location of the Golgi apparatus (Fig. 5a). Similar results (Fig. 5c) were obtained after incubating unerupted molars with galactose-^{3}H *in vitro* (A. Weinstock, 1969).

More recently, we have demonstrated by means of electron microscope radioautography the uptake of galactose-^{3}H label by Golgi saccules as early as $2\frac{1}{2}$ minutes after injection, indicating that galactose-^{3}H is incorporated into glycoprotein at this site (A. Weinstock and Leblond, 1971). At 5 minutes postinjection (Fig. 6), the Golgi-localized reaction is more intense than at $2\frac{1}{2}$ minutes. Most of the silver grains are located over the stacks of saccules rather than other Golgi elements. While the limits of resolution prevent a firm assignment of the grains to detailed parts of the Golgi, examination of numerous radioautographs with minimum development gave the impression that grains were distributed with the same frequency over any one of the four saccules constituting an average stack. Some grains could be observed over groups of intermediate vesicles and a few over condensing vacuoles. Quantitative analysis of grain counts in the electron microscope radioautographs show that at $2\frac{1}{2}$ and 5 minutes after injection, the largest distribution of silver grains is over the Golgi apparatus (Table I). These findings implied that the galactose-^{3}H, after entering the Golgi saccules, had been converted to UDP-galactose (Fig. 1) and then incorporated into glycoprotein (Krauss and Sarcione, 1964; Sarcione, 1964; McGuire *et al.*, 1965; Kalckar, 1965). The Golgi labeling would therefore result from galactose incorporation into glycoprotein. Galactose residues would have to be inserted into the proper sequence within the growing carbohydrate side chains of the incomplete glycoprotein, a step requiring the presence of the enzyme galactosyltransferase. This enzyme has been detected in Golgi fractions of liver (Fleischer *et al.*, 1969; Morré *et al.*, 1969), where the Golgi uptake of galactose label has also been demonstrated (Droz, 1966). Thus, galactose residues may be added to some carbohydrate side chains just prior to completion of enamel glycoprotein within the Golgi saccules.

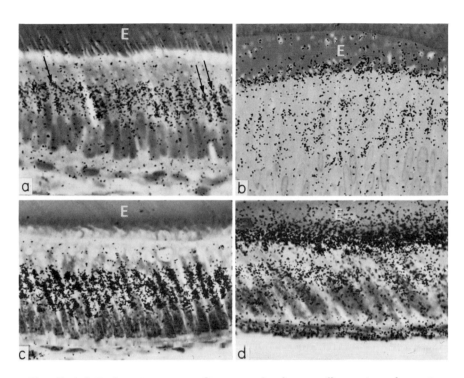

FIG. 5. (a) Light microscope radioautograph of a paraffin section of secretory ameloblasts obtained 5 minutes after injection of galactose-³H. ×630. The silver grains are localized in parallel rows over the supranuclear region, in correspondence with the location of the Golgi apparatus. [The enamel matrix (E) shows a slight reaction attributed to unspecific adsorption of label.] (From A. Weinstock and Leblond, 1971.) (b) Light microscope radioautograph of a 1-µ thick Epon section of secretory ameloblasts 20 minutes after injection of galactose-³H. ×585. Some silver grains are in rows over the Golgi regions and others are scattered over the cell, but the main accumulation of grains is over apical processes and nearby enamel matrix. The light areas seen near the top of the picture are tips of apical processes; they each show a few overlying grains. (From A. Weinstock and Leblond, 1971.) (c) Light microscope radioautograph of a paraffin section of secretory ameloblasts from an unerupted rat molar incubated for 5 minutes in a Krebs-Ringer solution containing galactose-³H. ×585. The silver grains are localized over the region of the cell corresponding to the location of the Golgi apparatus. The apical region of the cell and the enamel matrix are unlabeled [cf. (5a)]. (d) Light microscope radioautograph of a paraffin section of secretory ameloblasts from an unerupted rat molar incubated for 2 hours in a Krebs-Ringer solution containing galactose-³H. ×585. A strong reaction is present over the enamel matrix. Grains can also be observed over the Golgi region and scattered elsewhere over the cells.

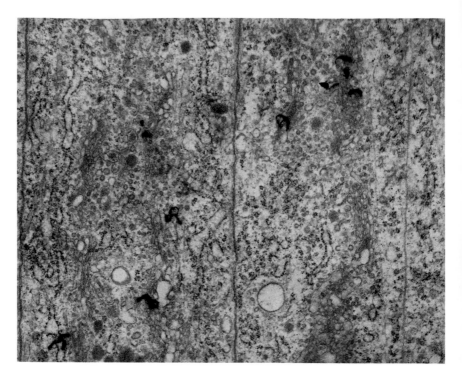

Fig. 6. Electron microscope radioautograph obtained 5 minutes after injection of galactose-³H. ×20,000. The silver grains are over the saccules of the Golgi apparatus in both the cell on the left and right. The rER is unlabeled except for a grain at lower left that overlaps a Golgi saccule and rER cisterna.

TABLE I

QUANTITATION OF SILVER GRAINS[a]

Time after galactose-³H injection (min)	No. of grains	Percentage of grains over				
		rER	Golgi	Secretory granules + condensing vacuoles	Matrix	Other structures
2½	145	9	75	12	—	4
5	273	13	66	17	—	4
10	261	19	45	29	—	7
30	1029	18	20	23	21	18

[a] From A. Weinstock and Leblond (1971).

There is evidence that fucose and perhaps glucosamine are also incorporated into glycoprotein within the Golgi apparatus of ameloblasts (A. Weinstock, 1969). Biochemical studies have shown that fucose-^{3}H serves as a reliable glycoprotein precursor since it is mainly incorporated into glycoproteins directly without being shunted along other metabolic pathways (Coffey et al., 1964; Bekesi and Winzler, 1967; Kaufman and Ginsberg, 1968). It can thus serve as a precursor to trace the fate of labeled glycoproteins over relatively long periods of time. Since fucose is usually located at the terminal end of the carbohydrate side chains in many glycoproteins (Dische, 1963; Spiro, 1969), the uptake of fucose would indicate that side chain elongation is completed within the Golgi apparatus. In addition, recent evidence indicates that sulfation of enamel matrix glycosaminoglycans also takes place within the Golgi apparatus (A. Weinstock and Young, 1972). On the other hand, preliminary results suggest that glucose (A. Weinstock and Leblond, 1971) and possibly mannose (A. Weinstock, 1969) may be taken up by the rough endoplasmic reticulum. Thus, the material entering the Golgi apparatus may consist of incomplete glycoprotein molecules (endogenous acceptor molecules) carrying some carbohydrates which include glucose and mannose residues. It is known that in the thyroid gland, the rough endoplasmic reticulum is the site of uptake of mannose (Whur et al., 1969), an "inner core" sugar, whose location in the carbohydrate side chains of thyroglobulin is close to the protein moiety.

By 10 minutes after injection of galactose-^{3}H a strong radioautographic reaction persists over the Golgi saccules but, in addition, numerous grains are detected over the condensing vacuoles and some secretory granules. The secretory granules in the apical processes and the enamel matrix are essentially label-free at this time. When radioautographs of amylase-incubated ameloblasts were examined, it was found that the amylase treatment did not seem to influence the radioautographic reaction (A. Weinstock and Leblond, 1971), indicating that it was not attributable to nearby glycogen granules. Quantitative analysis of grain counts showed a significant increase in the number of grains assigned to the condensing vacuoles at this interval (Table I). Even though the condensing vacuoles and secretory granules together occupy only 2.3% of the volume of the supranuclear cytoplasm, they contain 29% of its radioactivity at this time interval (Table I). Hence, glycoprotein synthesized in the Golgi saccules rapidly becomes segregated into condensing vacuoles. Indeed, that inner Golgi saccules evolve into condensing vacuoles has been demonstrated morphologically (A. Weinstock and Leblond, 1971).

At 20 minutes after galactose-^{3}H injection there is a persistence of the Golgi reaction, but more striking is the appearance of silver grains over the apical process[2] and enamel matrix (Fig. 5b). This observation has also been confirmed in *in vitro* studies in which the secretion of galactose-containing enamel glycoprotein has been demonstrated (Fig. 5d; A. Weinstock, 1969). Moreover, sulfate label, presumably in the form of sulfated glycosaminoglycan, is also secreted by ameloblasts and deposited in enamel matrix (Figs. 9a and 9b; see also Bélanger, 1955). These results demonstrate the migration of newly labeled material from its site of synthesis, the Golgi apparatus, to its site of secretion, the apical processes, and finally into the developing enamel. Indeed, electron microscope radioautography has shown the migration of labeled secretory granules from the Golgi apparatus to the apical process and enamel matrix (Fig. 7a). In the apical process, silver grains are predominantly situated over the numerous secretory granules which are gathered therein. The enamel matrix exhibits grains mainly over two specific regions that are less compact and often appear striated, that is, (1) the less dense regions above the ends of the apical processes, and (2) the tips of the enamel prongs projecting between the processes (cf. Figs. 2c and 3). These two zones of label deposition are termed *growth regions* since they are situated opposite the secretion zones of the cells and represent the newly formed enamel matrix (A. Weinstock and Leblond, 1971). The deposition of label in these two growth regions was also detected at 4 hours after injection of fucose-^{3}H (Fig. 7b), a glycoprotein precursor more stable than galactose-^{3}H over this period of time but behaving in a similar manner. It is tempting to speculate that the matrix secreted at the tips of the apical processes gives rise to the enamel rods per se, whereas the matrix secreted at the ends of the enamel prongs separating the processes corresponds to the interrod enamel.

The precise mode of discharge of the granule contents is incompletely understood at the present time. However, some images suggest, although not decisively, that secretory granules may release their content by exocytosis at the surfaces facing the two growth regions and perhaps into the associated membranous folds. An excess of membrane would result from such exocytosis, which may account for the formation of folds. It has been suggested that the presence of bristle-coated buds with long stems attached to the surface membrane and its folds indicates

---

[2] By 20 minutes postinjection and later, radioactivity is often detected in the portions of the apical processes located deep within the enamel matrix, as far in as the enamel–dentin junction (Fig. 5b). This observation may explain in part the apparent diffusion through enamel of newly synthesized enamel proteins (Young and Greulich, 1963; Greulich and Slavkin, 1965).

that excess membrane is released back into the cell in the form of bristle-coated vesicles (A. Weinstock and Leblond, 1971). These vesicles might be collected into the multivesicular bodies that are commonly found in the apical process. Whatever the mode of discharge, the appearance of radioactivity within the enamel of the growth regions demonstrates that the glycoprotein is released from secretory granules and deposited as enamel matrix. Since the linear subunits of the matrix contain glycoprotein, it is likely that the new glycoprotein molecules are assembled on to the free ends of the subunits adjacent to the plasma membrane, thus accounting for their continuous elongation during matrix formation.

In summary, the Golgi apparatus is the intracellular site in which galactose, and probably fucose, contribute to the formation of carbohydrate side chains of enamel matrix glycoprotein. Innermost Golgi saccules distribute the completed glycoprotein to condensing vacuoles, which later evolve into secretory granules. These rapidly migrate to the apical processes, where they discharge their glycoprotein content at specific secretory regions to form the developing enamel matrix.

IV. Dentin Matrix

A. Presence of Glycoproteins in the Organic Matrix of Dentin

Although collagen is the principal component of the organic matrix of dentin (Stack, 1955), the presence of carbohydrate has been known to exist for some time (Pincus, 1948, 1950; Rogers, 1949; Hess and Lee, 1952; Stack, 1955; Kumamoto, 1955). Some of the carbohydrate was shown to be in the form of chondroitin sulfate (Pincus, 1948, 1950; Hess and Lee, 1952; Stack, 1955), and chondroitin 6-sulfate has recently been found to be the predominant glycosaminoglycan (Clark et al., 1965). Kumamoto was able to identify glucuronic acid, galactose, glucose, mannose, xylose (1955), and fucose (1956) in hydrolysates of rat dentin, and later, information on the nature of the substances containing these sugar residues became available. Hexoses were found to be convalently linked to the collagen of bovine dentin, in the proportion of 2.2 per 1000 amino acid residues (Veis and Schlueter, 1964). These hexoses consist of galactose and glucose, with only trace amounts of other sugars (Veis, 1971). Dentin collagen therefore is a glycoprotein.

Recently, Veis et al. (1969) observed that an EDTA extract of fresh bovine dentin contained not only minerals but also several noncollagenous glycoproteins. Some of these glycoproteins were investigated

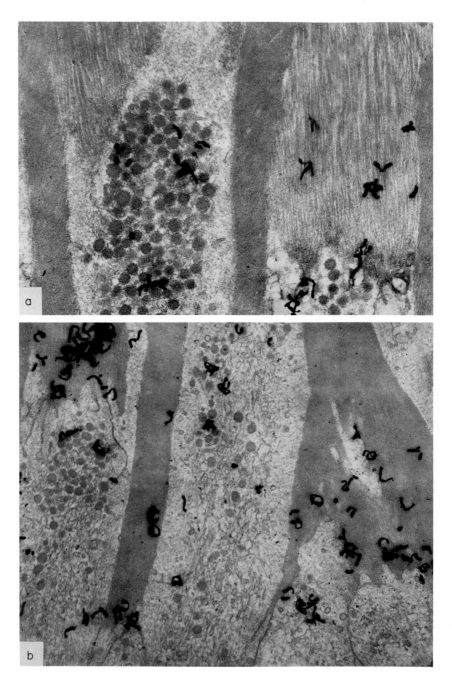

FIG. 7.

in detail and shown to contain 11% fucose by dry weight (Spector and Veis, 1968). A sialoglycoprotein containing fucose that has many features in common with bone sialoglycoprotein (Andrews *et al.*, 1967) has also been isolated from dentin (Zamoscianyk and Veis, 1966). At the present time, more is known about the sialoglycoprotein derived from bone.

B. Odontoblasts and the Elaboration of Dentin

1. *Cytology*

Dentinogenesis involves the elaboration of the organic predentin matrix which subsequently mineralizes to become mature dentin. The cells responsible for the elaboration of the predentin are the odontoblasts, columnar-type cells that are situated in a single layer along the periphery of the dental pulp adjacent to the predentin (Fig. 2a).

The ultrastructural aspects of dentinogenesis have been reported by a number of investigators (Watson and Avery, 1954; Quigley, 1959; Nylen and Scott, 1960; Scott and Nylen, 1960; Noble *et al.*, 1962; Bevlander and Nakahara, 1966; Frank, 1966; Takuma, 1967; Reith, 1968a,b; Garant *et al.*, 1968). The cytoplasm contains an abundant rough endoplasmic reticulum which occupies the bulk of the cytoplasm above the basally located nucleus. Situated in the cytocentrum is a well-developed Golgi apparatus (Fig. 9c) which possesses features in common with other collagen producing cells such as osteoblasts and fibroblasts. Mitochondria are scattered between the profiles of rough endoplasmic reticulum.

Extending apically from the terminal web is the odontoblastic process (Op in Fig. 8), a branched projection of cytoplasm that is embedded

---

FIG. 7. (a) Radioautograph of portions of the apical (Tomes') processes of two secretory ameloblasts and adjacent enamel matrix obtained 30 minutes after injection of galactose-^{3}H. ×26,400. From left to right: (1) an enamel prong separating apical processes; (2) an apical process containing a large number of secretory granules and facing a small portion of striated matrix (upper left); (3) another enamel prong; and (4) the distal end of an apical process with secretory granules at lower right, and, above it, a large portion of striated matrix. The silver grains are found in two locations: over the groups of secretory granules and over the regions of striated matrix, as shown at right. (From A. Weinstock and Leblond, 1971.) (b) Radioautograph of apical processes of secretory ameloblasts and adjacent matrix obtained 4 hours after injection of fucose-^{3}H. ×16,000. At this time, some silver grains remain over secretory granules. Most of the grains are over the two striated regions of enamel, that is, next to the distal ends of apical processes (upper left) and at the tips of the enamel prongs (lower left and right of figure). These labeled regions are located opposite the sites of secretion and are referred to as *growth regions*. (From A. Weinstock and Leblond, 1971.)

in the predentin and conspicuously devoid of most of the organelles normally present in the cell body proper. After EDTA- demineralization, the principal components of the processes appear to be microfilaments, microtubules, electron-dense elongated granules with limiting membranes, smooth-surfaced microvesicles, coated vesicles, and scattered glycogen-like particles (Fig. 11; A. Weinstock *et al.*, 1972). The elongated granules are similar in appearance to those detected in and around the Golgi zone, but they are somewhat denser. Those within the Golgi zone commonly contain parallel arrays of fine filaments that demonstrate a periodicity. A regular distribution of electron-dense particles is commonly observed in association with these filaments. These findings generally correspond to those of other investigators working with undemineralized specimens obtained from developing teeth of the rat (Reith, 1968b), and cat (Frank, 1970b). Very recent cytochemical evidence suggests that the filamentous content of the granules may be related to collagen (M. Weinstock, 1971b, 1972).

The base of the odontoblastic process is embedded in the predentin matrix which, in demineralized preparations, appears to consist of (1) a loose meshwork of collagen fibers exhibiting a wide range of cross-sectional diameters and (2) an interfibrillar material possessing little electron opacity (Fig. 11). The collagen fibers display the native banding pattern. In contrast, the bundles of collagen fibers of mature dentin seem to be more tightly packed and intimately associated with an electron-dense, granular material which obscures the banding pattern (Fig. 11; A. Weinstock *et al.*, 1972). This phenomenon can be seen to advantage at the junction of the predentin and the dentin, the site of the so-called calcification front. The collagen fibers that bridge the predentin–dentin interface display a coating material on those portions extending into the dentin, whereas those parts belonging to the predentin lack coating material (Figs. 10b and 11). Thus, after predentin becomes mineralized, the individual fibers of the collagen bundles seem to acquire a fine, granular, electron-dense, coating material.

2. Histochemical Detection of Glycoprotein

Early light microscope histochemical work using the periodic acid-Schiff (PAS) technique for the detection of glycoproteins (Leblond *et al.*, 1957) revealed the presence of glycoprotein in the matrix of dentin (Wislocki *et al.*, 1948) with only traces in the predentin (Greulich and Leblond, 1954). In 1955, Kumamoto suggested that the sugar residues extracted from the dentin matrix were responsible for its staining with PAS, although it was not known whether these residues were associated with collagen or the noncollagenous glycoproteins, or both.

More recently, ultrastructural investigations on glycol methacrylate–embedded odontoblasts (M. Weinstock, 1971a) using the acidified phosphotungstic acid technique (Rambourg, 1969) for the detection of glycoprotein have shown the staining of Golgi-associated vacuoles and elongated granules. The content of the granules demonstrated a periodicity. While precise information is lacking at the present time, the reactive elongated granules in the Golgi zone appear to be identical to those identified in the odontoblastic processes which also took up the stain. In addition, a heavily stained material was identified between and associated with the collagen fibers of the dentin, suggesting that mature dentin contained abundant glycoprotein. The collagen fibers of the predentin stained lightly, but in contrast to the dentin proper, the interfibrillar material was unreactive (M. Weinstock, 1971a). These findings are compatible with those of earlier investigators, using the PAS technique, namely, the positive staining of the dentin and the weak staining of the predentin. Our evidence suggests that the dense collagen-associated material of the dentin that is observed in routine demineralized preparations, as shown in Fig. 11, is responsible for the uptake of phosphotungstate and therefore is probably composed in part of glycoprotein. It should be noted that this material is detected only after "staining" with heavy metals such as uranium or lead in routine Epon preparations, or with phosphotungstate in glycol methacrylate preparations; the material is not visible in unstained preparations, indicating that it contains little or no residual mineral that may have escaped removal by EDTA. These findings demonstrate that relatively little detectable glycoprotein is present in the predentin matrix, whereas mature dentin is rich in glycoprotein.

2. Radioautography

Much of the radioautographic work on the elaboration of predentin and dentin has been carried out using collagen precursors such as glycine-³H or proline-³H. After injection of either tracer, the label first appears in the cytoplasm of the odontoblasts (Carneiro and Leblond, 1959; Leblond, 1963; Young and Greulich, 1963; Reith, 1968a; Frank, 1970b). Soon thereafter, the label can be traced to the collagen-rich predentin, indicating that newly synthesized collagen had been deposited there. As collagen continues to be deposited, the odontoblasts gradually become displaced toward the pulp.

More recently, radioautography has been applied to the problem of dentin glycoprotein biosynthesis. Inasmuch as fucose is incorporated into the carbohydrate moiety of glycoprotein fairly specifically without any significant conversion to other substances (Coffey *et al.*, 1964; Bekesi

and Winzler, 1967; Kaufman and Ginsberg, 1968), fucose-³H was selected to serve as a precursor for tracing dentin glycoprotein biosynthesis
in the rat incisor (A. Weinstock and M. Weinstock, 1971; A. Weinstock
et al., 1972). Thus, at 5 and 10 minutes after injection of fucose-³H,
light microscope radioautographs show silver grains localized over a

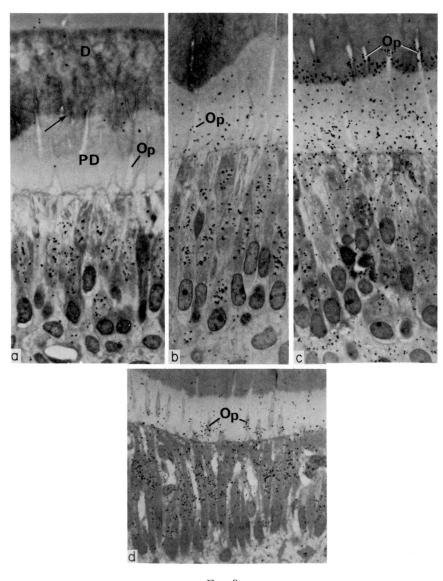

Fig. 8.

weakly stained region of the supranuclear cytoplasm of odontoblasts (Fig. 8a). This region corresponds to the location of the Golgi apparatus as confirmed by electron microscopy. In contrast, the apical cytoplasm of the cell, odontoblastic processes, predentin, and dentin are unlabeled at this time interval. By 35 minutes, some silver grains are located over the predentin region near the cells (proximal predentin), chiefly over the base of the odontoblastic processes (Fig. 8b). By four hours postinjection, the number of grains over predentin increases but most striking is the band of silver grains along the dentin side of the predentin–dentin junction (Fig. 8c). These data demonstrate that odontoblasts participate in the biosynthesis of fucose-containing glycoprotein and, as well, play a role in its transport and secretion. The glycoprotein is deposited in two locations within the dentin matrix: (1) the proximal predentin, and (2) the predentin–dentin junction.

In the electron microscope, the first site where silver grains are detected after fucose-^{3}H injection is the Golgi apparatus. Thus, as in other cell types that synthesize glycoprotein (Bennett and Leblond, 1970; A. Weinstock and Leblond, 1971), fucose, upon entering the odontoblast, is taken up into the Golgi apparatus. Since fucose has been shown to occupy a terminal position in the carbohydrate side chains of many glycoproteins (Dische, 1963; Spiro, 1969), its uptake by odontoblasts may signify the completion of carbohydrate side chain synthesis (elongation) and thus glycoprotein synthesis. Accordingly, it is likely that the Golgi apparatus not only participates in the attachment of sugar residues to forming glycoprotein but also is the site of completion of the fucose-containing glycoprotein of dentin. The protein moiety (endogenous acceptor molecules) would be synthesized in the rough endo-

---

FIG. 8. Light microscope radioautographs of odontoblasts (Figs. 8a–c from A. Weinstock *et al.*, 1972). (a) Five minutes after injection of fucose-^{3}H. ×880. Silver grains are localized over the supranuclear region of the cell, corresponding to the location of the Golgi apparatus. The predentin (PD) and dentin (D) are unlabeled. Arrow indicates the predentin–dentin junction. Op, odontoblastic process. (b) Thirty-five minutes after fucose-^{3}H injection. ×880. Silver grains are present over the odontoblastic processes and the predentin. The reaction over the Golgi region persists. (c) Four hours after fucose-^{3}H injection. ×880. Silver grains are concentrated over the dentinal side of the predentin–dentin junction, the site of the mineralization front. A reaction may also be seen along the sides of some dentinal tubules, within which the odontoblastic processes are located. The predentin shows a less discrete reaction, most of the silver grains occurring over the proximal portion close to the cells. (d) Twenty minutes after sulfate-^{35}S injection. ×640. Silver grains are localized mainly over the supranuclear cytoplasm in the region of the Golgi apparatus, and over the base of the odontoblastic processes.

plasmic reticulum (Reith, 1968a; Frank, 1970b; M. Weinstock, 1971a) prior to migrating to the Golgi apparatus.

The predominance of silver grains at 10 minutes and later over Golgi vacuoles (Fig. 9c), at 35 minutes over the elongated granules in the odontoblastic processes (Fig. 10a), and by 4 hours over the dentin matrix just beyond the predentin–dentin junction (Fig. 10b) suggests

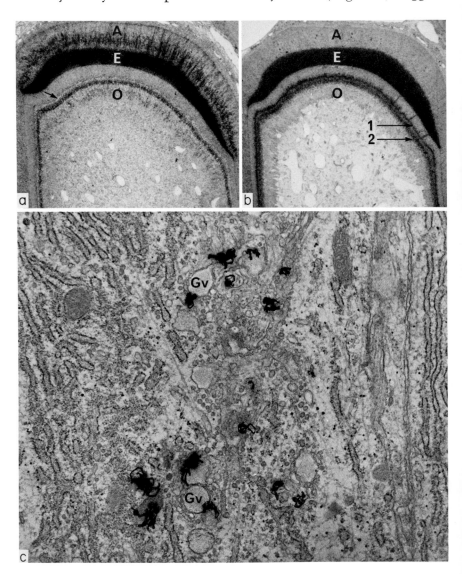

FIG. 9.

that newly synthesized glycoprotein is transported to the odontoblastic processes in the elongated granules derived from the Golgi apparatus and is then released into the matrix. The elongated granules may therefore be compared with the secretory granules of certain other secretory cells; indeed, morphological evidence suggests that they evolve from Golgi vacuoles (Fig. 9c), which are presumably analogous to condensing vacuoles.

The presence of fucose-^{3}H label in the predentin at 35 minutes (Fig. 8b) and in both predentin and dentin at 4 hours (Fig. 8c) may be explained in two ways. The first possibility is that the labeled glycoprotein was first deposited in the proximal predentin and some of it then diffused to the predentin–dentin junction where it began to accumulate. The alternative is that some newly labeled glycoprotein was released into the proximal predentin soon after injection, while some was transported along the odontoblastic processes to be subsequently discharged at the predentin–dentin junction. In fact, different fucose-containing glycoproteins might be released in these two locations. Since the predentin–dentin junction is also the site where radiocalcium is deposited (Kumamoto and Leblond, 1956) indicating that it corresponds to the calcification front, the deposition of a fucose-containing glycoprotein at this site suggests that glycoprotein may play a role in the initiation of mineralization.

With regard to the nature of the glycoproteins involved, significant amounts of fucose are known to exist in some of the noncollagenous

---

Fig. 9. (a) Light microscope radioautograph of an Araldite-embedded section through the growing end of an incisor obtained 2 hours after injection of sulfate-^{35}S. ×104. A strong supranuclear reaction over the Golgi region of ameloblasts (A) and over the enamel matrix (E) can be seen. A light reaction may be seen over the odontoblasts (O), and a dense band of silver grains may be observed over the predentin close to the odontoblasts. This reaction band does not extend as far as the predentin–dentin junction (arrow). (b) Light microscope radioautograph of an Araldite-embedded section through the growing end of an incisor obtained $2\frac{1}{2}$ days after injection of sulfate-^{35}S. ×104. The ameloblasts show little reaction, while the enamel matrix demonstrates an intense reaction throughout its thickness. The odontoblasts show only a weak reaction. The dentin exhibits a double band of silver grains: a narrow one within the dentin proper (arrow 1) and a broad one over the predentin (arrow 2). These two bands of silver grains are separated by a zone of weakly labeled dentin. (c) An electron microscope radioautograph of the Golgi region of an odontoblast, obtained 35 minutes after injection of fucose-^{3}H. ×19,200. The reaction is over the elements of the Golgi apparatus, with some silver grains adjacent to or overlying membrane-limited Golgi vacuoles (Gv) and over a developing elongated granule (top center, structure under silver grain to the right of Gv). Other elements of the cytoplasm are unlabeled. (Fig. 9c from A. Weinstock *et al.*, 1972.)

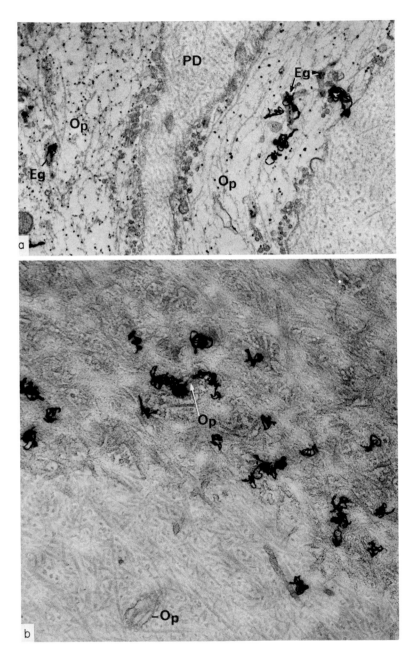

FIG. 10.

glycoproteins of dentin (Spector and Veis, 1968; Veis, 1971). The fucose label detected in the radioautographs, therefore, probably represents labeled noncollagenous dentin glycoproteins. In this regard, the electron-dense, granular material that is associated with the surface of dentin collagen fibers first appears at the site where fucose label accumulates at 4 hours (cf. Figs. 10b and 11), that is, the predentin–dentin junction. We believe that this material may represent morphological evidence of glycoprotein deposition at this location. It may be recalled that a PAS-positive reaction occurs in dentin with only a faint reaction in predentin (Greulich and Leblond, 1954), suggesting that as predentin transforms into dentin it acquires substantial amounts of a PAS-positive glycoprotein. The fucose-^{3}H label may therefore represent a specific fucose-containing glycoprotein that becomes associated with collagen at the onset of mineralization.

Very similar results have been obtained using sulfate-^{35}S as a precursor for dentin sulfated glycosaminoglycans (M. Weinstock, 1971a; A. Weinstock and Young, 1971). After leaving the Golgi region of odontoblasts, radiosulfate-labeled material enters the odontoblastic processes (Fig. 8d) and is detected in the predentin by 2 hours postinjection (Fig. 9a). At 4 hours, the radioautographic pattern is almost identical to that seen at this interval after fucose-^{3}H injection (M. Weinstock, 1971a). As time progresses (2$\frac{1}{2}$ days) a *double* band of label is observed in the matrix (Fig. 9b): a narrow one deep within the dentin (arrow 1 in Fig. 9b), and a wider one within the predentin (arrow 2 in Fig. 9b). These two bands appear to be separated by a relatively weakly labeled zone of dentin. This observation was unexpected insofar as it followed a single injection of sulfate-^{35}S. We believe that the narrow band of silver grains located deep within the dentin, that is, closest to the dentino-enamel junction, may correspond to the label originally de-

Fig. 10. (a) An electron microscope radioautograph of predentin including branches of an odontoblastic process, obtained 35 minutes after fucose-^{3}H injection. ×19,200. The silver grains are localized over the odontoblastic process (Op), where they frequently overlie membrane-limited elongated granules (Eg). The predentin (PD) shows no reaction in this micrograph; however, grains were observed over the predentin in other locations. (From A. Weinstock et al., 1972.) (b) An electron microscope radioautograph of the predentin–dentin junction obtained 4 hours after injection of fucose-^{3}H. ×19,200. The upper half of the micrograph represents dentin, and the lower half predentin. The silver grains are localized chiefly over the bundles of collagen fibers on the dentinal side of the predentin–dentin junction. Grains may also be seen associated with odontoblastic processes and their branches (Op) within the dentin. An electron-dense, fine granular material is associated with the collagen fibers of decalcified dentin but not with those of the predentin (cf. Fig. 11). (From A. Weinstock et al., 1972.)

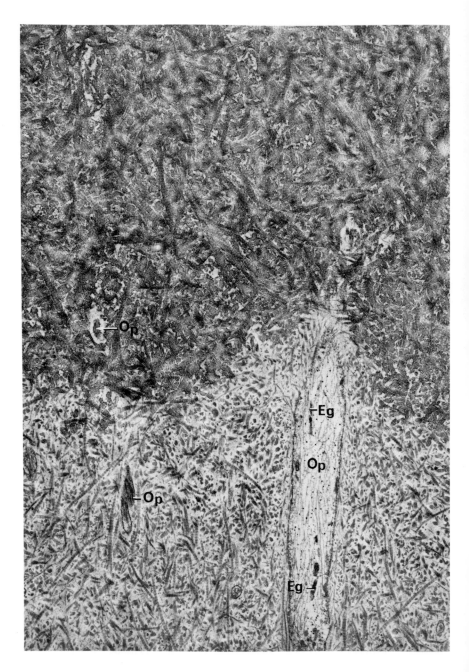

F<small>IG</small>. 11.

posited at the calcification front. Similarly, the band of label situated closer to the odontoblasts presumably resulted from the deposition of labeled sulfated glycosaminoglycans in the proximal zone of predentin, that is, close to the base of the odontoblastic processes. The weakly labeled zone of dentin separating these two bands of silver grains appears to have had its origin in the weakly labeled zone of predentin located next to the predentin–dentin junction, a zone which seems to acquire little labeled material (Fig. 9a). Indeed, at about 5 days after injection, the double band of silver grains persists deep within the dentin, the narrower band again appearing on the side closest to the dentino-enamel junction, and the wider one closer to the odontoblasts (Fig. 5 in Kennedy and Kennedy, 1957; A. Weinstock and Young, 1971). These findings illustrate that sulfate-^{35}S-labeled material, probably glycosaminoglycan, is deposited in two distinct zones: one corresponding to the site of the mineralization front, and the other in the predentin situated next to the odontoblasts. The explanation for this phenomenon may be akin to that described above for the deposition of fucose-containing glycoprotein by odontoblasts, i.e., selective diffusion, or the existence of two sites of secretion. Similarly, two types of sulfated glycosaminoglycans may be secreted, one for each zone of deposition.

V. Role of Glycoproteins in Enamel and Dentin

While the functional significance of glycoproteins in mineralizing matrices has not yet been fully elucidated, several important clues have been obtained to date.

Veis and co-workers (1969) have isolated phosphate-rich, noncollagenous glycopolypeptides from dentin and bone. The dentin glycopolypeptides are particularly rich in covalently bound phosphate, and both contain large quantities of aspartic acid and serine (see also Butler and Desteno, 1971). These acidic glycopolypeptides, possessing a negative net charge, are believed to be situated in a periodic fashion along

---

FIG. 11. A low power electron micrograph of deminearlized dentin from a rat incisor, demonstrating the junction of the mature dentin (upper half of micrograph) and the predentin (lower half of micrograph). A portion of an odontoblastic process (Op) containing microtubules, microfilaments, and membrane-limited elongated granules (Eg) may be seen at lower right. Obliquely sectioned branches of an odontoblastic process are visible at lower left and center. Note that the collagen fibers in mature dentin are intimately associated with an electron-dense material. In contrast, the collagen fibers of the predentin are not associated with this dense material. ×12,000.

the collagen subunits; moreover, the polypeptide moiety may be covalently bound to collagen via the carbohydrate moiety. In two types derived from dentin, it is postulated that galactose and glucose residues are linked to collagen hydroxylysine on one end and a phosphopeptide on the other (Carmichael and Veis, 1971; Veis, 1971). Since these and other glycopolypeptides are highly ionic in character, it has been suggested that they may serve as nucleation sites for the initial epitactic nucleation of calcium ions at specific regions within the collagen fibrils. This hypothesis receives additional support from recent experiments showing that bone sialoprotein has strong cation-binding properties (Peacocke and Williams, 1966; Chipperfield and Taylor, 1968). The radioautographic data presented herein suggests that a fucose-containing glycoprotein, perhaps similar to that found in bone (Andrews *et al.,* 1967), may be involved in the mineralization of dentin. The nature of the association between the fucose-containing glycoproteins and collagen remains to be determined.

For some time sulfated glycosaminoglycans have been implicated in the mineralization of enamel, dentin, and bone, as well as in pathological mineralization (Sobel, 1955). Nevertheless, the role of these high molecular weight anionic compounds in the calcification process is inconclusive. It has been proposed that they may be instrumental in the production of localized concentrations of calcium ions at the sites of mineral nucleation (Woodward and Davidson, 1968). Whatever their precise function, they appear to be synthesized and secreted in large quantities as matrix components for both the developing dentin and enamel, as well as bone (A. Weinstock and Young, 1972).

Despite the paucity of information concerning the mineralization of the enamel matrix, the identification of enamel glycopeptides that are rich in aspartic and glutamic acids and serine (Glimcher and Levine, 1966; Seyer and Glimcher, 1969) is presumptive evidence that, as in dentin and bone, anionic glycopeptides may serve as sites for the epitactic nucleation of mineralization. These glycopeptides are most likely bound at critical locations along the length of the individual matrix subunits in a manner favorable to the formation and growth of the large apatite crystals which are characteristic of enamel.

Acknowledgments

Most of this work was done in collaboration with Dr. C. P. Leblond, to whom I wish to express my gratitude. Appreciation is also expressed to Dr. H. Warshawsky, Dr. Beatrix Kopriwa, Dr. M. Weinstock and Miss Margaret Montague, all in the Department of Anatomy, McGill University, and Dr. R. W. Young (Department of

Anatomy, University of California, Los Angeles). Support was derived mainly by grants to the author from the Medical Research Council of Canada and in part from U.S.P.H.S. General Research Support Grant RR5304.

References

Andrews, A. T. DeB., Herring, G. M., and Kent, P. W. (1967). *Biochem. J.* **104**, 705.

Battistone, G. C., and Burnell, G. W. (1956). *J. Dent. Res.* **35**, 263.

Bekesi, J. G., and Winzler, R. J. (1967). *J. Biol. Chem.* **242**, 3873.

Bélanger, L. F. (1955). *J. Dent. Res.* **34**, 20.

Bélanger, L. F. (1956). *Anat. Rec.* **124**, 555.

Bennett, G., and Leblond, C. P. (1970). *J. Cell Biol.* **46**, 409.

Bevelander, G., and Nakahara, H. (1966). *Anat. Rec.* **156**, 303.

Burgess, R. C., and Maclaren, C. (1965). *In* "Tooth Enamel. Its Composition, Properties and Fundamental Structure" (M. V. Stack and R. W. Fearnhead, eds.), p. 74. John Wright and Sons, Bristol.

Burgess, R. C., Nikiforuk, G., and Maclaren, C. (1960). *Arch. Oral Biol.* **3**, 8.

Burnett, G. W., and Zenewitz, J. A. (1958). *J. Dent. Res.* **37**, 590.

Butler, W. T., and Desteno, C. V. (1971). *Program Abstr. Pap., 49th Gen. Sess., Int. Ass. Dent. Res., 1971* p. 74.

Carmichael, D. J., and Veis, A. (1971). *Program Abstr. Pap., 49th Gen. Sess., Int. Ass. Dent. Res., 1971* p. 74.

Carneiro, J., and Leblond, C. P. (1959). *Exp. Cell Res.* **18**, 291.

Chipperfield, A. R., and Taylor, D. M. (1968). *Nature (London)* **219**, 609.

Clark, R. D., Smith, J. G., and Davidson, E. A. (1965). *Biochim. Biophys. Acta* **101**, 267.

Chilley, J. W., Miller, O. N., and Sellinger, O. Z. (1964). *J. Biol. Chem.* **239**, 4011.

Deakins, M. (1942). *J. Dent. Res.* **21**, 429.

Dische, Z. (1963). *Ann. N.Y. Acad. Sci.* **106**, 259.

Droz, B. (1966). *C. R. Acad. Sci.* **106**, 259.

Eastoe, J. E. (1960). *Nature (London)* **187**, 411.

Eastoe, J. E. (1963). *Arch. Oral Biol.* **8**, 633.

Egyedi, H., and Stack, M. V. (1956). *N.Y. J. Dent.* **22**, 386.

Eylar, E. H. (1965). *J. Theor. Biol.* **10**, 89.

Fearnhead, R. W. (1960). *Nature (London)* **188**, 509.

Fearnhead, R. W. (1961a). *Arch Oral Biol.* **4**, Suppl., 24.

Fearnhead, R. W. (1961b). *In* "Electron Microscopy in Anatomy" (J. D. Boyd, F. R. Johnson, and J. D. Lever, eds.), p. 241. Arnold, London.

Fewer, D., Threadgold, J., and Sheldon, H. (1964). *J. Ultrastruct. Res.* **11**, 166.

Fleischer, B., Fleischer, S., and Ozawa, H. (1969). *J. Cell Biol.* **43**, 59.

Frank, R. M. (1966). *Arch. Oral Biol.* **11**, 179.

Frank, R. M. (1970a). *Arch. Oral Biol.* **15**, 569.

Frank, R. M. (1970b). *Arch. Oral Biol.* **15**, 583.

Garant, P. R., and Nalbandian, J. (1968). *J. Ultrastruct. Res.* **23**, 427.

Garant, P. R., Szabo, G., and Nalbandian, J. (1968). *Arch. Oral Biol.* **13**, 857.

Glimcher, M. J., and Levine, P. T. (1966). *Biochem. J.* **98**, 742.

Glimcher, M. J., Mechanic, G. L., Bonar, L. C., and Daniel, E. J. (1961). *J. Biol. Chem.* **236**, 3210.

Glimcher, M. J., Mechanic, G. L., and Friberg, U. A. (1964a). *Biochem. J.* **93**, 198.

Glimcher, M. J., Travis, D. F., Friberg, U. A., and Mechanic, G. L. (1964b). *J. Ultrastruct. Res.* **10**, 362.

Godman, G. C., and Lane, N. (1964). *J. Cell Biol.* **21**, 353.

Greulich, R. C., and Leblond, C. P. (1954). *J. Dent. Res.* **33**, 859.

Greulich, R. C., and Slavkin, H. C. (1965). *In* "The Use of Radioautography in Investigating Protein Synthesis" (C. P. Leblond and K. B. Warren, eds.), p. 199. Academic Press, New York.

Hess, W. C., and Lee, C. (1952). *J. Dent. Res.* **31**, 793.

Hwang, W. S. S., Tonna, E. A., and Cronkite, E. P. (1962). *Nature (London)* **193**, 896.

Hwang, W. S. S., Tonna, E. A., and Cronkite, E. P. (1963). *Arch. Oral Biol.* **8**, 377.

Jessen, H. (1968a). *J. Ultrastruct. Res.* **22**, 120.

Jessen, H. (1968b). *Arch. Oral Biol.* **13**, 351.

Kalckar, H. M. (1965). *Science* **150**, 305.

Kallenbach, E. (1970). *J. Ultrastruct. Res.* **30**, 38.

Kallenbach, E., Sandborn, E., and Warshawsky, H. (1963). *J. Cell Biol.* **16**, 629.

Karpishka, I., Leblond, C. P., and Carneiro, J. (1959). *Arch. Oral Biol.* **1**, 23.

Kaufman, R. L., and Ginsberg, V. (1968). *Exp. Cell Res.* **50**, 127.

Kennedy, J. S., and Kennedy, G. D. C. (1957). *J. Anat.* **91**, 398.

Krauss, S., and Sarcione, E. J. (1964). *Biochim. Biophys. Acta* **90**, 301.

Kumamoto, Y. (1955). *Rev. Can. Biol.* **14**, 265.

Kumamoto, Y. (1956). Ph.D. Thesis, McGill University, Montreal, Canada.

Kumamoto, Y., and Leblond, C. P. (1956). *J. Dent. Res.* **35**, 147.

Leblond, C. P. (1963). *Ann. Histochim.* **8**, 43.

Leblond, C. P. (1965). *In* "The Use of Radioautography in Investigating Protein Synthesis" (C. P. Leblond and K. B. Warren, eds.), p. 321. Academic Press, New York.

Leblond, C. P., Glegg, R. E., and Eidinger, D. (1957). *J. Histochem. Cytochem.* **5**, 445.

Levine, P. T., and Glimcher, M. J. (1965). *Arch. Oral Biol.* **10**, 753.

Losee, F. L., and Hess, W. C. (1949). *J. Dent. Res.* **28**, 512.

McGuire, E. J., Jourdian, G. W., Carlson, D. M., and Roseman, S. (1965). *J. Biol. Chem.* **240**, PC4112.

Marinozzi, V. (1967). *J. Microsc. (Paris)* **6**, 68a.

Marinozzi, V. (1968). *Electron Microsc. 1968, Proc. Eur. Reg. Conf., 4th, 1968* Vol. II, p. 55.

Marsland, E. A. (1952). *Brit. Dent. J.* **92**, 109.

Miller, E. (1972). *In* "Developmental Aspects of Oral Biology" (H. C. Slavkin and L. A. Baretta, eds.), Academic Press, New York (in press).

Moe, H. (1971). *J. Anat.* **108**, 43.

Morré, D. J., Merlin, L. M., and Keenan, T. W. (1969). *Biochem. Biophys. Res. Commun.* **37**, 813.

Neutra, M., and Leblond, C. P. (1966a). *J. Cell Biol.* **30**, 119.

Neutra, M., and Leblond, C. P. (1966b). *J. Cell Biol.* **30**, 137.

Noble, H. W., Carmichael, A. F., and Rankine, D. M. (1962). *Arch. Oral Biol.* **7**, 395.

Nylen, M. U., and Scott, D. B. (1960). *J. Indiana State Dent. Ass.* 39, 406.
Peacocke, A. R., and Williams, P. A. (1966). *Nature (London)* 211, 1140.
Pease, D. (1966). *J. Ultrastruct. Res.* 15, 555.
Peterson, M., and Leblond, C. P. (1964). *J. Cell Biol.* 21, 143.
Piez, K. A. (1961). *Science* 134, 841.
Pincus, P. (1948). *Nature (London)* 161, 1014.
Pincus, P. (1949). *Brit. Dent. J.* 86, 226.
Pincus, P. (1950). *Nature (London)* 166, 187.
Quigley, M. B. (1959). *J. Dent. Res.* 38, 558.
Rambourg, A. (1967). *C. R. Acad. Sci.* 265, 1426.
Rambourg, A. (1969). *J. Microsc. (Paris)* 8, 325.
Rambourg, A., and Leblond, C. P. (1967). *J. Cell Biol.* 32, 27.
Reith, E. J. (1960). *Arch. Oral Biol.* 2, 253.
Reith, E. J. (1961). *J. Biophys. Biochem. Cytol.* 9, 825.
Reith, E. J. (1963). *J. Cell Biol.* 18, 691.
Reith, E. J. (1968a). *J. Ultrastruct. Res.* 21, 383.
Reith, E. J. (1968b). *In* "Dentin and Pulp" (N. B. B. Symons, ed.), p. 19. Livingstone, Edinburgh.
Reith, E. J. (1970). *J. Ultrastruct. Res.* 30, 111.
Reith, E. J., and Coty, V. F. (1967). *Anat. Rec.* 157, 577.
Rogers, H. J. (1949). *Nature (London)* 164, 625.
Sarcione, E. J. (1964). *J. Biol. Chem.* 239, 1686.
Scott, D. B., and Nylen, M. U. (1960). *Ann. N.Y. Acad. Sci.* 85, 133.
Seyer, J., and Glimcher, M. J. (1969). *Biochim. Biophys. Acta* 184, 509.
Sobel, A. E. (1955). *Ann. N.Y. Acad. Sci.* 60, 713.
Spector, A. R., and Veis, A. (1968). *Abstr. 156th Meet., Amer. Chem. Soc.* p. 16.
Spiro, R. G. (1969). *N. Engl. J. Med.* 281, 991 and 1043.
Stack, M. V. (1954). *J. Amer. Dent. Ass.* 48, 297.
Stack, M. V. (1955). *Ann. N.Y. Acad. Sci.* 60, 585.
Takuma, S. (1967). *In* "Structural and Chemical Organization of Teeth" (A. E. W. Miles, ed.), Vol. I, p. 325. Academic Press, New York.
Veis, A. (1971). Unpublished results.
Veis, A., and Schlueter, R. J. (1964). *Biochemistry* 3, 1650.
Veis, A., Spector, A. R., and Carmichael, D. J. (1969). *Clin. Orthop. Related Res.* 66, 188.
Volpin, D., and Veis, A. (1971). *Biochem. Biophys. Res. Commun.* 44, 804.
Warshawsky, H. (1966). *Anat. Rec.* 154, 438.
Warshawsky, H. (1968). *Anat. Rec.* 161, 211.
Warshawsky, H. (1971). *Anat. Rec.* 169, 559.
Wassermann, F. (1944). *J. Dent. Res.* 23, 463.
Watson, M. L. (1960). *J. Biophys. Biochem. Cytol.* 7, 489.
Watson, M. L., and Avery, J. K. (1954). *Amer. J. Anat.* 95, 109.
Weinmann, J. P., Wessinger, G. D., and Reed, G. (1942). *J. Dent. Res.* 21, 171.
Weinstock, A. (1967). *Anat. Rec.* 157, 341.
Weinstock, A. (1969). Ph.D. Thesis, McGill University, Montreal, Canada.
Weinstock, A. (1970a). *Anat. Rec.* 166, 395.
Weinstock, A. (1970b). *J. Histochem. Cytochem.* 18, 875.
Weinstock, A. (1971). Unpublished results.
Weinstock, A. (1972). Program Abstr. Pap., *50th Gen. Sess., Int. Ass. Dent. Res.,* 1972 (in press).
Weinstock, A., and Leblond, C. P. (1971). *J. Cell Biol.* 51, 26.

Weinstock, A., and Weinstock, M. (1971). *Anat. Rec.* **169**, 450.

Weinstock, A., and Young, R. W. (1971). Unpublished results.

Weinstock, A., and Young, R. W. (1972). *Anat. Rec.* (in press).

Weinstock, A., Weinstock, M., and Leblond, C. P. (1972). *Calcif. Tissue Res.* **8**, 181.

Weinstock, M. (1971a). Unpublished results.

Weinstock, M. (1971b). *Abstr. Pap. 11th Ann. Mtg., Am. Soc. Cell Biol., 1971* p. 321.

Weinstock, M. (1972). *Z. Zellforsch.* (in press).

Whur, P., Herscovics, A., and Leblond, C. P. (1969). *J. Cell Biol.* **43**, 289.

Wislocki, G. B., Singer, M., and Waldo, C. M. (1948). *Anat. Rec.* **101**, 487.

Woodward, C., and Davidson, E. A. (1968). *Proc. Nat. Acad. Sci. U. S.* **60**, 201.

Young, R. W., and Greulich, R. C. (1963). *Arch. Oral Biol.* **8**, 509.

Zamoscianyk, H., and Veis, A. (1966). *Fed. Proc., Fed. Amer. Soc. Exp. Biol.* **25**, 409.

CHAPTER 4

Growth Hormone and Skeletal
Tissue Metabolism

MARSHALL R. URIST

I. Introduction

A large part of present knowledge of growth hormone comes directly
from observations on the skeletal system. For historical background,

the reader is referred to epochal experiments on skeletal development recalled in Chapter 21 by Asling and Evans (1956) of the first edition of this book. The painstaking studies of Asling and Evans and their associates at the University of California, affirmed by many research workers of the past fifteen years, are an important source of stimulation for a large group of new investigators. To make space for a review of literature on biochemical and metabolic studies of growth hormones and bone of recent years, permission has been granted by the editor to exclude morphological descriptions of skeletal maturation, body and bone disproportions, and craniofacial abnormalities. Important articles of the literature of the period from 1925 to 1950 and many recent papers expertly covered in review articles by Catt (1970), Asling (1965), McGarry *et al.* (1964), Li (1968), Theoleyre (1970), Wilhelmi (1955), and McLean and Urist (1968) are also excluded from the bibliography of this edition. This chapter summarizes selected contributions to experimental and clinical knowledge of growth hormone in hard tissue metabolism published in the period from 1950 to 1970.

Growth hormone (GH), also called somatotropin (STH), is the pituitary factor which promotes overall growth of the body, even when acting in the absence of other pituitary hormones (e.g., when injected into hypophysectomized animals). Growth hormone is the only one of the six anterior pituitary hormones that does not depend directly upon another endocrine gland for its action. All others—follicle stimulating hormone (FSH), luteinizing hormone (LH), prolactin (PL), adrenocorticotropic hormone (ACTH), and thyrotropic hormone (TH)—depend on a second endocrine organ to secrete another hormone for the physiologic effect. However, growth hormone has synergistic effects with other hormones and enhances their effects on many different target glands and tissues.

Growth is a highly complicated phenomenon. By definition, growth involves the laying down of new tissue. Measuring growth by weight increase alone is misleading since a weight increment may result from water retention, fat deposition, and a variety of other factors, as well as addition of new tissue. As growth is associated with protein anabolism, GH always induces nitrogen retention. Nitrogen retention is actually a result of protein synthesis and generally is associated with a decrease in the plasma NPN, urea nitrogen, amino acid nitrogen, and an increase in the tissue protein nitrogen. Since the hypophysectomized animal has a poor appetite and suffers at the same time from other hormonal deficiencies, the optimum effect of the growth hormone can be demonstrated in hypophysectomized animals only under certain well-defined circumstances. For example, nitrogen retention and deposition of body protein must be studied under conditions of paired feeding in order to control factors related to nonhormonal nutritional conditions of the body before and after treatment.

Not all growth phenomena are under strict hypophyseal control. Mitotic activity and regeneration of liver following partial hepatectomy, for example, show only slight impairment in hypophysectomized animals as compared to the intact ones. The same is true of fracture healing. However, the size of the liver increases disproportionately in relation to the rest of the body in animals treated with growth promoting pituitary extracts. In some species, at least, growth and development of newborns continue for several weeks in the absence of pituitary and only from the fourth week on does its deficiency manifest itself.

The mode of action of GH is not known. As a rule, the concept of growth implies permanent addition of differentiated tissues and excludes temporary additions to bulk and weight such as would result from seasonal development of the gonads or accumulation of fat or glycogen. Thus, increase in linear dimensions offers the safest criteria for detection of body growth, particularly over a specified interval of time for an experimental bioassay study. And inasmuch as the growth in length of a bone takes place in the epiphyseal cartilage, roentgenologic, histologic, and radiochemical measurements on its proximal epiphyses of the tibia of a rat is the standard area for measurement of growth hormone. Of the three measurements, radiosulfate incorporation is the most precise, sensitive, and specific (Collins *et al.*, 1961).

II. Chemical Properties, Including Species Differences

Growth hormone is a single polypeptide chemical entity of high activity. The isoelectric point is estimated to be at pH 6.8 and the molecular weight has been found to be 44,250 (Li, 1957). When growth hormone is subjected to enzymic hydrolysis under strictly controlled conditions, smaller molecules are obtained which still have the same activity as the starting material; this suggests that the activity does not depend upon the integrity of the growth hormone protein but resides in only a portion of the whole molecule.

Li (1968) reviewed research establishing a primary sequence of amino acids of human growth hormone (HGH). Smaller in size than growth hormones of any other species, HGH is composed of a single chain of 188 amino acids without carbohydrate substituents. In man, the amino acid chain probably exists with a large and small loop formed from intramolecular disulfide bonds. Unlike the disulfide bonds of insulin and the neurohypophyseal hormones, the disulfide bonds of HGH are not essential for biologic activity.

Using a strategy employed for synthesis of ribonuclease by the solid phase method, Li and Yamashiro (1970) recently synthesized HGH. Spectrophotometric measurements on the synthetic protein indicated a tyrosine-tryptophan ratio of 7.5 as compared to the known value of 8. Amino acid analysis of an acid hydrolysate gave:

$$Lys_{12.8}His_{1.8}—Arg_{9.7}Asp_{25.5}Thr_{9.2}Ser_{17.8}Glu_{22.0}Pro_{5.9}Gly_{9.9}Ala_{7.8}Cys_{4.3}—$$
$$Val_{9.2}Met_{1.5}Ile_{7.2}Leu_{30.1}Tpr_{3.6}Phe_{12.4}$$

These values were comparable with the analysis of HGH treated with HF and Na–NH$_3$:

$$Lsy_{9.9}His_{2.5}Arg_{10.0}Asp_{23.3}Thr_{9.9}Ser_{27.1}—Glu_{28.7}Pro_{8.1}Gly_{9.3}Ala_{7.1}Cys_{3.1}$$
$$Val_{7.6}Met_{1.2}Ile_{6.7}Leu_{24.7}—Tyr_{6.4}Phe_{11.9}$$

A few months after the Li and Yamashiro (1970) synthesis of HGH, Niall (1971) proposed that because the structure of HGH is about the same as that of human prolactin (HPL), the number of amino acids should be increased from 188 to 190. Leucine and arginine should be added at the end of the aberrant sequence. The facts, however, are that even with two amino acids missing, the biologic activity is present, and that assuming HGH and HPL are identical in structure, the action of HGH does not depend upon the integrity of the total sequence of the HGH molecule.

Growth hormone from other primates resembles HGH in many physical properties but immunologic differences increase with the degree of phylogenetic separation. These immunologic differences indicate differences in amino acid sequence similar to those that have been described for insulin and ACTH from various species. Growth hormones from pig, whale, sheep, and cow pituitaries are believed to have significantly larger molecular weight than HGH. Bovine hormone has one amino end group and two carboxyl end groups which suggest that this hormone exists as a branched chain. These hormones show little or no immunologic cross-reactivity when tested in most immune systems. The larger size of most of the nonprimate GH has suggested to Li (1968) that the inactivity in human beings and the immunologic unrelatedness is dependent upon a core structure that is enclosed in a cloak of amino acids which does not contribute to the biologic activity of the core. When bovine growth hormone is subjected to various enzymic digestions, as much as 24% of the weight of growth hormone may be removed before there is loss in biologic activity in rats. The residual core material has biologic activity in man and cross-reacts with antibodies reactive with HGH.

Briefly stated, monkey pituitary growth hormone is effective in both monkey and man, but human growth hormone pituitary is only effective in man. Monkey and human growth hormone differ chemically from beef growth hormone. Beef, sheep, horse, and pig hormone differ chemically but all appear to be active in the rat, the most commonly used test animal. Knobil *et al.* (1956) injected hypophysectomized monkeys with allogeneic GH and reinstated epiphyseal growth not obtainable with beef GH. Growth hormone prepared from fish pituitaries is inactive in the rat whereas beef growth hormone is active in fish. These studies are interpreted as suggestive of a common nucleus responsible for growth hormone activity (Knobil and Greep, 1959). There is some suggestion that there are important structural differences that do not pertain to the active core. The outer structure of the growth hormone molecule would be responsible for many of the species-specific characteristics (Wilhelmi, 1955). Synthetic HGH reacts immunologically with rabbit antiserum to HGH as revealed by the agar diffusion test. When synthetic HGH is assayed by the rat tibia test for growth promoting activity and pigeon crop sac test for lactogenic activity, the levels are 10 and 5%, respectively, in comparison with native hormone. Now that HGH has been synthesized (Li and Yamashiro, 1970), the core-activity hypothesis can be subjected to rigorous experimental tests. The possibility still exists that the effector sites in the epiphyseal plate are more selective in the primates than in the rat in terms of a molecular lock and key mechanism (Wilhelmi, 1955).

Human pituitary is particularly rich in growth hormones and is resistant to autolysis after death. The yield is 4–10 mg of hormone per gram, and between 4 and 10% of the dry weight of human pituitaries is HGH. Octogenarians have nearly as much HGH in the pituitary as a rapidly growing child.

III. Assay Methods and Plasma Levels

Radioimmunoassay for growth hormone is remarkably accurate because ^{131}I-labeled growth hormone has high specific activity and minimal denaturation. The validity of the method is supported by finding no detectable hormone after total hypophysectomy and the complete identity of the slope of the reaction of plasma extracts and purified hormone in test systems. With radioimmunoassay, the level of circulating HGH in a well-rested adult, prior to breakfast, is less than 3 mμg/ml of plasma.

With moderate exercise, higher values are found. The tendency of plasma HGH level to rise after exercise is greater in women than in men, and a rise occurs in plasma HGH in many individuals 2–4 hours after a meal and during prolonged fasting beyond one night.

In the first days of life very high levels of HGH may be observed, but there is great variability among individual infants. After 2 weeks of age, lower mean levels are found. In older children the circulating fasting plasma concentration of HGH is not greatly different from that reported for adults. Information obtained from isolated measurements tells little about total secretion of hormones during a day. Turnover of growth hormone in the plasma is rapid; the half-life is only about 25 minutes. Hypoglycemia induces prompt secretion of growth hormone.

In normal individuals, GH influences the level of the blood sugar and vice versa. A fall in blood sugar as small as 10 mg % was sufficient to activate growth hormone secretion. Agents which inhibit the utilization of glucose by tissues stimulate the secretion of growth hormone. Hypothyroidism in the rat greatly reduces growth hormone content of the pituitary and the concentration of the hormone in the plasma (Glick *et al.*, 1965). Control of GH secretion is a highly active field of chemical research. In sleep, when plasma glucose is not fluctuating, and insulin has fallen to a very low level, GH is released (Quabbe *et al.* 1971). About two hours later, plasma fatty acids may rise but insulin does not rise in response to nocturnal GH release. Protein depletion initiates compensatory elevation in plasma GH. Vander Laan (1971) regards acromegaly as a disease in which the brain perceives the individual as malnourished. Levodopa, a drug used in patients with parkinsonism, stimulates GH release (Boyd *et al.*, 1970).

A. AMINO ACID INFUSION TEST

Simulating the effects of ingestion of a large quantity of protein, intravenous infusion of amino acid stimulates release of HGH. The level of plasma HGH rises promptly to levels comparable to those observed after insulin hypoglycemia. The response is less consistent in males than in females. A fasting-resting woman is particularly responsive, but high levels of plasma amino acid produced by intravenous infusion of a dose of 0.5 mg/kilo of neutralized arginine within 30 minutes is essential. The blood is collected at 30 minute intervals for 2 hours. A rise, greater than 10 mμg of HGH per milliliter of plasma, is normal. Pretreatment with 3 mg of stilbestrol per day for 2 days will heighten the response. Measurement of HGH is done only by radioimmunoassay, using antiserum to HGH and radioiodinated GH tracer to establish the saturation analysis system. In general, differences in GH titer in response to arginine infusion must be interpreted with caution and are of diagnostic value chiefly in patients with acromegaly (Catt, 1970).

B. Observations on Sites of Action of Growth Hormone

Although the response of the epiphyseal cartilage to hypophysectomy in the rat is consistent and sensitive enough to use for assay work, the site of action of GH on epiphyseal cartilage cells is not known (Daughaday and Mariz, 1962; Daughaday and Reeder, 1966). Sulfate incorporation by epiphyseal cartilage is reduced 30–40% of normal by hypophysectomy, but it is restored within 24 hours by administration of pituitary growth hormone. Addition of growth hormone directly to an *in vitro* incubation of a hypophysectomized rat cartilage, has little stimulating effect. Normal serum is capable of stimulating cartilage directly, whereas serum from hypophysectomized rats is inactive. Still, growth hormone may not act directly on cartilage but may exert its effect through a sulfation factor which is directly active. Tritiated thymidine uptake is also stimulated by a factor contained in normal rat serum but absent in the serum of hypophysectomized rats. This factor is probably identical to the sulfation factor (Daughaday and Kipnis, 1966).

The stimulation of mitogenesis in epiphyseal cartilage under influence of GH is accompanied by similar responses in pancreas, intestinal mucosa, adrenal cortex, liver, and adipose tissues (Murakawa and Raben, 1968). ^{3}H-thymidine uptake during DNA synthesis is quantitatively accelerated in growth cartilages even *in vitro* and is a reaction that is reliable in HGH assay work. Human growth hormone produces a four- to fivefold increase in ^{3}H-thymidine uptake above values obtained in hypophysectomized rats (Breuer, 1968). *In vivo*, the response is low in fetal and weanling rats, high in the premature growing rats, and again low in rats in the long postmature periods of life. Provided that serum containing the sulfation factor of Daughday and Kipnis (1966) is used for the incubating medium, these levels of responsiveness are the same in systems *in vitro* as in the living rat. If the sulfation factor, an intermediary agent in the local action on cartilage, is absent, *in vitro* assay methods are unsatisfactory (Heins et al., 1970). Weltenhall et al. (1969), using labeled precursors, chemically defined media, and postnatal bone tissue, demonstrated stimulation of growth by insulin but not by GH (as measured by collagen and chondroitin sulfate synthesis) and concluded that the reaction to GH may be mediated by insulin and other agents as well as by a sulfation factor. Nevertheless, this factor mediates both the action of GH on muscle as well as cartilage metabolism (Salmon and DuVall, 1970). Van Wyk *et al.* (1971), making important progress on chemical identification of the sulfation factor (SF) and other constituents of acromegalic plasma, suggest SF is protein with a molecular weight of 8000, bound to a larger carrier protein.

Work-induced growth of muscle occurs from both synthesis of protein and decrease in the average rate of protein catabolism. In GH-treated hypophysectomized rat, muscle mass, as measured by uptake of ^{3}H-leucine, increases owing to increase in the rate of synthesis, but there is no change in the normal rate of protein catabolism (Goldberg, 1969). This balance in protein metabolism is lost only by muscles atrophied from cortisone treatment or degeneration, or similar disorders, and would not be expected to be restored by GH.

Little is known of the effect of GH on the biochemical reactions of collagen synthesis. Growth hormone increases the rate of synthesis of soluble collagen, determined by total activity of ^{14}C-hydroxyproline in skin and bones following injections of ^{14}C proline into rats. The uptake is followed by increased urinary excretion of hydroxyproline, presumably reflecting the increase in rate of catabolism of soluble collagen. Growth hormone does not change the soluble to insoluble collagen when expressed per unit of soluble collagen (Aer *et al.*, 1969).

As a rule, hormones interact with a component of the cell membrane and initiate a chain of reactions, the products of early events acting as inducers of subsequent events. A hormone thus activates a built-in chain of reacting substances, and at any one time only a part of the whole system may be in motion. Adenosine-3′,5′-phosphate (cyclic AMP) seems not to act as an intracellular mediator for GH (Butcher *et al.*, 1970), but other systems must be present in cells to amplify its effects. Growth hormone can produce a general effect on protein synthesis within 15 minutes, presumably without intervention of gene mechanism of cell regulation. Korner (1970) observed that an effect of GH on the rate of synthesis or degradation of messenger RNA or of ribosomes is unlikely, although it does enhance the activity of isolated ribosomes *in vitro*. Talwar *et al.* (1970) noted that GH influences the rate of RNA synthesis, and the main locus of its action is on the membranous structures of the cell. When tissue is incubated with GH for 2–10 minutes and examined by the fluorescent antibody technique using rabbit antigrowth hormone plus goat antirabbit globulin serum, the hormone appears in the membranous structures of adipose or endothelial cells. Glucose and amino acids are incorporated rapidly in cell suspensions and homogenates exposed to GH for only a few minutes.

The epiphyseal plate of the hypophysectomized rat is sensitive enough to respond to GH-like substances as well as GH itself. Spargana, a tapeworm, secretes GH-like substance and restores epiphyseal growh of infested hypophysectomized rats (Mueller, 1968; Mueller and Reed, 1968). Injections of the plasma of infested hypophysectomized rats stimulates uptake of radiosulfate by costal cartilage. The GH equivalents are as high as 100 $\mu g/ml$ of plasma, far greater than the quantity in normal rat plasma and about the same as obtained from a single pituitary gland of a rat (Steelman *et al.*, 1970). A worm factor stimulates the hypophysectomized rat to produce the sulfation factor in the absence of GH (Garland *et al.*, 1971).

IV. Experimental Models, Target Tissues, and Deficiency of Growth Hormone

Nearly every tissue in the body may be considered a target tissue for the effect of GH, but some tissues are more responsive than others. One of the prime targets for GH is the *bone growth apparatus*, the epiphyseal plate, and particularly the zone of cell proliferation adjacent to the layer of rows of mother cells (Ross and McLean, 1940). During the period of growth, the epiphyseal plate maintains a constant thickness and maintains an equilibrium between proliferating cartilage, hypertrophic cartilage, calcified cartilage, and endochondral bone. This structure is extremely sensitive to the level or titer of growth hormone in the circulating plasma. When the titer falls from hypophysectomy and deficiency of growth hormone, the epiphyseal plates decrease in thickness and become sealed by a plate of lamellar bone. When growth hormone therapy is instituted in the rat, a species that grows slowly throughout adult life, the growth apparatus is restored by proliferation of cartilage, increase of thickness of the epiphyseal plates, resorption of the lamellar bone-seal, and continuation of growth of the diaphyses in length.

A. HYPOPHYSECTOMY

The classic experimental model on growth hormone is the hypophysectomized rat. With the technique devised by P. E. Smith (1930) and special measures to feed a diet high in protein from natural sources and supplements of the essential vitamins and minerals, the rat will survive hypophysectomy very well. Paired feeding of measured quantities of the diet to normal and hypophysectomized rats is essential for low morbidity and mortality and for a consistently reproducible standard animal model. Replacement therapy with thyroxin and sex hormones

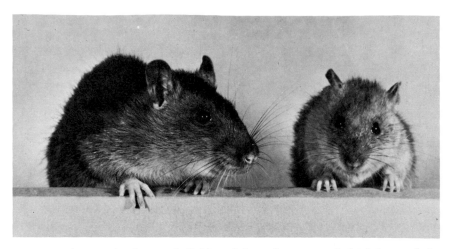

FIG. 1. Photograph of normal (left) and hypophysectomized (right) rat of the Long-Evans strain at 3 months of age. Note the markedly smaller size of the head and paws of the GH-deficient rat. Reproduced from the *Atlas of Skeletal Development of the Rat* with permission of the American Institute of Dental Medicine, San Francisco, Calif.

to compensate for the loss of thyrotropic hormone and gonadotropins is necessary in any experimental design which requires a high level of precision. Two easily detectable responses to deficiency of GH in immature rats are (1) decline in the rate of increase in body weight with growth and (2) decrease in thickness of the epiphyseal plates (Figs. 1 and 2).

B. ENDOCHONDRAL OSSIFICATION IN HYPOPHYSECTOMIZED RATS

The abnormities of endochondral ossification in the hypophysectomized rat are illustrated in Figs. 3 and 4A and 4B. The plates are from copy No. 112 of a limited edition of Becks and Evans' (1953) atlas of skeletal development of the Long-Evans rat of the Institute of Experimental Biology, University of California. Hypophysectomy causes cessation of proliferation and maturation of the growth cartilages, and as a result the epiphyseal plates decrease in thickness. The vascular tufts from the marrow which normally invades the hypertrophic vacuolated cells disappear and the metaphyseal trabecular bone is resorbed without replacement or reconstruction. Eventually, calcification of the juxtamedullary portion of the cartilage ensues and deposition of lamellar bone plates finally seals epiphyseal plate off from the marrow. This lamellar bone-seal closely resembles that observed in growth stasis from other causes. Among the other conditions which similarly seal the epiphyses are normal aging, phosphorus poisoning, thyroidectomy, vitamin A deficiency, riboflavin deficiency, protein deficiency, caloric restriction, and radiation injury. The radiographic "lines of arrested growth," observed in children recovering from an acute infectious disease, is indicative of a similar abnormality in the pattern of epiphyseal bone growth.

In the hypophysectomized rat, internal remodeling of bone is much less affected by GH deficiency than epiphyseal endochondral ossification. Anderson and McKeen (1969) injected [85]Sr into GH-treated hypophysectomized, untreated hypophysectomized, and normal rats, and measured whole body radioactivity over an interval of 6 weeks. No significant difference in [85]Sr retention or weight of the whole tibias was noted among groups of animals, but the net gain in weight was always significantly greater in normal and GH-treated hypophysectomized rats than in untreated hypophysectomized rats. Hence, the increase in weight from treatment with GH was chiefly in nonosseous tissues and not associated with measurable alterations in rate of turnover of mineralized bone tissue. These seemingly negative data testify to the fact that the layer of interdigitating calcifying cartilage and primary spongiosa is a specific target while bone remodeling sites are unspecific targets of action of GH. Similar data obtained on patients treated with HGH will be discussed in Section V.

C. REPLACEMENT THERAPY

Growth hormone replacement therapy must be evaluated with the aid of a preparation of animal GH or HGH of maximum physicochemical and biologic purity. For a valid test, growth hormone must be of a single molecular species as demonstrated by electrophoresis and free from contamination with other pituitary hormones. Evans *et al.* (1943) considered a minimal effective dose of the order of magnitude of 10 μg of GH (free from any detectable inclusion of othe anterior pituitary hormones), but at least 5 μg of GH administered daily over a period of 4 days is necessary for a valid test. Evidence of the effects on the skeleton is obtained from gross measurements of the length of the bone, radiographic measurements of the thickness of the epiphyseal plate, and histologically detectable resorption of the bone-seal between metaphysis and epiphysis.

Administration of the GH of the anterior lobe of the pituitary promptly repairs the defect in growth of hypohysectomized rats. The animals are responsive to the effect of GH whether the injections are commenced

Normal – 71 days

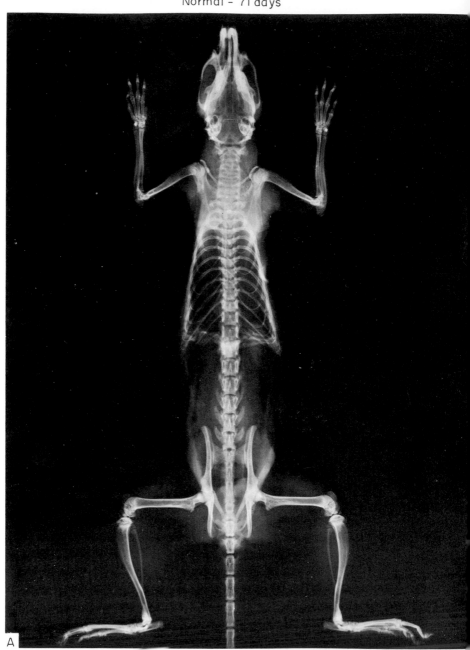

A

Fig. 2A.

Hypophysectomized
77 days postoperative

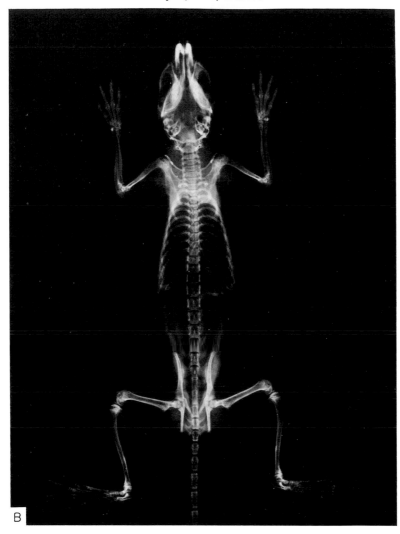

Fɪɢ. 2B.

Fɪɢ. 2. (A) Roentgenogram of the whole skeleton of the normal individual at about 10 weeks of age, when the growth of the Long-Evans rat begins to decrease in rate. (B) Roentgenogram of the skeleton of a hypophysectomized rat at about 10 weeks of age. Note the 30% smaller diameter and length of the bones; the metaphyses are 50% as long as normal; the epiphyseal lines are barely perceptible; and the overall radiodensity of both flat and long bone structure is low. Reproduced by permission of the American Institute of Dental Medicine, San Francisco, Calif.

Normal - 71 days

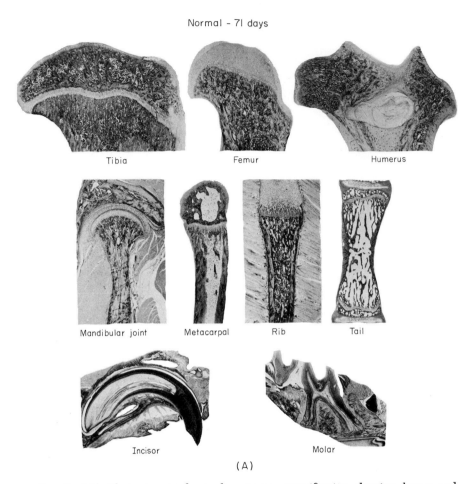

(A)

FIG. 3. (A) Photomicrographs in low power magnification showing bones and teeth of a normal rat at 10 weeks of age. Note the thickness of the epiphyseal plates of the long bones and quantity of trabecular bone in ribs and tail vertebra.

shortly after the operation or whether the delay is a year or longer (Becks *et al.*, 1946). Although the majority of experiments have been made on rats hypophysectomized when 28 days old, age at the time of hypophysectomy is not a factor; rats hypophysectomized when as young as 6 days of age and as old as 6–7 months have been shown to be responsive to administration of the growth hormone.

Growth hormone administration restores the histologic appearance of epiphyseal cartilage plates to that characterizing young, actively growing bones. Promptly (in 5 days or less), chondrogenesis is reawakened,

Hypophysectomized
77 days postoperative

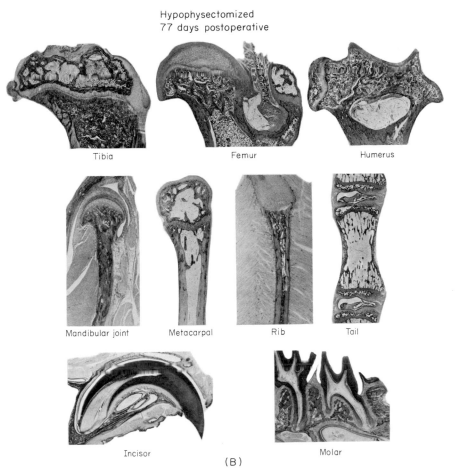

Tibia   Femur   Humerus

Mandibular joint   Metacarpal   Rib   Tail

Incisor   Molar

(B)

FIG. 3. (B) Photomicrograph of bones and teeth from a hypophysectomized rat of about 10 weeks of age. Compared with the specimens from the rat shown in (A), the overall dimensions of the epiphyses are smaller, the epiphyseal plates are thinner, the trabecular bone tissues are attenuated, while the ratio of diameter of shaft to thickness of cortical bone is not significantly different. Figure 3 reproduced by permission of the American Institute of Dental Medicine, San Francisco, Calif.

vascular tufts from the marrow again invade the vacuolated cells and even resorb the lamellar bone-seal if one was present. The trabecular bone structure of the metaphysis is redeposited by palisades of newly differentiated osteoblasts. The cortical bone, as one may eventually see by differential staining, develops layers of metachromatic-formed new bone concentrically round layers of old eosinophilic bone. The widening of the epiphyseal cartilage plate is, within a broad range of dosages, proportional to the quantity of hormone administered (Becks *et al.*, 1941). The epiphyseal plate method of assay of the potency of hormone

Tibia

Proximal epiphysis – normal

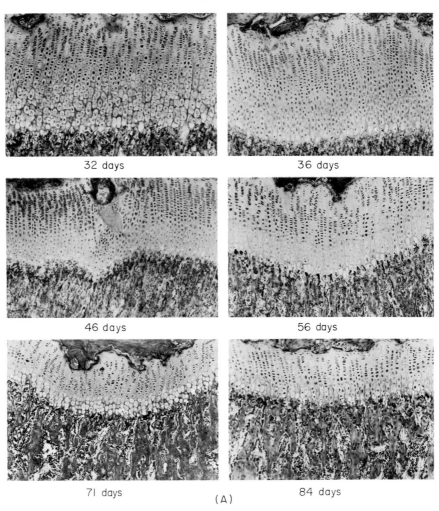

FIG. 4. (A) Photomicrographs in higher power magnification showing the normal structure of the epiphyseal plate of the proximal end of the tibia at successive intervals of time between 32 and 84 days of age in the Long-Evans strain of rats. Note the progressive decrease in thickness of the zones of hypertrophy and vesiculation of chondrocytes.

Tibia

Proximal epiphysis – hypophysectomized

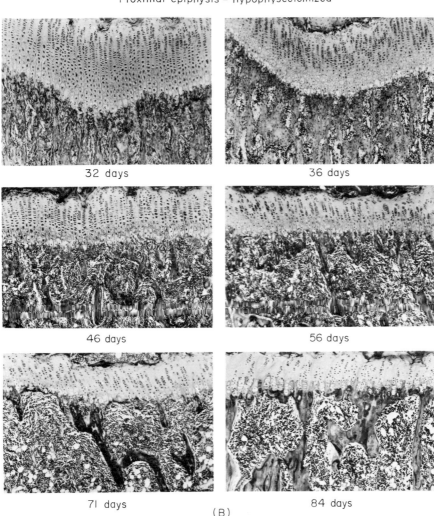

32 days

36 days

46 days

56 days

71 days

(B)

84 days

FIG. 4. (B) Photomicrographs of a series of sections of the proximal end of the tibia of hypophysectomized rats, at the same intervals of time as shown in (A). Note the pronounced decrease in the zone of cell hypertrophy within a 4-day period between 32 and 36 days, the loss of about 30% of the thickness of the epiphyseal plate within the 24-day interval between 32 and 56 days of age, the epiphyseal plate sealed off from the metaphysis at 71 days of age, and the thick malformed bone trabeculae of the metaphysis at 84 days.

Tibia

Normal   Hypophysectomized

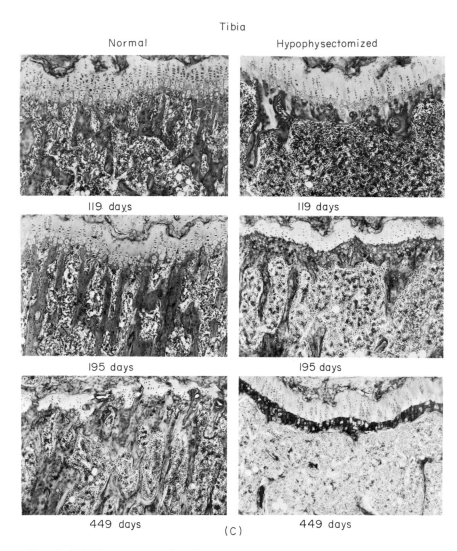

119 days   119 days

195 days   195 days

449 days   449 days
                              (C)

FIG. 4. (C) Photomicrographs of the normal (left) and hypophysectomized (right) rats at intervals of 119, 195, and 449 days. Note the progress of replacement of trabecular bone with bone marrow and development of the characteristic lamellar bone seal of the epiphyseal plate of the hypophysectomized rats. Normally, the rat tibia continues to grow slowly in length long after sexual maturity; parts of the epiphyseal plate are resorbed and bars of bone bridge the gap between metaphysis and epiphysis at about 400 days of age. In the hypophysectomized rat, the epiphyseal plate is not resorbed or replaced by bone but simply enclosed in a dense mass of avascular lamellar bone. Figure 4 reproduced by permission of the American Institute of Dental Medicine, San Francisco, Calif.

preparations is sensitive to as little as 5 μg of hormone given over a 4-day period (Greenspan *et al.*, 1949).

The synergistic effect on the thyroid gland and thyroxin augments the action of GH. Accordingly, thyrotropic hormone acts synergistically with GH (Marx *et al.*, 1943). Although appreciable (but subnormal) growth may be maintained when thyroxin is administered immediately after hypophysectomy (at 28 days of age), this growth does not continue very long (Asling *et al.*, 1954). Histologically, after 14 months the proximal tibial epiphyseal cartilage plates show the same inactivity and atrophy as does untreated hypophysectomized controls. Thyroxin is not a growth-promoting hormone per se, since one of the established criteria for such a hormone is that administration over a prolonged period should result in sustained growth of the hypophysectomized rat.

In hypophysectomized animals, ^{3}H-thymidine labeling experiments demonstrate that a number of labeled cells are reduced to about 20% of normal for animals of the same age. Although the cells are dividing more infrequently, the proliferation zone in the columns of cartilage cells is reduced to only about ¾ of the usual length. After administration of growth hormone there is a delay of as much as 16 hours, and the maximum response may occur as late as 48 hours. The cause of the lag is not known, but it generally occurs in nonskeletal tissue or in any site in which a stimulus is necessary to initiate cell division. In hypophysectomized animals both before and after growth hormone is administered, there is no change in the labeling profile; the distribution of cells along the columns of proliferating chondrocytes is the same. Growth hormone, or its active derivative, affects all cells of the epiphyseal plate, and not just the row mother cells preferentially (Kember, 1971; Asling and Nelson, 1962). However, Rigal (1964) noted that *in vitro* labeling with tritiated thymidine is confined to the row mother cell or proliferating zones of epiphyseal cartilage excised from a rabbit injected with growth hormone. Additional studies are necessary to characterize the factors controlling interaction between endothelial cells and epiphyseal cartilage under the influence of growth hormone. Hansson and Thorngren (1971) are increasing the precision of the epiphyseal plate bioassay method with the use of an oxytetracycline labelling technique.

Labeling experiments do not explain how hypophysectomy reduces the rate of cell division in the cartilage plate with little change in the length of the proliferation zone or how rickets produces little decrease in the length of the proliferation zone but a large increase in the cell hypertrophy zone. Some of the changes in the epiphyseal plate produced by hypophysectomy resemble those seen in aging rats; the intercolumnar matrix increases in quantity along with a corresponding reduction in the number of columns of cells. Hypophysectomy produced a marked decrease in the incorporation of proline-^{14}C and ^{35}SO$_4$ into costal cartilage (Daughaday, 1968). Cartilage slices from hypophysectomized rats take up little or no ^{35}SO$_4$, but growth hormone reinstitutes sulfate metabolism *in vitro*. The very presence of growth hormone in rat serum can stimulate uptake of ^{35}SO$_4$, presumably by increasing the rate of sulfate incorporation into chondroitin sulfate in cartilage. Growth hormone also enhances the conversion of proline to hydroxyproline in surviving tissues *in vitro*. Growth hormone increases the rate of DNA synthesis (Daughaday and Reeder, 1966) and enhances RNA synthesis and increased formation of polysomes (Korner, 1965). Other hormones share with GH the capacity to accelerate protein synthesis, as, for example, thyroid, adrenal cortical steroid, insulin, and sex hormones. Because of great differences in organ structure and variable rates of growth of the individual bones, experiments on growth-promoting endocrine agents must be very carefully planned to be conclusive (Cheek and Hill, 1970).

D. Human Dwarfism and Human Growth Hormone Replacement Therapy

Deficiency of HGH in childhood produces pituitary dwarfism. Before birth and in early infancy, deficiency of pituitary function does not impair growth (Grunt and Reynolds, 1970). Without any brain or pituitary, anencephalic monsters can grow to very large or normal size (Cheek and Hill, 1970; Naeye and Blanc, 1971). In early childhood and before the end of the fourth year, HGH deficiency becomes apparent by the grossly visible immature facial features and body proportions. Facial wrinkles give the appearance of presenility mixed with immaturity. Low fasting bloor sugar and abnormally high glucose tolerance may occur. The bone age, as determined by roentgenograms of the wrist, is always less than the chronological age. The primary teeth appear on time, but eruption of secondary teeth is delayed. In most cases of pituitary dwarfism, the etiology is either entirely obscure or inherited by an autosomal recessive mechanism, or by some acquired defect in a hypothalamic center regulating HGH secretion such as Hand Schüller-Christian disease and brain tumors. The diagnosis is unequivocally established only by radioimmunoassay and amino acid infusion tests. True, pituitary dwarfism is rare. The differential diagnosis must include Russel dwarfs, premordial dwarfs

(Lorrain-Livi), hypothyroidism, gonadal aplasia, malnutrition, mongolism, constitutional idiopathic retardation of growth, achondroplasia, Laurence-Moon-Biedl syndrome, neurofibromatosis, congenital heart disease, congenital hemolytic anemias, and progeria (Daughaday, 1968).

After injection of HGH into a pituitary dwarf, as differentiated from any other kind of dwarf, nitrogen balance becomes strongly positive; plasma urea and urine urea values promptly fall. Although the levels of daily nitrogen retention gradually decrease with continuous growth hormone treatment, it is still adequate to maintain greatly increased growth rate. Plasma levels of hydroxyproline rise, suggesting increased rate of conversion of proline to hydroxyproline and deposition of new collagen (Daughaday and Mariz, 1962). Sodium, chloride, potassium, magnesium, and phosphorus are retained concomitant with positive nitrogen balance. Calcium may be retained by the body despite increased calciuria. This is explained by increased gastrointestinal absorption of calcium. Plasma phosphorus levels may or may not rise after growth hormone administration in dwarfism. When HGH raises plasma phosphorus levels, the effect is to increase kidney tubular reabsorption of phosphate ions (Corvalain et al., 1962). The urinary hydroxyproline excretion also rises sharply (Jason et al., 1962). Serum alkaline phosphatase is little changed. The long-term administration of growth hormone does not produce diabetes unless very large doses are administered. Infusion of HGH very promptly blocks the ability of insulin to increase glucose removal by muscle tissue. Human growth hormone possesses an intermediate blood sugar lowering action; it alters the central nervous system metabolism directly or indirectly in such a way as to cause pituitary dwarfs to become much more active and alert.

African pigmies are genetic dwarfs with no deficiency in immunologically active HGH, but they show less response to the hormone than either normal or hormone-deficient subjects. Low levels of response of end-organ biosynthetic mechanisms may be responsible for genetic dwarfism. Antigen antibody and other blocking reactions are other possibilities for investigation in genetic forms of dwarfism (Merimee et al., 1968).

E. Regeneration of Bone

Hypophysectomy retards the healing of ordinary undisplaced long bone fractures. Apituitary dwarf mice produce only unmineralized soft callus and delayed union of fractures of the tibia (Hsu and Robinson, 1969). Large defects in the calvarium heal in normal weanling rats but not hypophysectomized rats; nearly normal repair occurs in hypophysectomized rats treated with growth hormone (Simpson *et al.*, 1953). Large diaphyseal defects not repaired by normal mature dogs are repaired by mature dogs treated with bovine growth hormone (Zadek and Robinson, 1961).

Shepanek (1953) treated normal mice with 5.0 mg of GH daily and noted enlargement of callus trabecular bone mass; union was inhibited rather than hastened by treatment with GH. Koskinen (1959) measured fracture healing in normal rats by correllated roentgenographic, ^{32}P autoradiographic, and line diagram histologic techniques and concluded that procine GH alone increased the volume of callus while GH plus thyroxin produced union 2 weeks earlier than in untreated controls. Udupa (1966) and Lindohm *et al.* (1967) corroborated Koskinen's observations on rats. Koskinen (1963, 1967) also treated 64 patients with thyroxin and procine GH for anticipated delay or nonunion and reported beneficial results in some instances. Misol *et al.* (1971) reported delayed union in a fracture of the femur in a 26-year-old man who had subnormal levels of plasma growth hormone, and they suggested that HGH therapy is justifiable in such cases. Thus, experimental and clinical studies suggest that the availability of synthetic HGH might bring important benefits to patients with bone defects from injury or disease.

Anterior pituitary secretions, as noted previously, are essential for regeneration of whole limbs, including bone in adult urodeles. Hypophysectomy inhibits regeneration in the adult newt but not in the larval amphibian. The whole process of limb regeneration is restored by whole gland implants, crude extracts, and purified GH and ACTH hormones (Schmidt, 1960). Regeneration of the deer's antler is profoundly influenced by sex hormones (Goss, 1969) and as such is prevented by hypophysectomy and withdrawal of FSH or by castration. The effects of hypophysectomy in the buck, under adequate testosterone replacement therapy, require further study.

F. Lower Vertebrates

Cells comparable to GH hormone secreting cells in the pituitary glands of mammals are present in the pituitary of fish. Accordingly, it is reasonable to suppose that the same cells secrete GH or prolactin-like GH in all species from cyclostomes to man.

In fishes, gill, kidney, and integumentary membranes regulate calcium total ion concentrations and osmotic equilibrium. Pituitary hormones, possibly prolactin or GH, influence ion regulatory mechanism. Parathyroids (which are absent) or ultimobranchial bodies—calcitonin-secreting glands—(which are present) are not involved. Pang *et al.* (1971) described hypocalcemic tetany in the hypophysectomized teleost in calcium-free, but not calcium-rich, sea water. Thus, gill membranes regulate calcium fluxes in sea water (in which the levels of calcium are normally 10 mM/l) but need the pituitary hormones to defend the organism against hypocalcemia in calcium-free sea water or fresh water (in which the levels of calcium are normally only 0.7 mM/l). Which pituitary hormone is responsible for control of calcium ion concentrations is not clear. The possibility that a pituitary hormone, as yet undiscovered, may regulate calcium separately from sodium to maintain calcium homeostasis when the fish is a fresh water habitat, warrants further investigation.

Hypophysectomy prevents limb regeneration in fish, but neither the character of the hormones involved nor their sites of action has been elucidated (Goss, 1969). In reptiles and birds, prolactin has growth-promoting properties. In teleost fish, as noted above, prolactin is identified more easily by its effects on osmoregulation and resistence to environmental stress than by promotion of growth (Bern and Nicol, 1968). In urodeles, prolactin stimulates limb regeneration (Waterman, 1965). In hypophysectomized newts, in which administration of ACTH or cortisone can restore regeneration of limbs, it appears that the pituitary is required only insofar as it stimulates secretion of glucocorticoids from adrenals (Schmidt, 1960). These observations point out the difficulty of separating unspecific from specific effects of pituitary hormones in lower vertebrates.

V. Excessive Action of Growth Hormone

Excessive secretion of growth hormone is frequently associated with eosinophilic adenoma, a tumor of the pituitary gland. In immature individuals this tumor produced gigantism, in adults acromegaly. The characteristic feature of acromegaly is enlargement of the terminal parts of the body—nose, mandible, fingers, toes—with an increase in diameter of the long bones. Overgrowth of the skeleton is a constant reaction to administration of growth hormone in excess of normal requirements for long periods of time. In a short-term (30 days) experiment, in which the hormone was administered to normal growing, female rats, starting at 81 days of age, 1 mg of GH per day stimulated growth in body and tibia length in excess of normal, and widened the epiphyseal cartilage plate (Asling *et al.*, 1948, 1950). Evans and Simpson (1931) produced gigantism in gonadectomized as well as intact rats. The intact males receiving the hormone exceeded their controls in body length by over 9%; the corresponding females exceeded their controls by 15%. Gonadectomized rats were surprisingly responsive; in fact, the response seemed even greater in ovariectomized rats.

Gigantism generally can be produced to the degree that most of the skeletal dimensions exceed normal by 12–16% in immature as well as mature hypophysectomized female rats. In immature rats, in which the pituitary is removed at 28 days of age, the hormone can be injected for $14\frac{1}{2}$ months starting 12 days after hypophysectomy (Simpson *et al.*, 1949) (as little as one-fifth to one-tenth the dose given to adult rats) and still produces gigantism. Such rats, while exceeding normality in weight, maintain normality in length and in dimensions of the individual bones. In mature hypophysectomized rats, the dose of hormone given over a period of 13 months may closely approximate that given the intact rats and still produce gigantism (Moon *et al.*, 1951). Hypophysectomized GH-treated rats often exceed in some skeletal dimensions even the intact giant rats (Asling *et al.*, 1955).

Harris and Heaney (1969) treated adult dogs of both sexes with bovine GH, 0.5 mg/kg/day for 84 days, and increased the mass of skeletal tissue without inducing acromegaly or diabetes. The increase was measured by tetracycline labeling and mineral accretion using ^{45}Ca kinetic techniques. Formation, not resorption, occupied almost every endosteal bone surface, and the estimated increase in skeletal mass was 63% compared with less than 5% in control periods in corresponding bones. Absorption of calcium from the diet was more than doubled under the influence of GH. Previously, Marx and Rheinhardt (1942), using radiostrontium uptake measurements, were unable to detect a stimulating effect of GH on accretion of bone. On the assumption that endocrine deficiencies cause osteoporosis and that postmenopausal women might have lower than usual output of growth hormone (either resting and after hypoglycemia), Harris and Heaney (1969) suggested that HGH might be an effective therapeutic agent for postmenopausal osteoporosis. A therapeutic trial of HGH in a patient with senile osteoporosis produced only negative results (Urist *et al.*, 1963). More recently, five patients with severe senile osteoporosis showed no depression of the GH titer (Urist and Heuser, 1971). Inasmuch as senility alters the molecular conformation of intracellular enzymes (Root and Oski, 1969), there is the possibility that bone cells have a low level of end organ response to normal HGH secretion in idiopathic or senile osteoporosis. Aging also reduces the response of cells to the sulfation factor, which mediates the effect of GH (Heins *et al.* 1970).

Reinhardt and Li (1953) produced chronic arthritis in knees and ankles of gonadectomized-adrenalectomized rats under prolonged treatment with growth hormone. Joint deformities developed in both intact and hypophysectomized rats, and most constantly in the vertebral column, knee, and ankle joints. The incidence and the degree of deformity was much greater in hypophysectomized rats than in intact rats similarly treated. M. Silberberg *et al.* (1964) described the ultrastructure of GH-induced arthropathy in mice; GH increases the rate of development of coarse endoplasmic reticulumn, Golgi vesicles, glycogen bodies, and other organelles of the chondrocyte, but it breaks the cell down after about 4 weeks. The intercellular collagen fibers become disoriented and frayed, producing the so-called asbestos transformation characteristic of acromegalic arthropathy and osteoarthritis of advanced age. Through these changes, GH treatment produces arthrosis within 2 weeks in adult animals (R. Silberberg and Hasler, 1971). Grossly, these deformities are comparable to those found in human acromegalic joint disease (Waine *et al.*, 1945; Kellgren *et al.*, 1952; Bluestone *et al.*, 1971).

The kyphosis and the characteristic overgrowth of bone on the anterior aspect of the vertebral bodies, described by Erdheim (1931), are characteristic features of human acromegalic osteoarthropathy. These features of acromegaly in the human are similar but not exactly the same as in the skeleton of the rat. The paws become thickened both laterally and dorsoventrally in mature individuals treated chronically with growth hormone but the phalanges do not elongate beyond normal. The thickening seems chiefly in skin and subcutaneous connective tissues. Epiphyseal fusion occurs during the treatment if it has not already taken place before the hormonal injections began. The incisor malocclusion of mandibular prognathism is not demonstrable in the rat, perhaps because of the special features of incisal occlusion in rodents, whose incisors form and erode continuously throughout life. However, there is overgrowth and deformity of the mandibular zone of endochondral ossification (that cartilage of the condyle subjacent to the temporomandibular joint), actually the squamosomandibular articular cartilage. Some malocclusion of the molar teeth, by antero-displacement of the mandibular molars as a result of the excessive condylar growth, is demonstrable. The bony attachments of the temporal and suboccipital muscles are unusually large. Kurtz *et al.* (1970) treated rats with 1 IU/day for 10 days and noted reactivation of the cartilage in the palatal suture and mandibular symphysis. The chondrocytes increased in number and hypertrophied osteoclasts destroyed the zone of calcified cartilage; no changes were visible in the adjacent bone structure. Thus, GH produced an easily detectable growth-promoting effect on cartilaginous closing sutures and symphyses. Prominences of the appendicular skeleton, such as the deltoid tuberosity of the humerus, are markedly overgrown in GH-treated rats.

VI. Interaction with Other Hormones

A. Thyroidectomy and Thyroid Replacement Therapy

The hypophysectomized animal has a low level of oxidative processes owing to secondary hypothyroidism. Administration of thyroid hormone improves the growth-promoting effect of growth hormone both morphologically and metabolically. Thyroid alone, however, does not induce growth in the hypophysectomized animals. The response of an hypophysectomized rat's epiphyseal growth zone is somewhat misleading in this respect inasmuch as a widening obtained by treatment with thyroxin is similar, albeit quantitatively inferior, to that obtained with growth hormone. Removal of thyroid hormone also results in a deficient pituitary function, one of the first signs of which is degranulation of the acidophils, the presumptive source of growth hormone. Evans *et al.* (1939) described growth retardation following thyroidectomy at 35–45 days of age much like that which follows hypophysectomy. Thyroidectomized–hypophysectomized rats had body lengths still shorter than those only thyroidectomized. The epiphyseal cartilage plate regression after thyroidectomy corresponds in all essential features to those observed after hypophysectomy (Becks *et al.*, 1942a,b).

Thyroidectomized growing rats gain about 140% over their original body length in 2 months, while intact rats gain 300%. The greatest part of these gains is achieved before the rats are a month old (Ray *et al.*, 1950). Some excess of growth of thyroidectomized rats over that of rats hypophysectomized and observed at comparable ages is to be expected. Thyroid hormone is known to be relatively long lasting, and the full effect of its deprivation (including pituitary hypofunction) might not be developed immediately after thyroidectomy, whereas growth hormone has a very short survival time and would be expected to disappear promptly after hypophysectomy. With the above reservations, the effect of the two deficiencies on skeletal growth is quite similar. The similarity is reflected in a stereotyped atrophy of histologic structure of the proximal tibial epiphyseal cartilage plate when rats operated upon at an early age are compared. In both GH and thyroid hormone deficiencies the plates remain wider and the abnormalities of the epiphyseal ossification center are greater in young than in older rats (Asling and Evans, 1956).

Reinstating growth after thyroidectomy differs in some respects from that after hypophysectomy; thyroxin will stimulate active growth in thyroidectomized rats. Concurrently, pituitary function is restored. As attested by evidence from gonads and adrenals, gonadotropic and adrenocorticotropic hormones again come into good supply from endogenous sources. The repair of pituitary structure, and particularly the regranulation of acidophils (Koneff *et al.*, 1949), make it likely that the growth from administration of thyroxin can be attributable to an endogenous supply of growth hormone. Thus, many of the conditions necessary for a growth hormone-thyroxin synergism are restored simply by the administration of thyroxin.

The response of rats to hypophysectomy and thyroidectomy combined, and to replacement therapy, has been studied by Evans *et al.* (1939) in rats approximately 40 days of age when operated upon. It has also been studied by Ray *et al.* (1954) who performed thyroidectomy on the first day of life and hypophysectomy on the twentieth day of age. The presence of each gland complicated the analysis of results obtained when administering products of the other. Thyroxin administration has negligible effects on growth in a hypophysectomized rat. Still, analysis of the results of growth hormone administration is complicated by variability in response and the delicate condition of these test rats. Fortunately, some individuals tolerate the experiment well enough to demonstrate that concurrent administration of growth hormone and thyroxin stimulates vigorous growth and even surpasses the growth rate of intact rats.

B. Pancreas and Insulin Therapy

Insulin is another factor influencing the protein–anabolic action of growth hormone. In the completely depancreatectomized dog receiving no insulin, the growth hormone fails to induce nitrogen retention. If such a dog is treated with small amounts of insulin (not even enough to control diabetes completely), growth hormone produces its characteristic nitrogen sparing protein–anabolic effect. Such findings suggest that some insulin must be present to permit growth hormone to act as a protein anabolizer. In the Houssay depancreatectomized–hypophysectomized cat, growth hormone fails to induce nitrogen retention in the absence of insulin. Optimum nitrogen retention is reached only when the insulin does not induce true growth in cat, but the results in rodents are contradictory even with the use of the tibia growth effect. Antenatally, insulin acts in the absence of GH (Naeye and Blanc, 1971). Human growth hormone has an insulin-like effect immediately and an anti-insulin effect late after administration by injection (Goodman and MacDonald, 1969). A synergistic effect similar to that of insulin has been reported with glucagon.

In hypophysectomized rats, as noted previously, administration of GH increases the total body protein and decreases the total body fat. Some of these effects of GH on skeletal tissue can also be reproduced with insulin, but the major increase in body constituents with insulin takes place in the body fat rather than the protein. The primary metabolic action of growth hormone has not yet been definitely localized. The rate of conversion of amino acids to blood urea and to urinary urea is decreased. Entrance of amino acids into the cell is accelerated by growth hormone because there is a prompt fall in the plasma level of amino acids. Hypophysectomy leads to a fall of the hepatic RNA synthesis with a decrease not only of the number of ribosomes but also in the amount of messenger and soluble RNA. When growth hormone is given to the hypophysectomized rats there is a stimulation of all RNA synthesis. While these results have established definite effects of growth hormone on the subcellular protein synthesizing machinery, they fail to pinpoint the specific locus of growth hormone action (Daughaday, 1968).

C. Adrenal Glands and ACTH Therapy

In castrated rats, adrenocorticotropic hormone (ACTH) depressed growth of body weight (Moon, 1937). As demonstrated later in intact male rats, ACTH impairs bony growth markedly (Evans *et al.*, 1943; Becks *et al.*, 1944). In hypophysectomized rats, a direct antagonism to the effects of pituitary growth hormone is shown by injecting ACTH concurrently with a potent growth hormone preparation (Marx *et al.*, 1943). In the tibia, the proximal epiphyseal cartilage plate becomes narrow with many irregularities in cell columns. Osteogenesis is slow (Becks *et al.*, 1942b). These effects are not attributable to reduced food intake because the rats treated with both hormones actually consume more food than those given only growth hormone. In spite of marked growth inhibition, skeletal maturation is not delayed by ACTH treatment.

The extent to which ACTH participates in the pituitary gland's regulation of normal skeletal development through its opposition to the stimulating effect of growth hormone requires further investigation. Adrenal corticosteroid therapy retards growth in children by suppression of the hypothalamic pituitary-adrenal axis, but the effect is not entirely attributable to insufficient secretion of HGH. The deleterious effects on growth of children with Still's disease can be mitigated by intermittent administration of cortisone (Sturge *et al.*, 1970). In the future, supplements of synthetic HGH may become available to counteract some of the side effects of cortisone on bone.

D. Sex Glands, Sex Hormone Therapy, and Osteoporosis

Pituitary control of skeletal development through the action of gonadotropic hormones was presented by Asling and Evans (1956) and might be brought up to date by a few brief statements. Sex hormones do not initiate skeletal growth but only augment the action of growth hormone in hypophysectomized rats. Species differences are very important in the pituitary gland–sex hormone influence upon formation and development. Gardner and Pfeiffer (1943) observed no inhibition of estrogen-induced endosteal bone formation in hypophysectomized mice, while Kibrick *et al.* (1942) observed that in rats hypophysectomy inhibited the intramedullary ossification normally induced by estrogen. In birds, estrogen produces still another reaction in which the intramedullary ossification of selected long bones occurs even after hypophysectomy. In human beings, estrogen produces neither endosteal nor intramedullary bone. These seemingly diverse results demonstrate that the action of sex hormones on osteogenesis in the rat at least depends upon the cellular activity in growth apparatus. Factors responsible for inhibition of bone resorption and growth by estrogen in the rat but not in the mouse, or bird (Urist *et al.*, 1948), are not known.

In human beings, sex hormones stimulate secretion of HGH. Franz and Robkin (1965), Merimee *et al.* (1966), Buckler (1969), and Bacon *et al.* (1969) observed release of HGH in response to estrogen treatment, and Martin *et al.* (1968) reported a similar release in response to androgen treatment (1968). Sperling *et al.* (1970) viewed the arginine infusion test as a dependable means of stimulation of HGH release and confirm the above-noted effects of estrogen but not androgen. In response to the amino acid infusion, pubertal girls secrete more HGH than prepubertal children of both sexes, and even pubertal boys.

Attempts to apply the amino acid infusion test to disorders of bone are now in progress by several research groups. R. W. Smith (1967) supplied the impetus with an observation that the postmenopausal female has a reduced HGH response to hypoglycemia. Henneman *et al.* (1960) reported increases in absorption of calcium and net positive calcium balance following injections of GH.

In an investigation supported by the Endocrine Study Section of the National Institutes of Health, U. S. Public Health Service, human growth hormone became available in 1961 for treatment of patients with severe osteoporosis. Urist and associates (1963) administered by intramuscular injection 2 mg of HGH per day to a patient under intensive investigation in the hospital for a period of 75 days for: (1) metabolic balance studies for calcium, phosphorus, and nitrogen; (2) radioisotope kinetic measurements with ^{47}Ca-, ^{85}Sr-, and ^{131}I-labeled serum albumin; and (3) bone biopsy. The patient was 71 years of age and able to walk only with the aid of two canes because of muscle atrophy secondary to multiple compression fractures of the dorsal and lumbar vertebrae. The diagnosis of osteoporosis was established by clinical and laboratory studies which were negative for osteomalacia, malabsorption syndrome, hyperparathyroidism, Paget's disease, multiple myeloma, and malignancy. In this patient, exhibiting the most common form of pathologic osteoporosis in the United States, HGH produced 2 g of positive nitrogen balance but the calcium and phosphorus balances were either unchanged or slightly negative (Fig. 5A). Radioisotope osteograms, urinary excretion, and whole body counting revealed that the rate of accumulation of mineral was the same as in normal subjects (Figs. 5B–5D). The rate of resorption was slightly higher than the rate of accretion. Biopsies after tetracycline labeling of the bone, before and following administration of growth hormone, showed the same quantity of lamellar new bone as in nonosteoporotic untreated controls.

Table I summarizes the results of studies with injections of HGH compared with injections of chondroitin sulfates A and C (Osseofac, Squibb), extracted from bovine bone matrix, but without any growth stimulating properties. High growth hormone evokes a consistently reproducible increase in nitrogen retention in aged individuals with osteoporosis, but the effect is the same as in normal aged individuals.

An intravenous injection containing 5 μCi of ^{47}Ca-, 5 μCi of ^{85}Sr-, and 1 μCi of ^{131}I-labeled serum albumin was administered during the period of treatment with daily injection of polysaccharides and again during the period of treatment with HGH. Osteograms of the midshaft of the tibia showed a slow change in rate of uptake, rising over a period of more than 1 hour; on treatment with human growth hormone, the rate of accumulation was the same as in nonosteoporotic normal subjects, where the accumulation of radioisotopes reaches a plateau in 15 minutes. Other areas of the skeleton responded in the same way as the tibia. The daily loss of ^{85}Sr in the urine during treatment with polysaccharide, especially during the first 3 days, was less than with human growth hormone. One-half of the ^{85}Sr was excreted in 5 days on polysaccharide treatment; on human growth hormone, the same percentage of the dose was excreted in only 2 days; ^{47}Ca was always much better retained in the skeleton than ^{85}Sr. The 50% excretion point was reached after 18 days on placebo treatment but only 5 days on human growth hormone; strontium is not reabsorbed as efficiently as calcium by the kidney tubules.

When relative values of the exchangeable pool and calcium excretion rate are calculated on the basis of urinary clearance of strontium, the values are not absolute but can be used to compare one case with another (Table I). The size of the exchangeable calcium pool (on the basis of the osteogram) was the same during the entire period of treatment, but the bone accretion rate was not greater than in normal subjects with human growth hormone. Because calcium balance was unchanged, it is necessary to assume that the higher rate of accretion may be associated with a higher rate of resorption. This is reflected in the urinary excretion curves (Fig. 5C). The daily loss of ^{85}Sr in the urine on polysaccharide treatment was slightly less during the first 10 days than with the growth hormone. Thereafter, more ^{85}Sr was lost per day on polysaccharides, suggesting a higher rate of resorption of bone which had been labeled with the isotope. Thus, the ^{85}Sr excreted during the early days comes mainly from soft tissue and from ^{85}Sr deposited on preexisting bone salt crystals by exchange rather than by incorporation into newly forming crystals (accretion). Only at later times could the daily loss be derived from slow resorption of mineral crystals which contained ^{85}Sr laid down earlier by accretion. Although difficult to interpret, radio isotope turnover studies show no reason to assume HGH will increase skeletal accretion in patients with senile osteoporosis.

The major effect of HGH upon the normal nonosteoporotic skeleton is to increase the rate of bone formation which also leads to increased rate of bone remodeling. Fraser and Harrison (1960) regarded these effects as secondary to increased activity of parathyroid glands because growth hormone alters the renal and intestinal transport of calcium and phosphate in addition to having direct effects on the skeleton. The renal effects of growth hormone are opposite to those of parathyroid hormone (PTH), causing increased retention of phosphate. This makes for tendency toward hypocalcemia which is corrected by increased secretion of parathyroid hormone. Increased secretion of parathyroid hormone promotes increased calcium absorption from intestine. In this respect the effect of PTH is synergistic to that of the growth hormone because positive calcium balance would increase bone turnover. Slightly elevated plasma phosphate levels are also characteristic of the state of a high level production of growth hormone. Nordin (1966) reviewed and evaluated the conflicting data in the clinical literature and summarized present knowledge as follows: GH raises plasma calcium, reduces parathyroid

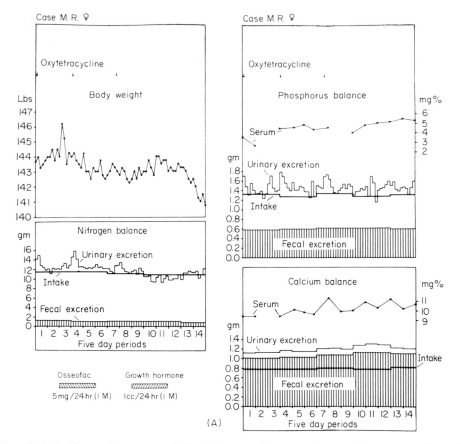

(A)

FIG. 5. (A) Charts showing metabolic balance studies in a 71-year-old woman with senile osteoporosis. The patient lost weight and was in continuous negative calcium, phosphorus, and nitrogen balance. Placebo treatment with injections of bone polysaccharides (Osseofac, Squibb) did not restore equilibrium. Human growth hormone produced nitrogen retention but did not correct negative calcium and phosphorus balances. (B) Radioisotope osteogram showing the changes in rate of uptake of an intravenous injection of ^{85}Sr and ^{47}Ca in the patient referred to in (A). The upper curve (first study) represents the reaction of the tibia during a period of treatment with intramuscular injections of polysaccharides. The lower curve (second study) represents the response to treatment with human growth hormone. These results with HGH are the same as obtained in untreated nonosteoporotic subjects and corroborate results with bovine GH in experimental animals reported by Anderson and McKeen (1969). (C) Graph showing urinary excretion of ^{85}Sr and ^{47}Ca in patient referred to in (A) and (B). The total loss of ^{85}Sr isotope during the first 3 days was only 23% on placebo polysaccharide therapy (first study). The net effect of the treatment on the loss of calcium in the urine over a period of 3 weeks is about the same on placebo and HGH. (D) Charts illustrating the retained amounts of ^{85}Sr and ^{47}Ca as measured by whole body counting in the patient referred to in (A) to (C). At all times, the amounts of both isotopes retained by the skeleton were slightly greater during treatment with the placebo (first study) than with human growth hormone (second study). The time required to lose 40% of the ^{85}Sr was 5 days for the first study as compared with 2 days for the second. These observations reveal no preferential effect of growth hormone on deposition of new tissue in the skeleton, and, if anything, less effect than an unspecific placebo. Figures (A) to (D) reproduced with permission of Urist et al. (1963) and Amer. Ass. Advance Sci., Washington, D.C.

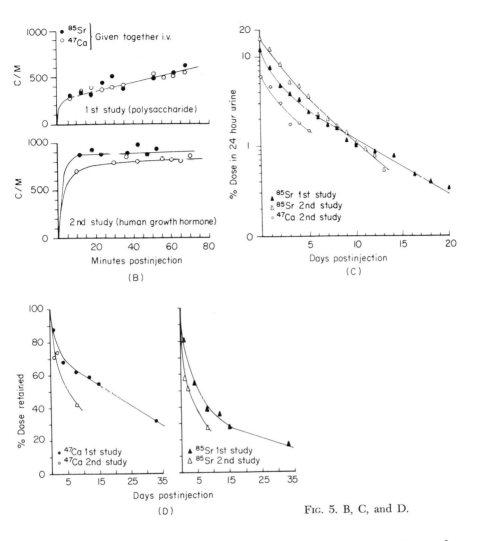

FIG. 5. B, C, and D.

activity, raises plasma phosphate, increases urinary calcium. Hypercalciuria would cause negative calcium balance and possibly lead to osteoporosis.

Inhibition of bone resorption (as determined by positive calcium balance) conceivably could be produced in patients with osteoporosis by administration of estrogens. The question arises whether this response is secondary to effects upon secretion of growth hormone. According to Buckler (1969), both men and women of all ages show an increase in GH production in response to large doses of estrogen. Other mechanisms not dependent upon GH production may also explain the action of estrogen on patients with osteoporosis, as, for example: (1) suppression of parathyroid hormone production, (2) decrease in sensitivity of bone tissue and/or kidney to the adverse effects of parathyroid hormone (Young and Nordin, 1967), (3) decrease in the tendency to bone loss

TABLE I

Summary of Results of Intravenous Injections of a Mixture of
^{85}Sr and ^{47}Ca in a 71-Year-Old Osteoporotic Treated with
Placebo (Polysaccharides) and HGH

	Treatment	
Determinations	Placebo	Human growth hormone
Tibia osteogram	Both ^{47}Ca and ^{85}Sr still rising after 70 minutes	Both ^{47}Ca and ^{85}Sr leveled off after 15 minutes
Knee osteogram	Both ^{47}Ca and ^{85}Sr still rising after 70 minutes	Both rising after 70 minutes but less steeply
Urinary excretion (3 days)	Sr, 23%; Ca, 15%	Sr, 37%; Ca, 14%
Total excretion (total body counting): time to lose first 50% of dose	Sr, 5 days; Ca, 18 days	Sr, 2 days; Ca, 5 days
Exchangeable calcium pool[a]		
From ^{85}Sr data	1.9 gm	1.5 gm
From ^{47}Ca data	—	5.9 gm
Accretion rate for calcium[a]		
From ^{85}Sr data	0.06 gm/day	0.04 gm/day
From ^{47}Ca data	—	0.22 gm/day

[a] Calculated by the method of Bauer *et al.* (1955).

from the acidosis which accompanies physiologic secondary hyperparathyroidism, (4) restored response of bone to balanced calcitonin-parathyroid hormone production following the menopause, and (5) retardation of the adverse effects of parathyroid hormone on bone marrow mastocytosis (Frame and Nixon, 1968). The level of response of the adult human skeleton either to HGH or estrogen is too small to restore bone mass in osteoporotics to a degree demonstrable by roentgenography. Since the cause of pathologic osteoporosis in human beings is not known, and since excessive HGH may aggravate rather than retard the disorder, HGH must be considered another unspecific modality and therefore indicated only in selected patients under investigation in metabolic wards (Urist, 1970).

The osteoporosis of acromegaly is an inconstant and puzzling entity. Some observers suggest the cause is hypersecretion of both ACTH and GH (Snapper, 1957). Chronic suppression of calcitonin production is a possibility. Some writers suggest the cause is premature aging (M. Silberberg and Silberberg, 1942; Fourman, 1955).

E. Calcitonin

The rate of secretion of calcitonin is influenced only indirectly but not necessarily insignificantly by GH. According to Milhaud and Moukthar (1965) the calcitonin content of the C cells of the thyroid is comparable in hypophysectomized and normal rats. Zileli *et al.* (1968) observed secretion of calcitonin in the urine of rats injected with guinea pig GH; thyro-parathyroidectomy prevented this effect of GH on production of calcitonin. Care *et al.* (1969) perfused the thyroid glands of pigs with hypercalcemic blood and noted secretion of calcitonin for 4 hours in intact pigs but only 1.3 hours in hypophysectomized pigs. Salzer and Lischka (1970) contended that hypophysectomy, first reduces the size of the nuclei of C cells of the thyroid in rats, and second, produces slower and weaker defense against hypercalcemia (produced by injections of calcium chloride). Whether GH increases secretion of calcitonin and inhibits bone resorption, or decreases secretion of calcitonin and increases bone resorption (as in acromegaly) or has no effect is not altogether clear, but a GH effect on resorption seems essential for longitudinal growth of bones. Indeed, GH may be necessary to maintain the proper balance of thyroid, parathyroid, and calcitonin-hormone activity that accounts for internal remodeling (resorption and reformation) of bone.

VII. Tissue Culture

Growth hormone is secreted into media by tissue organ cultures of pituitaries from human (Thompson *et al.*, 1959) and rodents (Smolders, 1939; Gaillard, 1942; Verdam, 1946). Explanted rat (Verdam, 1946) and chick (Hay, 1958) bones do not elongate beyond control bones when supplements of bovine GH are added to the media. Embryonic chick cartilage anlage show uptake of ^{35}S-labeled chondroitin sulfate in greater quantities and grow longer in the presence of supplements of GH in the media (Ito *et al.*, 1959, 1960a,b). Embryonic chick somites also synthesize increased quantities of polysaccharides when GH is added to a standard culture media (Lash and Woodhouse, 1960). Nogami and Urist (1971), using chemically defined media containing both GH and thyroxin, described differentiation of mesenchymal cells into chondro-osseous tissues but not bone or bone marrow. These observations demonstrate that GH acts on skeletal tissues and sustains growth of cartilage *in vitro*. In view of the species specificity of the chemical structure of GH, autologous and allogeneic GH might produce responses different from those obtained with bovine xenogeneic GH, particularly in systems reported to yield negative results.

VIII. Summary

From the demonstrations of growth hormone (GH) by Evans and associates (reviewed by Asling and Evans, 1956) in the third decade of this century, there emerged a twenty-year period of intensive research on the physiology of GH deficiency and replacement therapy. In the fifth and sixth decades, the mainstream of research effort was directed toward the biochemistry, bioassay, mode of action, and metabolism of GH. The beginning of the seventh decade was heralded by the synthesis of HGH by Li and Yamashiro (1970).

Human growth hormone is a chain of 188 to 190 amino acids, with a molecular weight of about 44,000. Beef, sheep, horse, and pig GH differ from HGH and from each other chemically, but all may have a common core structure, and all are active in the rat, the most commonly used test animal. Octogenarians have almost as much HGH in the pituitary as rapidly growing individuals, but the tissues of immature individuals respond more rapidly and completely.

Hypophysectomy of immature animals retards chondrogenesis; proliferation and maturation of chondrocytes ceases and the thickness of the epiphyseal plates diminishes precipitously; vascular loops are unable to perforate the zone of preparatory calcification, osteoblasts differentiate slowly, and the quantity of metaphyseal bone declines. The normal proportions of calcified cartilage to primary spongiosa to metaphysis is maintained only when both GH and thyroid hormones are present. While the effects of these two hormones are difficult to separate, growth hormone sustains the rate of growth of the bones in length while thyroxin controls differentiation and maturation of chondrogenetic and osteogenetic tissues. Treatment of hypophysectomized rats with thyroxin alone produces rapid premature closure of the epiphyseal lines. Treatment of thyroidectomized rats with growth hormone produces rapid proliferation of epiphyseal cartilage, but the cells fail to hypertrophy or invite ingrowth of osteoprogenitor cells for differentiation of osteoblasts. Immature hypophysectomized rats fail to develop normal ossification centers.

Growth hormone accelerates the rate of proliferation of cartilage in the epiphyseal plates. Skeletal growth can be restored to normal in hypophysectomized rats (or even stimulated to excess) by injection of growth hormone in adequate amounts. The extent of skeletal retardation is independent of the age at the time of hypophysectomy. The equivalent of 2–3 weeks of further long bong growth occurs in immature rats even after hypophysectomy or thyroidectomy; maturation but not growth can be restored to normal by administration of thyroid hormone. No other hormone overcomes the effects of GH deficiency. In thyroidectomized rats, thyroxin also stimulates growth, but as much by its action of restoring pituitary function as by its own action. Unlike thyroid hormone, GH does not control skeletal maturation.

The mode of action is not known but GH appears to interact with constituents of cell membrane and activate a chain of reactions in pre-existing cell machinery. Growth hormone may increase mitogenesis four-fold and accelerate RNA synthesis without any effect on the rate of protein catabolism. A sulfation factor, insulin, and presumably other factors in serum are intermediary agents in the action of GH on growth cartilages *in vitro*.

Growth hormone is essential for the normal rate of regeneration. The treatment of delayed and nonunion of fractures with HGH is open to question. The effects of HGH on patients with osteoporosis are not clear. Restoration of growth in pituitary dwarfism is well established by clinical and metabolic balance studies. The development of sensitive methods of measurement of HGH in plasma, and the availability of synthetic HGH, provide the momentum for important progress in this decade of research on GH in health and disease in man and other animals.

References

Aer, J., Holme, J., and Kivirkko, J. K., *et al.* (1969). *Biochem. Pharmacol.* **17**, 1173–1178.
Anderson, J. J. B., and McKeen, J. D. (1969). *Fed. Proc., Fed. Amer. Soc. Exp. Biol.* **28**, No. 2, (abstr. 2804) p. 760.
Asling, C. W. (1965). *Rev. Suisse Zool.* **72**, 1.
Asling, C. W., and Evans, H. M. (1956). *In* "The Biochemistry and Physiology of Bone" (G. H. Bourne, ed.), 1st ed., pp. 671–704. Academic Press, New York.
Asling, C. W., and Nelson, L. E. (1962). *In* "Radioisotopes and Bone" (F. C. McLean, P. Lacroix, and A. M. Budy, eds.), pp. 191–195. Blackwell, Oxford.
Asling, C. W., Becks, H., Simpson, M. E., Li, C. H., and Evans, H. M. (1948). *Anat. Rec.* **101**, 23.
Asling, C. W., Simpson, M. E., Li, C. H., and Evans, H. M. (1950). *Anat. Rec.* **107**, 399.
Asling, C. W., Simpson, M. E., Li, C. H., and Evans, H. M. (1954). *Anat. Rec.* **119**, 101.
Asling, C. W., Simpson, M. E., Moon, H. D., Li, C. H., and Evans, H. M. (1955). *In* "The Hypophyseal Growth Hormone, Nature and Actions" (R. W. Smith, O. H. Gaebler, and C. N. H. Long, eds.), pp. 154–177. McGraw-Hill, New York.
Bacon, G. E., Lowery, G. H., and Knoller, M. (1969). *J. Pediate.* **75**, 385.
Bauer, G. C. H., Carlsson, A., and Lindquist, B. (1955). *Kungl. Fysiogr. Sällsskap Lund Förhandl.* **25**, 1.
Becks, H., and Evans, H. M. (1953). "Atlas of the Skeletal Development of the Rat." Amer. Inst. Dent Med., San Francisco, California.
Becks, H., Kibrick, E. A., Marz, W., and Evans, H. M. (1941). *Growth* **4**, 437.
Becks, H., Kibrick, E. A., and Evans, H. M. (1942a). *J. Exp. Zool.* **89**, 297.
Becks, H., Ray, R. D., Simpson, M. E., and Evans, H. M. (1942b). *Arch. Pathol.* **34**, 334.

Becks, H., Simpson, M. E., Li, C. H., and Evans, H. M. (1944). *Endocrinology* **34**, 305.

Becks, H., Simpson, M. E., Evans, H. M., Ray, R. D., Li, C. H., and Asling, C. W. (1946). *Anat. Rec.* **94**, 631.

Bern, H. A., and Nicol, C. S. (1968). *Recent Progr. Horm. Res.* **24**, 681.

Bluestone, R., Bywater, E. G., Hartog, M., Holt, J. L., and Hyde, S. (1971). *Ann. Rheum. Dis.* **30**, 243.

Boyd, A. E., Leboritz, H. E., and Pfeiffer, J. B. (1970). *N. Engl. J. Med.* **283**, 1425.

Breuer, C. B. (1968). *Endocrinology* **85**, 989.

Buckler, J. M. (1969). *Clin. Sci.* **37**, 765.

Butcher, R. W., Robinson, G. A., and Sutherland, E. W. (1970). *Contr. Process. Multicell. Org., Ciba Found. Symp.* pp. 64–85.

Care, A. D., Anderson, L. L., Cooper, C. W., Oxenwender, S. L., and Phillipo, M. (1969). *J. Endocrinol.* **43**, 679.

Catt, K. J. (1970). *Lancet* **1**, 933.

Cavallero, C. (1946). *Ciba Found. Colloq. Endocrinol.* [*Proc.*] **9**, 266.

Cheek, D. B., and Hill, D. E. (1970). *Fed. Proc., Fed. Amer. Soc. Exp. Biol.* **29**, 1503.

Collins, E. J., Lyster, J. C., and Carpenter, O. S. (1961). *Acta Endocrinol.* (*Copenhagen*) **36**, 51–56.

Corvailain, A. N., Abramow, M., and Bergans, A. (1962). *J. Clin. Invest.* **41**, 1230.

Daughaday, W. H. (1968). *In* "Textbook of Endocrinology" (R. H. Williams, ed.), 4th ed., pp. 27–84. Saunders, Philadelphia, Pennsylvania.

Daughaday, W. H., and Kipnis, D. M. (1966). *Recent Progr. Horm. Res.* **22**, 49.

Daughaday, W. H., and Mariz, J. K. (1962). *J. Lab. Clin. Med.* **59**, 741.

Daughaday, W. H., and Reeder, C. (1966). *J. Lab. Clin. Med.* **68**, 357.

Dupont, B., Hoyer, I., Borgeskob, S., and Herup, J. (1970). *Acta Med. Scand.* **188**, 25.

Erdheim, J. (1931). *Virchows Arch. Pathol. Anat. Physiol. K. M.* **281**, 197.

Evans, H. M., and Simpson, M. E. (1931). *Amer. J. Physiol.* **98**, 511.

Evans, H. M., Simpson, M. E., and Pencharz, R. I. (1939). *Endocrinology* **25**, 175.

Evans, H. M., Simpson, M. E., and Li, C. H. (1943). *Endocrinology* **33**, 237.

Fourman, P. (1955). *Proc. Roy. Soc. Med.* **48**, 571.

Frame, B., and Nixon, R. K. (1968). *N. Engl. J. Med.* **279**, 626.

Franz, A. G., and Robkin, M. T. (1965). *J. Clin. Endocrinol. Metab.* **25**, 1470.

Fraser, R., and Harrison, M. T. (1960). *Ciba Found. Colloq. Endocrinol.* [*Proc.*] **13**, 135.

Gaillard, P. J. (1942). *Actual Sci. Ind.* **932**, pp. 1–101.

Gardner, W. V., and Pfeiffer, C. A. (1943). *Physiol. Rev.* **23**, 139.

Garland, J. T., Ruegamer, W. R., and Daughaday, W. H. (1971). *Endocrinology* **88**, 924.

Glick, S. M., Roth, J., Yalow, R. S., and Berson, S. A. (1965). *Recent Progr. Horm. Res.* **21**, 241.

Goldberg, A. L. (1969). *J. Biol. Chem.* **244**, 3217.

Goodman, H. M., and MacDonald, G. J. (1969). *Horm. Metab. Res.* **1**, 290.

Goss, R. J. (1969). "Principles of Regeneration." Academic Press, New York.

Greenspan, F. S., Li, C. H., Simpson, M. E., and Evans, H. M. (1949). *Endocrinology* **45**, 455.

Crunt, G. A., and Reynolds, D. W. (1970). *J. Pediat.* **76**, 112.

Hansson, L. I., and Thorngren, K. G. (1971) *Is. J. Med. Sci.* **7**, 377.

Harris, W. H., and Heaney, R. P. (1969). *Nature* (*London*) **233**, 403.

Hay, M. F. (1958). *J. Physiol.* (*London*) **144**, 490.

Heins, J. N., Garland, J. T., and Daughaday, W. H. (1970). *Endocrinology* **87**, 688.

Henneman, P. H., Forbes, A. P., Moldawer, M., Dempsey, E. F., and Carroll, E. L. (1960). *J. Clin. Invest.* **39**, 1223.

Hsu, J. D., and Robinson, R. A. (1969). *J. Surg. Res.* **9**, 535.

Ito, Y., Takamura, K., and Endo, H. (1959). *Endocrinol. Jap.* **6**, 68.

Ito, Y., Takamura, K., and Endo, H. (1960a). *Proc. Int. Congr. Endocrinol.*, *1st, 1960* p. 227.

Ito, Y., Takamura, K., and Endo, H. (1960b). *Endocrinol. Jap.* **7**, 327.

Jason, H. E., Fink, C. W., Wise, W., and Ziff, M. (1962). *J. Clin. Invest.* **41**, 1928.

Kellgren, J. H., Ball, J., and Tutton, G. K. (1952). *Quart. J. Med.* **21**, 405.

Kember, N. S. (1971). *Clin. Orthop. Related Res.* (in press).

Kibrick, E. A., Simpson, M. E., Becks, H., and Evans, H. M. (1942). *Endocrinology* **31**, 93.

Knobil, E., and Greep, R. O. (1959). *Recent Progr. Horm. Res.* **15**, 1.

Knobil, E., Morse, A., and Greep, R. O. (1956). *Anat. Rec.* **124**, 320.

Koneff, A. A., Scow, R. O., Simpson, M. E., Li, C. H., Evans, H. M. (1949). *Anat. Rec.* **104**, 465.

Korner, A. (1965). *Recent Progr. Horm. Res.* **21**, 205.

Korner, A. (1970). *Contr. Process. Multicell. Org., Ciba Found. Symp.* pp. 68–107.

Koskinen, E. V. S. (1959). *Ann. Chir. Gynaecol. Fenn.* **86–92**, 1.

Koskinen, E. V. S. (1963). *Acta Orthop. Scand.* **62**, 1.

Koskinen, E. V. S. (1967). *In* "Callus Formation Symposium on the Biology of Fracture Healing" (S. T. Krompecher and E. Kerner, eds.), pp. 315–322. Akadémiai Kiadó, Budapest.

Kurtz, R. C., Furstman, L., and Burnick, A. A. (1970). *Amer. J. Orthodontol.* **573**, 599.

Lash, J. W., and Woodhouse, M. W. (1960). *Proc. Int. Symp. Endocrinol., 1st, 1960* Vol. 1, p. 249.

Li, C. H. (1957). *Fed. Proc., Fed. Amer. Soc. Exp. Biol.* **16**, 774.

Li, C. H. (1968). *In* "Growth Hormone" (A. Pecile and E. Muller, eds.), pp. 3–28.

Li, C. H., and Yamashiro, D. (1970). *J. Amer. Chem. Soc.* **92**, 26.

Lindholm, R., Lindhom, S., and Paasimaki, J. (1967). *Acta Orthop. Scand.* **38**, 115.

McGarry, E. E., Beck, J. C., Ambe, L., and Nayak, R. (1964). *Recent Progr. Horm. Res.* **20**, 1.

McLean, F. C., and Urist, M. R. (1968). *In* "Bone," 3rd ed. Univ. of Chicago Press, Chicago.

Martin, L. G., Clark, J. W., and Conner, T. B. (1968). *J. Clin. Endocrinol. Metab.* **28**, 425.

Marx, W., and Rheinhardt, W. O. (1942). *Proc. Soc. Exp. Biol. Med.* **51**, 112.

Marx, W., Simpson, M. E., Li, C. H., and Evans, H. M. (1943). *Endocrinology* **33**, 102.

Merimee, T. J., Burgess, J. A., and Rabinowitz, D. (1966). *J. Clin. Endocrinol. Metab.* **26**, 791.

Merimee, T. J., Remoin, D. L., Cavalli-Sforza, L. C., Rabinowitz, D., and McKusick, U. A. (1968). *Lancet* **2**, 194.

Milhaud, G., and Moukthar, K. (1965). *C. R. Acad. Sci.* **260**, 3179.

Misol, M. D., Samaan, N., and Pousetti, I. V. (1971). *Clin. Orthop. Related Res.* **74**, 206.

Moon, H. D. (1937). *Proc. Soc. Exp. Biol. Med.* **37**, 34.

Moon, H. D., Simpson, M. E., Li, C. H., and Evans, H. M. (1951). *Cancer Res.* **11**, 535.

Mueller, J. F. (1968). *J. Parasitol.* **54**, 795.

Mueller, J. F., and Reed, P. (1968). *J. Parasitol.* **54**, 51.

Murakawa, S., and Raben, M. S. (1968). *Endocrinology* **83**, 645.

Naeye, R. L., and Blanc, W. A. (1971). *Arch. Pathol.* **91**, 140.

Niall, H. D. (1971). *Nature New Biology* **230**, 90.

Nogami, H., and Urist, M. R. (1971). *Exp. Cell. Res.* **63**, 404.

Nordin, B. E. C. (1966). *In* "Calcified Tissues" (H. Fleisch, H. J. J. Blackwood, and M. Owen, eds.), pp. 226–241. Springer-Verlag, Berlin and New York.

Pang, K. T., Griffith, R. W., and Pickford, G. E. (1971). *Proc. Soc. Exp. Biol. Med.* **136**, 85.

Quabbe, H. J., Helge, H., and Kubicki, S. (1971). *Acta Endocrinol. (Copenhagen)* **67**, 767.

Ray, R. D., Simpson, M. E., Li, C. H., Asling, C. W., and Evans, H. M. (1950). *Amer. J. Anat.* **86**, 479.

Ray, R. D., Asling, C. W., Walker, D. G., Simpson, M. E., Li, C. H., and Evans, H. M. (1954). *J. Bone Joint Surg., Amer. Vol.* **36**, 94.

Reinhardt, W. O., and Li, C. H. (1953). *Science* **117**, 295.

Rigal, W. M. (1964). *Proc. Soc. Exp. Biol. Med.* **117**, 794.

Root, A. W., and Oski, F. A. (1969). *J. Gerontol.* **24**, 97.

Ross, E. S., and McLean, F. C. (1940). *Endocrinology* **27**, 327.

Salmon, W. D., Jr., and DuVall, M. R. (1970). *Endocrinology* **87**, 1168.

Salzer, G. M., and Lischka, M. (1970). *Horm. Metab. Res.* **2**, 369.

Schmidt, A. J. (1960). *In* "Cellular Biology of Vertebrate Regeneration and Repair," p. 252. Univ. of Chicago Press, Chicago.

Shepanek, L. A. (1953). *Surg., Gynecol. Obstet.* **96**, 200.

Silberberg, M., and Silberberg, R. (1942). *Amer. J. Pathol.* **18**, 1141.

Silberberg, M., Silberberg, R., and Hasler, M. (1964). *J. Bone Joint Surg., Amer. Vol.* **46**, 766.

Silberberg, R., and Hasler, M. (1971). *Arch. Pathol.* **21**, 241–255.

Simpson, M. E., Evans, M. M., and Li, C. H. (1949). *Growth* **13**, 151.

Simpson, M. E., Van Dyke, C., Asling, C. W., and Evans, H. M. (1953). *Anat. Rec.* **115**, 615.

Smith, P. E. (1930). *Amer. J. Anat.* **45**, 205.

Smith, R. W., Jr. (1967). *Fed. Proc., Fed. Amer. Soc. Exp. Biol.* **26**, 1737.

Smolders, F. F. M. (1939). *Acta Neer. Morphol. Norm. Pathol.* **2**, 97.

Snapper, I. (1957). "Bone Disease in Medical Practice." Grune & Stratton, New York.

Sperling, M. A., Kenny, F. M., and Drash, A. L. (1970). *J. Pediat.* **77**, 462.

Steelman, S. L., Morgau, E. R., Caccaro, A. J., and Glitzer, M. S. (1970). *Proc. Soc. Exp. Biol. Med.* **133**, 269.

Sturge, R. A., Beardwell, C., Hartog, M., Wright, D., and Ansel, B. M. (1970). *Brit. Med. J.* **3**, 547.

Talwar, G. P., Jailhani, B. L., Sharma, S. K., Sopori, M. L., Pandian, M. R., Sundharadas, G., and Rao, K. N. (1970). *Contr. Process. Multicell. Org., Ciba Found. Symp.* pp. 108–122.

Theoleyre, M. (1970), *Ann. Endocrinol.* 31, 100.

Thomspon, K. W., Vincent, M. M., Jensen, F. C., Price, R. T., and Shapiro, E. (1959). *Proc. Soc. Exp. Biol. Med.* 107, 565.

Udupa, K. N. (1966). *J. Surg. Sci.* 1, Suppl., 168.

Urist, M. R. (1970). *In* "Osteoporosis" (U. S. Barzel, ed.), pp. 3–37. Grune & Stratton, New York

Urist, M. R., and Heuser, G. F. (1971). Unpublished observations.

Urist, M. R., Budy, A. M., and McLean, F. C. (1948). *Proc. Soc. Exp. Biol. Med.* 68, 324.

Urist, M. R., MacDonald, N. S., Moss, M. J., and Skoog, W. A. (1963). *In* "Mechanisms of Hard Tissue Destruction," Publ. No. 75, p. 385. *Amer. Ass. Advance Sci.*, Washington, D.C.

Vander Laan, W. P. (1971). *Calif. Med.* 115, 38.

Van Wyk, J. J., Hall, K., vanden Brande, L., and Weaver, R. P. (1971). *J. of Clin. Endocrinol. Metab.* 32, 389.

Verdam, H. D. (1946). Dissertion, Rijksuniversiteit, Leiden.

Waine, H., Bennett, G. A., and Bauer, W. (1945). *Amer. J. Med. Sci.* 209, 671.

Waterman, A. J. (1965). *Amer. Zool.* 5, 237.

Weltenhall, R. E. H., Schwartz, P. L., and Bornstein, J. (1969). *Diabetes* 18, 280.

Wilhelmi, H. E. (1955). *In* "The Hypophyseal Growth Hormone," Nature and Actions" (R. W. Smith, O. H. Gaebler, and C. N. H. Long, eds.), pp. 59–69. McGraw-Hill, New York.

Young, M. M., and Nordin, B. E. C. (1967). *Lancet* 2, 118.

Zadek, R. E., and Robinson, R. A. (1961). *J. Bone Joint Surg., Amer. Vol.* 43, 1261.

Zileli, M. S., Kanra, G., Urunay, G., Guner, T., Cagar, T., and Cagar, S. (1968). *Experientia* 21, 960

CHAPTER 5

Vitamin A and Bone

N. A. BARNICOT AND S. P. DATTA

I. The Chemistry of Vitamin A

The fat-soluble vitamins A_1 and A_2 appear to be entirely animal products, one or the other occurring in all vertebrates. They are obtained in the diet either preformed in foods of animal origin, or they are formed in the animal body by the conversion of the carotenoid provitamins of which β-carotene is the most active. The efficiency of the conversion of the carotenoids into vitamin A and the amount of carotenoids absorbed as such into the animal tissues vary considerably in different species and between breeds in the same species.

Vitamin A_1 is a highly unsaturated primary alcohol of the following formula:

$$H_3C\diagdown C \diagup CH_3$$

H₃C   CH₃   CH₃   CH₃
   \ / | |
    C | |
H₂C   C—CH=CH—C=CH—CH=CH—C=CH—CH₂·OH
    | ‖
H₂C   C
    \ / \
     C   CH₃
     H₂

The free alcohol, its esters, the corresponding aldehyde (retinene), various vitamin A ethers, vitamin A acid, and dimethylamino vitamin A are all active biologically. The corresponding hydrocarbon, axerophthene, is also active although this has been disputed (Goodwin, 1951). According to Zechmeister (1944) vitamin A can exist in four possible stereoisomeric forms because bonds 3 and 5 are unhindered. This isomerism appears to have an important bearing on the action of vitamin A in the visual processes, but to date no indications have been given of any isomeric specificity in relation to other actions of the vitamin.

In mammals and birds the main stores of vitamin A are found in the liver with smaller amounts in the kidneys, lungs, adrenals, and adipose tissue. In fishes, apart from stores of the vitamin in the liver, considerable quantities of the vitamin are found in the intestinal tissues, which may even supersede the liver as the main storage site.

It is only in relation to the visual processes that the metabolic role of vitamin A is known in any detail. A recent review of this subject is presented by Wald (1968).

II. Hypovitaminosis A

A. Effects on Tissues Other Than Bone

Apart from night blindness, which is caused by interference with the visual pigment systems detailed above and which is a well-marked and clear-cut symptom of vitamin A deficiency, the changes found are principally in the epithelial structures (see Bourne, 1953, for a general review). The various epithelia of the body undergo metaplastic change, the more differentiated epithelia regress to the simpler stratified type and those which are normally stratified become more cornified. The earliest changes are found in the respiratory system, marked desquamation occurring in the nares, the trachea, and the bronchi. Early changes are also found in various glands, particularly in the ducts of the salivary glands and the pancreas. The skin becomes rougher and hyperkeratinized, and sweating is interfered with by blockage of the ducts and other changes in the sweat glands. Changes in the sebaceous glands lead to degeneration of the hair follicles.

Classically the most obvious sign of vitamin A deficiency is xerophthalmia, which is characterized by keratinization of the surface layer of the corneal epithelium, the lining epithelium of the eyelids, and the conjunctiva. Atrophy of the tubules and keratinization of the ducts of the lachrymal glands leading to desiccation of the eye also occur. It is, however, only in severe deficiency that marked changes occur in the structure of the retina.

B. Effects on Bone

It is mainly in the dog that investigations have been made into the effects of vitamin A deprivation on the skeleton, although the rat and other animals have also been studied.

1. Hypovitaminosis A in the Dog

An extremely detailed and extensive description of the bony changes in dogs because of vitamin A deficiency has been given by Mellanby as the result of a masterly and thorough investigation of the question over a number of years. The results have been summarized in a Croonian lecture of the Royal Society (Mellanby, 1944) and in a monograph (Mellanby, 1950). Reference should be made to these works for details of the numerous original publications.

The discovery of the effects of hypovitaminosis A on bone resulted from the investigation of the extensive nervous lesions occurring in puppies reared on a vitamin A–deficient diet. These lesions included degeneration of both the cochlear and the vestibular divisions of the 8th cranial nerve; degenerations of the 2nd cranial nerve and the 1st and 2nd divisions of the 5th cranial nerve were also prominent. The changes in the cranial nerves were almost always confined to the afferent fibers. In the spinal nerves also the degenerations were mostly in the posterior roots, and in the cord itself changes were most marked in the ascending afferent fibers.

It was in relation to the lesions of the 8th nerve that the connection between the nervous degeneration and skeletal changes was first found. Histological preparations of the labyrinthine capsule of normal and vitamin A–deficient dogs showed masses of newly formed bone in the modiolus and the internal auditory meatus of the deficient animals. This new bone was interfering with and destroying both divisions of the 8th nerve (Fig. 1). It was soon found that abnormal bone growth and overgrowth was not confined to the internal auditory meatus but that there was a great thickening of many of the skull bones and several other cranial nerves were being affected by these bony changes.

The nerve bundles of the 1st cranial nerve were affected by swelling of the cribriform plate and the optic nerve was often degenerated because of bone overgrowth. Similar changes leading to blindness have been described in vitamin A–deficient cattle (L. A. Moore, 1939). The 5th nerve was also greatly affected by bony hypertrophy around the petrous ridge. The 7th nerve was often compressed, but being a motor nerve, appeared to be more resistant to degeneration. The 9th, 10th, and 11th cranial nerves, which pass through the jugular foramen, showed no degeneration because this foramen was not narrowed although the length of the canal was increased by thickening of the temporal and occipital bones. The same was true of the 12th nerve emerging through the hypoglossal canal.

Thickening of the vertebrae, particularly in the cervical region, led to narrowing of the spinal canal and pressure degeneration in the spinal cord, especially of the dorsal columns. The vertebrae had a coarse appearance resulting from blunting of sharp edges and flattening of curved surfaces (Fig. 2).

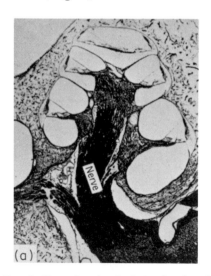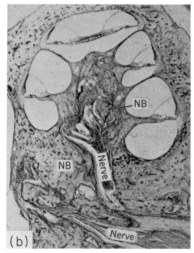

FIG. 1. Hypovitaminosis A in the dog. Photomicrographs (×12.5) of sections of cochlea and surrounding bone of two littermate dogs of the same age: (a) +A diet and (b) —A diet. Note: Great narrowing of internal auditory meatus and compression of nerve by bone overgrowth (NB) in —A animal b.

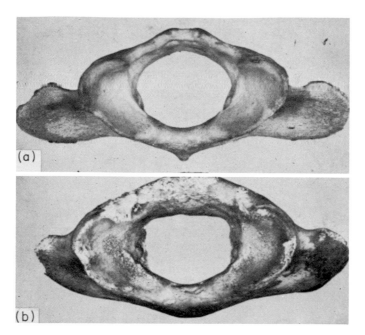

Fig. 2. Hypovitaminosis A. Photographs of atlas vertebrae of two littermate dogs of the same age: (a) +A diet and (b) −A diet. *Note:* (1) The overall sizes of the comparable vertebrae are not greatly dissimilar. (2) The vertebra of the −A animal is coarse and blunted and has lost its delicate outline. (3) The spinal canal in the vertebra of the −A animal is smaller than that of the +A. (Reproduced by courtesy of the late Sir Edward Mellanby, and the editors of the *Proceedings of the Royal Society,* London.)

In the skull as a whole the posterior fossa was reduced in size by hypertrophy of the supraoccipital and temporal bones. The basioccipital was also thickened, but the parietals were only slightly affected and the frontals even less so. These bony changes distorted the brainstem and squeezed the posterior part of the cerebellum through the foramen magnum. The facial bones, especially the mandible, zygomatic-temporal, and malar, were also thickened and lacking in modeling; the pelvic bones were affected in the same way.

In the femur the marrow cavity was reduced by thickening of the wall of the shaft which was largely cancellous rather than compact and showed incompletely developed Haversian systems. However, no changes were seen in the epiphyses or in growing cartilage generally. This is in contrast to Wolbach's (1946) findings in vitain A–deficient rats. He described cessation of endochondral ossification in the epiphyseal plate, leading to the formation of a densely calcified bony partition. These changes were like those seen in inanition, but in vitamin A deficiency they occurred before growth of other tissues was seriously affected. The discrepancies between Mellanby's and Wolbach's results are discussed further below.

2. Hypovitaminosis A in the Rat

The changes in the nervous system in rats on a vitamin A–deficient diet have been described in detail by Wolbach and Bessey (1941) and their relation to disorders of bone growth discussed (Wolbach and Bessey, 1941; Wolbach, 1946). The nervous lesions were thought to be wholly of mechanical origin, being caused by a disproportionate growth of the central nervous system in relation to the surrounding bony case.

There was overcrowding of the cranial cavity, resulting in distortion of the brain, dislocation of the brain toward the foramen magnum with herniation of the cerebellum into the venous sinuses of the dura at the sites of the arachnoidal drainage structures. In the spinal canal there was also overcrowding and distortion of the spinal cord with herniations of the nerve roots into the intervertebral foramina and into the bodies of the vertebrae. Rats in which the growth had been stunted by a diet deficient in quantity but not in quality, or by a diet deficient in riboflavin or pyridoxine, did not show this disproportion between the central nervous system and its bony investment.

This general retardation of bone growth had previously been described (Hess *et al.*, 1921; Wolbach and Howe, 1925). The skeleton was thought however to be normal, although bony overgrowth in relation to the bony capsule of the labyrinth was seen in rats and guinea pigs. In the inner table of the skull, immediately adjacent to the sutures, bone formation in excess of that found in normal rats of the same age was described, although this growth conformed in general to the normal pattern. The bony arch which forms the spinal canal was thinner than normal, and evidence of the normal growth sequence by which the ventral side of the canal enlarges was absent.

Clovell (1940) has described thickening of the periosteal layer of bone in the middle ear and exostoses in the internal auditory canal in rats kept for 52 days on a vitamin A–deficient diet.

3. Hypovitaminosis A in Rabbits

Perlman and Willard (1941) have tested cochlear function in vitamin A–deficient rabbits by determining the threshold curve for contraction of the tensor tympanic muscle over the range 128–4096 cps. None of the depleted animals was deaf by this test, and only slight differences in the threshold were observed before and after depletion of vitamin A. Such differences as were seen were within the experimental error.

Vestibular function was note tested, but some unsteadiness in gait and some increase in extensor tone with occasional torsion of the neck were seen.

The bony changes observed were extensive hypertrophy of the cranial aspect of the otic capsule including the internal auditory meatus and the posterior fossa surface. The internal auditory canal was lengthened and narrowed with compression and stretching of the nerve and Scarpa's ganglion. In spite of the pressure on the 8th cranial nerve, good cochlear function was retained.

Perlman (1949) has described the bony changes in vitamin A deficiency and recovery. After 5 months on the vitamin A–free diet the deficiency was severe, the corneal changes were gross, and the conditions of the animals very poor. In such animals new bone formation was uniformly found on the cerebral aspect of the temporal bone although changes in the 8th cranial nerve fibers and ganglion cells were variable. New bone also narrowed the cochlear aqueduct, but none was found in relation to the endolymphatic duct or sac. No serious labyrinthitis was observed.

If vitamin A was fed to these deficient animals there was no reversal of new bone formation. The bone however became more compact and the large islands of vascular connective tissue in the bone were replaced by compact bone. Degenerative changes in the nerve fibers and ganglion cells were also not reversed.

In addition to the bony changes on the posterior fossa aspect of the temporal bone there were definite changes throughout the bone. Islands or buds of vascular connective tissue appeared to be invading the old bone of the capsule. These islands were not lined by multinucleate osteoclasts but rather by cells with a single nucleus resembling osteoblasts although no osteoid was seen. In the recovery experiments these islands of connective tissue were replaced by bone.

4. Hypovitaminosis A in Man

In spite of the extensive literature on vitamin A deficiency in man, which includes several series of reports of postmortem examinations, very little information is available on skeletal changes.

Sweet and K'ank (1935) reported the occurrence of headaches in their cases and found signs of rickets. Wilson and Du Bois (1923) reported that the line between cartilage and bone at the costochondral junctions was irregular and in one postmortem examination they found that the middle ear was normal.

Blackfan and Wolbach (1933) reported a large series of postmortem cases. Radiographic evidence of increased density of the metaphyseal margin of long bones was obtained in four cases. In one case of an infant of 8 months a histological examination of a costochondral junction and one vertebra showed complete arrest of bone growth with atrophy of proliferating cartilage.

Deafness has not been reported as being associated with vitamin A deficiency in man (Perlman and Willard, 1941).

Gerlings (1947) has described three cases of oxycephaly. In one case a histological and gross anatomical examination of the skull showed hyperotosis of the temporal bone with narrowing of the internal auditory canal. The 8th cranial nerve was compressed and the ganglion partially atrophied. Gerlings commented on the similarity of the findings to those of Mellanby (1944) in vitamin A–deficient dogs. Apart from the similarity in these findings there is no evidence of hypovitaminosis A being concerned in oxycephaly in man.

5. *Hypovitaminosis A in the Chick and the Duck*

Wolbach and Hegsted have described vitamin A deficiency in the chick (1952a) and in the duck (1952c). Evidence of great disproportion in the growth of the central nervous system and the axial skeleton was found in the cranial cavity and the spinal canal. There were obvious signs of compression and distortion of the cranial contents and herniations of the brain into the anterior confluence of the longitudinal sinus with the veins from the surface of the brain, the nose, and the orbits. The medulla was compressed and molded into the foramen magnum, and its dorsal surface showed the imprint of the first cervical vertebra. Evidence of compression of the spinal cord was seen at all levels. There was no gross evidence of injury to the spinal roots, but it must be remembered that in the chick the spinal cord extends the entire length of the spinal canal and the nerve roots leave the cord at right angles.

The most obvious effect of vitamin A deficiency on the growth of long bones was on the epiphyseal cartilage sequences and endochondral bone growth. The tunneling of the epiphyseal cartilage was irregular and less extensive than normal. The zone of proliferating cartilage cells was less clearly demarcated and mitoses were absent. The intercellular matrix increased, and a broad zone of moderately enlarged cells in noncalcified matrix was formed. Cells of mature size surrounded by a calcified matrix constituted a narrow and irregular zone on the diaphyseal side where tunneling was present.

Appositional bone growth was retarded earlier than in mammals on a deficient diet. Periosteal and endosteal osteoblasts were fewer and smaller than in the restricted-diet controls. Much less cancellous bone was present in the metaphyseal region, and the adjacent cortical bone was thinner and less dense than normal. In all bones resorption where remodeling should occur ceased, as shown by a great scarcity of osteoclasts.

Retardation and suppression of endochondral ossification was very striking in the vertebrae. The bodies of the vertebrae were very deficient in cancellous bone, and the cortical bone was thin and wholly devoid of compact bone.

C. The Influence of the Diet on the Severity of the Hypovitaminosis A

In the Mellanby's experiments with dogs the hypertrophied bone which distorted the normal shape of the brain was cancellous in structure and the interstices full of fatty marrow; frequently, there was a diminution in compact bone. The microscopic structure of the bone appeared to be normal, and there was no osteoid tissue or other abnormalities resembling those in rachitic bones. The diet which the dogs were receiving was thought to be adequate in phosphorus, but the possibility existed that the hypertrophy of the cancellous bone might in some way be related to a relative lack of calcium in the diet. Experiments were therefore undertaken in which additional calcium, as $CaCO_3$, was given to animals on both the normal and the vitamin A–deficient diet. This addition of calcium was found to have the effect of making the bone more compact in both the deficient and the control animals, but the bone in the deficient dogs was still hypertrophied. Thus, the part played by calcium in these effects was only secondary.

Wolbach (1946) regarded the inhibitory effect of vitamin A deficiency on endochondral bone growth of the bones of the base of the skull, with the consequent distortion and failure of the bony case to increase adequately in size, as the prime cause of the degenerative changes in the central nervous system. In Mellanby's experiments, however, the changes in the endochondral cranial bones were only slight, and he did not consider them to be responsible for the changes in bone shape and size (Mellanby, 1950). Wolbach's rats were on a synthetic diet, completely devoid of vitamin A; they continued to grow until the sixth week of age, stationary weight or loss of weight being usual in the ninth week. There is thus some difficulty in deciding whether the cessation of endochondral bone growth, which is a common feature in young rats in inanition, is in fact brought about by the specific vitamin A deficiency. Mellanby has repeated on a small scale Wolbach's experiments, with a diet and under conditions as nearly the same as possible, and has found that even when supplements of vitamin A were given, growth was still subnormal. The histological findings were similar to Wolbach's. Animals fed on Mellanby's deficient diet (diet No. 43) did not cease growth so soon, the epiphyseal changes were less severe, and they did not show the diaphyseal disc. This diet contained oatmeal and therefore traces of carotene, but nevertheless many of the changes associated with cessation of growth and vitamin A deficiency were seen; thus, there is interference with endochondral ossification and slight overgrowth of periosteal bone.

Mellanby also reared rats on a normal diet to the age of 3–5 weeks and then placed them on the deficient diet (No. 43). In these animals endochondral ossification was almost normal, but there was a great overgrowth of periosteal bone. These results were similar to those of the dog experiments where conditions were similar.

It appears therefore that the main discrepancy betwen Wolbach's results and those of Mellanby may be attributed to differences in the age of the animals when deficiency starts and the degree of inanition which develops. The earlier in life the vitamin A reserves are exhausted the more likely is the supervention of inanition and cessation of epiphyseal growth; periosteal growth however continues at most stages of deficiency. When deficiency develops at a later age the effects on epiphyseal growth are much less marked and periosteal bone overgrowth much more prominent. It is, however, clear that the one abnormal change in bone produced by vitamin A deficiency, whatever the age of the animals, is that affecting periosteal bone.

D. THE MECHANISM OF ACTION OF VITAMIN A DEFICIENCY ON BONE GROWTH

There are two different actions to be considered in the experiments of Mellanby with dogs. There is first the actual laying down of superfluous bone in some parts, such as in the internal auditory meatus (Fig. 1). Here bone is present in a position where it is not normally to be found at all. In these cases we may consider that there is an abnormal activity of the osteoblasts. In many cases however there is not so much a bone overgrowth but the failure, relative or complete, of absorption of previously formed bone. Thus, in the overall dimensions of the skull there is not so much an increase in the outside measurements as a diminution in the inside measurements. Similar considerations apply to the spinal canal (Fig. 2).

That these ideas are substantially correct has been demonstrated by Mellanby who has shown that there is a difference in the number and activity of the osteoclasts on the inner side of the skull bones, that is, the part of the bone adjacent to the central nervous system, between normal and vitamin A–deficient animals. Sections of the basioccipital bones in normal and vitamin A–deficient animals (Fig. 3) show that in normal animals there are abundant osteoclasts on the surface of the bone nearest the brain, directly in contact with the bone under the periosteum; there are practically no osteoclasts in the same position in the sections from vitamin A–deficient animals. There are, however, many more osteoclasts on the marrow surface of the same area of bone in the section from the deficient animal than there are in the normal control. Thus, the position of the osteoclasts seems to have been reversed. Similar changes and reversal of the position of the osteoclasts from the inner surface of the bone to the marrow surface are seen in the vertebrae. It may be pointed out that in the normal animals where the osteoclasts are on the inner surface of the bones they appear to be very active as judged from their lying in bone lacunae, which they have obviously hollowed out, in contrast to the relatively inactive state in which they are flattened against the bone surface.

Thus, it would appear that in the normal animal the increase in the

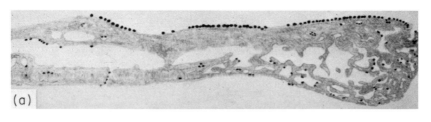

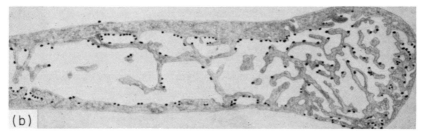

Fig. 3. Hypovitaminosis A in dog. Semidiagrammatic drawings of the basioccipital bones of two littermate dogs of the same age: (a) +A diet and (b) −A diet. Osteoclasts are indicated by black dots. *Note:* (1) Thickening of bone in (b) as compared with (a). (2) In (a) there is a large number of osteoclasts on the surface of the bone adjacent to the brain (upper surface in diagram). In (b) they are absent from this region but are abundant on the marrow surface of the same portion of bone. There seems to have been a reversal of the position of the osteoclasts. (Reproduced by courtesy of the late Sir Edward Mellanby and the editors of the *Proceedings of the Royal Society,* London.)

size of the central nervous system is being accommodated by removal of bone from the inner surface of the bony case, and its deposition on the outer surface, consequently enlarging the capacity. In vitamin A deficiency this mechanism breaks down because of the changed position of the area of osteoclasis in the bone.

While these changes in osteoclastic activity in deficient dogs are undoubtedly responsible indirectly for many of the destructive changes in the central nervous system, they are not the whole cause. Thus, in some bones there is obviously a great increase in osteoblastic activity at certain sites with the laying down of excessive amounts of new bone, as in the internal auditory meatus and in the petrous bone.

From these experiments of Mellanby it may be concluded that vitamin A acts as a specific chemical controller of the activities of osteoblasts and osteoclasts. The exact way in which this control is exercised is, however, unknown.

E. Recovery Changes on the Restoration of Vitamin A Intake

If vitamin A was added to the diets of dogs that had been on a deficient diet for some time but in whom growth had not ceased, recovery was initiated. The ataxia and incoordination of movement was reduced and almost disappeared in early cases but not as completely in late cases. The pressure effects on the brainstem and cerebellum were relieved and their shape became more normal. Other effects on the central nervous system were reversed, except for the deafness which persisted.

From histological studies it was seen that the administration of vitamin A caused a return of osteoclastic and osteoblastic activity to the surfaces of the bone where they are normally found. The reaction was often very vigorous; great numbers of very active cells were to be seen, as if there was an attempt to restore the normal shape of the malformed bone as rapidly as possible. The changes in cellular activity were not anarchic but orderly and they occurred even in regions adjacent to destroyed nerves or nerve tissue.

III. Hypervitaminosis A

A. Historical Survey

The earliest publication suggesting a toxic action of excessive amounts of vitamin A appears to be that ot Takahashi et al. (1925) who found that if rats were given a vitamin A–rich fish oil concentrate (Biosterin) in large doses they died within a few days or weeks, showing emaciation, loss of hair, paralysis of the hind limbs, and internal hemorrhages. Drigalski (1933), using a different proprietary preparation, confirmed this result. The first investigators to report skeletal lesions, however, were Collazo and Rodriguez (1933); they administered approximately 60,000 IU of vitamin A daily to young rats, in the form of a fish oil concentrate (Vogan), and noted that, among other symptoms, the animals suffered from fractures of the distal limb bones. Their observation was confirmed by Bomskov and Sievers (1933) and Davies and Moore (1934). The latter used a distillate rich in vitamin A and their work, therefore, marks some progress toward the identification of vitamin A itself as the causative agent; this was a point of some importance since preparations rich in vitamin A generally contained in addition considerable amounts of vitamin D, which might reasonably be suspected as a possible cause of skeletal changes. The work of Vedder and Rosenberg (1938), claiming that the severity of the bone damage was not closely correlated with the amount of vitamin A in the various preparations which they used, raised doubts concerning the importance of vitamin A in producing these effects. In 1945, however, T. Moore and Wang were able to demonstrate that the same skeletal lesions occurred if young rats (48–86 g initial weight) were daily given 50,000 IU of crystalline vitamin A acetate, dissolved in arachis oil; neither they nor previous authors succeeded in producing fractures in older animals. In the same year Pavceck et al. (1945) obtained fractures in rats given vitamin A in the alcohol form, and Rodahl (1950) confirmed the effect using oily solutions of the crystalline acetate.

B. Experimental Hypervitaminosis A in the Rat

The majority of workers have used the rat as an experimental animal and since information about the effects of hypervitaminosis A is greatest for this species, we shall deal with work on the rat at some length, reserving discussion of the results on other animals for a later section.

1. Dosage

The majority of workers have administered the vitamin by mouth, but as Rodahl (1950) showed, prolonged and repeated application to the skin can be effective. The dosage required to produce severe symptoms, including fractures, has generally been found to be about 25,000–50,000 IU/day for a period of 1–3 weeks. Under these conditions, the animals cease to gain weight and ultimately die. Rodahl (1950), who has investigated the dosage relations most thoroughly, found that a dose of 50–100 IU/g body weight was sufficient to interfere with the growth of young animals but did not produce skeletal lesions even after several weeks. He found, contrary to many other workers, that adult rats could be affected in the same way as young animals if the dosage was the same on a body weight basis, namely, in the region of 500 IU/g body weight.

The relative potency of different crystalline derivatives of vitamin A, from the point of view of the effects of excess on the bones, has not received much attention. Wolbach and Maddock (1951) stated that vitamin A methyl ether is less potent than either the acetate or the alcohol and that, in relatively short experiments, vitamin A phenyl ether is without effect.

2. Skeletal Lesions in the Rat

a. Macroscopic. A number of workers, for example, T. Moore and Wang (1945), Wolbach (1947), and Rodahl (1950), have published radiographs of the limbs of hypervitaminotic rats. In Figs. 4 and 5 we have reproduced similar pictures from unpublished material of our

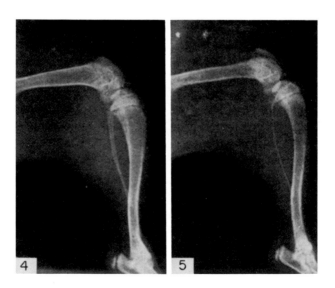

Fig. 4. Radiograph of the femur, tibia, and fibula of a normal rat; pair-fed control to that in Fig. 5.

Fig. 5. Radiograph of the femur, tibia, and fibula of a hypervitaminotic rat for comparison with pair-fed control in Fig. 3; 50,000 IU vitamin A per day for 1 week. Note narrowing of the lower end of the shaft of the femur and upper end of the tibia and reduction in diameter of the fibula.

own showing the hind limb of a young animal which had received 50,000 IU of vitamin A daily for a week (Fig. 5) in the form of a whale oil concentrate (kindly supplied by Dr. Kare Rodahl); the corresponding region in a pair-fed control, matched in initial weight, is shown for comparison (Fig. 4). The lengths of the femora and tibiae in the two animals are almost the same. In the hypervitaminotic animal, the antero-posterior diameter of the tibia is reduced at the proximal end, which is the most actively growing region, and the shadow of the cortical bone in the region of the tibial crest is more diffuse. The tibia is also more curved on its posterior aspect in the proximal half of the bone. The fibula is very much reduced in diameter and the marrow cavity is no longer discernible. The reason for this is well shown by Wolbach's (1947) diagrams of two superimposed growth stages of the tibia and fibula (Fig. 6); the remodeling of the bones as they increase in length involves removal of material from the posterior aspect of the tibia and the anterior aspect of the fibula, thus increasing the diameter of the region between the two bones. It is evidently an increase in the intensity of the resorptive processes at just these sites, without corresponding increase in the bone length and in the absence of normal rates of bone deposition on the opposite surfaces which leads to this characteristic

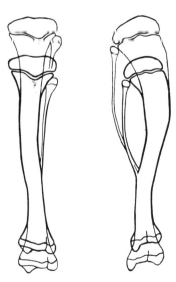

Fig. 6. Diagrams to illustrate the remodeling of the tibia and fibula of the rat during growth viewed from the anterior aspect (left) and in profile (right). The thick line shows the bone at a younger stage than that outlined by the thinner line. (Reproduced by courtesy of the late Dr. S. B. Wolbach and the editors of the *Journal of Bone and Joint Surgery.*)

change of shape. Turning to the femora, the most obvious difference is that in the hypervitaminotic animal, the shaft, owing to narrowing at its distal end, becomes a parallel-sided cylinder; this again appears to result from relatively greater resorption on the anterior aspect which is subject to resorptive remodeling in the normal growth sequence. The epiphyseal line is narrower in the hypervitaminotic animal, and, at the distal end of the femur, is only just discernible. In young animals given moderate excess of vitamin A for 6 weeks or more, the whole shaft of both tibia and femur may become much reduced in diameter so that the marrow cavity is, in places, almost obliterated as may be seen in Wolbach's (1947) photographs. When fractures occur they are most frequent in the tibia, generally near the level of the proximal one-third of the bone, but they may also occur in the humerus and forearm.

Certain features of hypervitaminosis A can be studied to advantage in macerated skeletons; the general shape of the bones can be more easily appreciated, particularly in some regions of the skeleton where superposition of structures renders the interpretation difficult in X-rays. Details of surface texture under the binocular dissecting microscope permit areas of resorption and active bone deposition to be located. We found in our own material that almost all regions of the skeleton are affected to a greater or lesser extent in severely hypervitaminotic animals. In some situations where resorption of thin sheets of bone is normally occurring, intensification of this process in the treated animals leads to perforations, which are very easily detected in macerated specimens. An example is given in Figs. 7 and 8, which show the scapulae of an affected animal and its pair-fed control; both the supraspinous and infraspinous fossae are perforated in the former and the acromion also shows resorption. Pathological changes are also very evident in the mandible (Figs. 10 and 11); an extensive area of resorption over the insertion of the masseter muscle leads to perforation of the tooth sockets and exposure of the roots of the molars. At the posterior end (Fig. 11) resorption of the anterior aspect of the coronoid process is intensified, as may be seen by the more ragged contour, and because of this, together, in all probability, with decreased bone deposition on its posterior aspect, the shape is altered.[1] There is also evidence of resorption on the anterior aspect of the articular process, in the region of the incisor apex anterior to the inferior dental foramen and on the angular process, leading in both cases to perforation. In the macerated bones of rapidly growing animals it is often possible to distinguish areas of active bone deposition because of the more chalky, opaque appearance of the bone and the

[1] See, however, Baer (1954).

regular arrangement of its fine foramina; in hypervitaminotic animals such areas tend to be more translucent and the foramina fewer and less regular, suggesting, in agreement with Irving (1949), that osteoblastic activity is relatively inhibited. Inspection of macerated material suggests, in agreement with Wolbach, that resorption of bone in hypervitaminotic animals is most intense in regions where resorption is already occurring in normal remodeling; furthermore, the area of resorption is extended from these sites. This is clearly seen, for example, on the anterior aspect of the femur at its distal end; in the normal growing animal, resorption as indicated by bone texture is mainly confined to the immediate level of the metaphysis but in severely hypervitaminotic animals this area is extended up the shaft and the whole of the distal two-thirds has a rough texture. In the forelimb intensification and extension of resorption is most evident at the actively growing ends of the bones, that is, the ends adjacent to the elbow. Resorption is not restricted to endochondral bones, as the findings for the mandible show, and some membrane bones of the skull, particularly the interparietal, show evidence of thinning by endosteal resorption.

b. Microscopic Structure of the Bones. The histology of the bones in hypervitaminosis A has been dealt with by several workers, notably Strauss (1934), Wolbach (1947), and Rodahl (1950). A systematic account of the histological sequences at various levels of vitamin A intake and at various stages in the development of acute hypervitaminosis remains to be made, however; the present account is based on the work of the authors mentioned above, supplemented by a limited amount of material of our own.

The main changes which have been described are as follows: The epiphyseal line becomes reduced in thickness owing to continued erosion of the hypertrophic zone from the diaphyseal aspect without compensating multiplication of cells in the proliferative zone. In the guinea pig, a species in which the cartilage of the epiphyseal line is completely destroyed as part of the normal growth sequence, this process leads to premature closure of the epiphysis if the dosage of vitamin A is high enough. In the rat, the cartilage is not entirely removed either in normal growth or in hypervitaminosis A. Inhibition of the normal increase in weight accompanied by decreases in the longitudinal growth of the long bones (van Metre, 1947) is an early sign of excessive vitamin A overdosage and doubtless partly results from decreased food consumption. To this extent it is likely to be a nonspecific effect. Essentially similar changes in the epiphyseal line can be induced by the administration of many other biologically active compounds in toxic quantities.

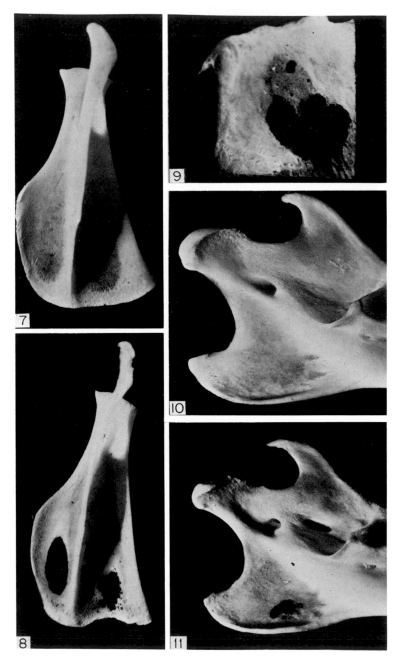

Wolbach (1947, and in other publications) believed that the skeletal lesions in hypervitaminosis A essentially result from interference with the organizing activity of the cells of the epiphyseal cartilage. It is difficult to agree that a simple speeding up of the normal mechanisms controlling the shape of the bone is an adequate explanation since this could only result in a more rapid differentiation, whereas the changes in shape which we have described indicate unbalanced resorptive and osteogenic processes. Evidence for the "organizer" function of the epiphyseal cartilage is reviewed by Lacroix (1947). Dissolution of the cartilage matrix comparable to the remarkable changes described by Fell and Mellanby (1950) in the embryonic bones of chicks cultured *in vitro* in media containing excess of Vitamin A does not seem to have been observed in experiments on the intact animal, either birds or mammals.

We have already mentioned the intensification and extension of resorption in certain regions of the skeleton, which can be inferred from the shape changes of the bones and from close examination of the bone texture in macerated specimens; histologically, such areas show numerous osteoclasts on the periosteal aspect of the cortical bone. The cellular layer of the periosteum is unusually thick and mitoses are occasionally seen in the numerous spindle-shaped mesenchymal cells which occupy it. The capillary vessels are engorged, and there is often evidence of blood extravasation even in the absence of fracture. These small hemorrhages, both in the periosteum and in other organs, have been remarked by many workers, and some have been led to compare the lesions in hypervitaminosis A with those in scurvy on this account. In regions where osteoclasts are numerous, the layer of cortical bone may be very

FIG. 7. The effects of hypervitaminosis A. Scapula of normal rat. Pair-fed control to that in Fig. 8.

FIG. 8. Scapula of hypervitaminotic A rat for comparison with pair-fed control, Fig. 6. 50,000 IU/day given as whale oil concentrate for 1 week. Perforation of subscapular and suprascapular fossae and resorption on the acromion process.

FIG. 9. Fragment of parietal bone of a mouse after 14 days' grafting to the cerebral hemisphere of a normal littermate, showing perforation at the site of implantation of a fragment of crystalline vitamin A acetate. (Reproduced from Barnicot 1950, by courtesy of the *Journal of Anatomy*, London.)

FIG. 10. Articular end of the mandible of a normal rat; pair-fed control to that shown in Fig. 11.

FIG. 11. Articular end of the mandible of a hypervitaminotic rat for comparison with its pair-fed control, Fig. 10. Resorption at the anterior aspect of the coronoid process, the upper border of the articular process; perforation in the fossa of the angular process and in the region of the incisor root anterior to the inferior alveolar foramen. (Photographs by the late F. J. Pittock.)

thin, as may be seen from Fig. 12, a and b illustrating projection draw-ings of the upper half of the tibia in a severely hypervitaminotic animal and a pair-fed control. In regions where this thinning of the cortex is most severe, there is often a layer of pale-staining osteoid on the corresponding endosteal surface. This simultaneous periosteal resorption and endosteal bone deposition is well shown in Wolbach's (1947) publi-cation, a figure from which is reproduced in Fig. 13. The pale-staining, reticulate structure and the numerous osteoblasts and osteocytes of this new bone resemble the early stage of callus formation; insofar as the staining reaction can be taken as a guide, it may be supposed that calci-fication of this bone is defective. Abundant callus may be observed at sites of fracture in hypervitaminotic animals. In addition to resorption of bone periosteally there is some reduction in metaphyseal trabeculae. No striking abnormalities are to be seen in the marrow tissue. The effects of

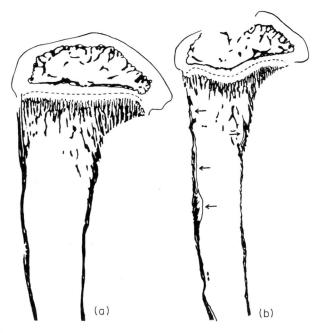

FIG. 12. (A) Projection drawing of the upper end of the tibia of a pair-fed con-trol rat to that shown in B. Fully ossified bone indicated in black; the level of the function between the zone of cell columns and of hypertrophic cells of the epiphy-seal plate is indicated by a dotted line. (B) Projection drawing of the upper end of the tibia from a hypervitaminotic rat which had received 50,000 IU vitamin A per day for a week, for comparison with pair-fed control in Fig. 12. The metaphyseal region is narrowed. The cortical bone of the shaft is reduced in thickness on both the anterior (left) and posterior (right) aspects, and in places indicated by arrows there is deposition of osteoid (white).

hypervitaminosis A on the microscopic structure of the cortex of the rat tibia are also shown in Figs. 14 and 15.

C. Experimental Hypervitaminosis A in Other Species

Ypsilanti (1935) failed to produce fractures in mice by administering various vitamin A concentrates by subcutaneous injection, but Rodahl (1950) obtained skeletal lesions and hemorrhages in this species when he gave 60–600 IU/g body weight by mouth. Bone changes could also be produced by applying the concentrates to the skin. Rodahl also found that lesions essentially similar to those described in the rat could be produced in guinea pigs and rabbits if the dose was of the same order of magnitude on a body weight basis. Maddock *et al.* (1949) have described the lesions in two littermate dogs, 2 months old, which were given 300,000 IU/day/kg body weight. Decline of the weight curve, compared with their control littermates did not occur until the fifty-eighth and sixty-third day of the experiment. The long bones showed closure of the epiphyseal line and periosteal resorption and hemorrhage; the fibula, as in the rat, was greatly reduced in diameter.

Some work has been done on hypervitaminosis A in birds. Rodahl (1950) administered 260 IU/g body weight per day orally to young cockerels and although he noted a decline in weight and a generally miserable appearance after a few days, he did not record any skeletal abnormalities. Wolbach and Hegsted (1952b), however, found skeletal changes in 7-day-old chicks which had been given 660–900 IU/g body weight for 30 days or more. The long bones of the hind limbs showed narrowing of the epiphyseal cartilage owing to more advanced tunneling of the cartilage from the diaphyseal aspect; more osteoclasts were said to be present on the trabeculae and cortical bone adjacent to the epiphyseal cartilage, but fractures were not observed, and the cortical bone of the shaft, although reduced in total thickness in comparison with controls, was denser in structure in the sense that there were fewer Haversian systems. The same authors (1953) found similar but less pronounced changes in young ducks. It appears, therefore, that periosteal bone resorption culminating in fracture is not a feature of hypervitaminosis A in birds as it is in mammals.

D. Hypervitaminosis A in Man

1. Acute Vitamin A Poisoning

It has been known for some time from the experiences of polar explorers and from the lore of the polar Eskimo, that toxic symptoms might develop as a result of eating the livers of certain Arctic animals

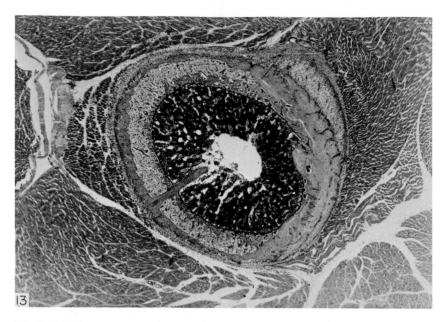

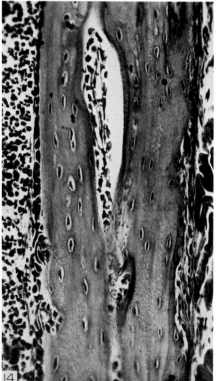

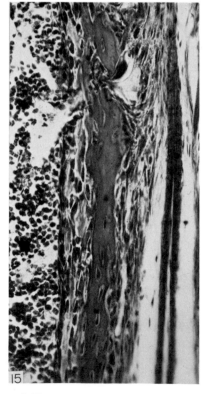

Figs. 13, 14, and 15.

218

such as the polar bear and the bearded seal, *Erignathus barbatus*. Rodahl and Moore (1943) found that the livers of these animals contained very large amounts of vitamin A; the consumption of a pound would provide 7,500,000 IU of vitamin A which, from experience in animal experiments, might well be a toxic dose. The symptoms in man start within a few hours of the meal of liver, and include severe headache, vomiting, extreme lassitude, and irritability; in some cases, peeling of the skin of the face or of the entire body might occur after 24 hours. Subsequent work by Rodahl (1949) confirmed the suspicion that the toxic agent in the livers was vitamin A.

2. *Chronic Hypervitaminosis A*

The condition of acute vitamin A poisoning is less relevant from the present point of view than are the various reports of chronic vitamin A poisoning. This condition has been observed mainly in young children 2–3 years old, who have unwittingly been given doses of potent fish oil preparations amounting to as much as 600,000 IU vitamin A daily for periods of a year or more. The first case of this kind was described by Josephs (1944); since then more than 20 cases have been described in the United States. Caffey (1951) has described and discussed seven cases, with radiographs of the bones, and the findings of a number of other authors seem to be essentially the same. The symptoms, which appear only some months after the start of the excessive vitamin A consumption, include anorexia, irritability, pruritus, and tender swellings over the limbs, with difficulty of movement. The X rays reveal smooth hyperostoses on the middle region of the shafts of some of the long

---

Fig. 13. Transverse section of the humerus of a hypervitaminotic rat which had received 1250 IU of vitamin A daily from the twenty-first to the twenty-eighth day of age. Note thick layer of endosteal osteoid on the left side where the original shaft bone is much reduced in thickness. (By courtesy of the late Dr. S. B. Wolbach and the *Journal of Bone and Joint Surgery*.)

Fig. 14. Photomicrograph of a portion of the cortex of the shaft of the tibia on its posterior aspect approximately one-third of the length from the upper end; pair-fed control to animal shown in Fig. 15. The marrow tissue is seen on the left-hand side; there are large osteoblasts on this surface of the bone. Some osteoclasts and an irregular contour are noted on the periosteal surface and the periosteum is thin ($\times 220$).

Fig. 15. Photomicrograph of the same region of the tibia as in Fig. 14 but from a hypervitaminotic animal which had received 20,000 IU vitamin A per day as whale oil concentrate for 1 week. There is a layer of osteoid on the endosteal surface (left); the original cortical bone of the shaft is only about one-quarter the thickness of the control. Osteoclasts are seen in the periosteum, which is unusually thick and contains spindle-shaped cells and enlarged capillaries ($\times 220$). (Photomicrographs by Mr. J. Armstrong, Anatomy Dept., University College.)

bones; the ulnae and metatarsals appear to be the most commonly affected sites, but Bair (1951) has described a case in which some of the skull bones were also involved. The serum calcium and phosphorus is generally normal but the serum alkaline phosphatase is somewhat elevated. The plasma vitamin A has been found on several occasions to be raised from normal levels of 50–150 IU/100 ml to 400–2000 IU/100 ml. On cessation of the excessive vitamin intake the bone lesions disappeared within a few months. The reports of these cases do not suggest that skeletal resorption of the type seen in experimental hypervitaminosis A occurs; the dosage on the body weight basis, however, is in general considerably less than the level known to produce these resorptive changes in animals. On the other hand, hyperostoses resembling those in human cases have not, as far as we know, been described in animals given more moderate excess of vitamin A over prolonged periods of time.

E. Biochemical Findings in Experimental Hypervitaminosis A

1. Calcium and Phosphorus

The fractures which are such a striking feature of experimental hypervitaminosis A in the rat led several investigators to inquire whether the skeleton was imperfectly calcified in this condition. Bomskov and Sievers (1933), T. Moore and Wang (1945), and Rodahl (1949, 1950), found, however, no significant changes in the mineral content of the bones. The fractures presumably result, then, from the cortical bone in certain regions becoming very thin as a result of resorption, but the bone that remains is normally calcified; the osteoid, which we have mentioned as occurring on some parts of the marrow surface of the cortex, if indeed it is deficient in mineralization, is presumably too small in amount to influence the overall analysis.

Major changes in the levels of blood calcium or phosphorus, such as occur in experimental hyperparathyroidism, have not been found in hypervitaminotic rats, but Maddock et al. (1949) noted a terminal rise of blood calcium in the dog.

2. Vitamin A Level in the Blood and Tissues

Since the capacity of the liver to store vitamin A is very great, and most of the vitamin in the body is contained in this organ, it is interesting to consider whether in animals showing symptoms of hypervitaminosis A the level of the vitamin in the blood is raised. The liver stores themselves are very much increased on large doses of vitamin A. Davies and Moore (1934) found, for example, that a rat, which was given a total of 1,413,000 Blue Units (approximately 4,000,000 IU) of vitamin A over a period of 33 days and which died showing fractures, had 60,000 Blue Units/g in the liver as compared with a range of 500–100 Blue Units/g in animals on a maintenance diet; the vitamin A content of certain other organs such as the lung and kidney was also raised considerably. However, it did not appear that the level of the liver store and the severity of the symptoms were closely correlated; another animal which died with bone fractures had very much lower amounts of vitamin A in the liver. The authors suggested that symptoms of hypervitaminosis only occur when the ingestion and absorption of the vitamin exceeds the animal's capacity for elimination and storage. Walker *et al.* (1947) found that in rats given large amounts of halibut liver oil the plasma vitamin A level was increased about ten times in some cases and that animals with these high plasma levels showed bone fractures. In attempting to understand the control of the level of vitamin A in the blood, the particular chemical form in which the vitamin occurs appears to be important; according to Gray *et al.* (1940), the liver vitamin is mainly in the form of esters, but about 10% of vitamin A alcohol is always present. Clausen *et al.* (1942) stated that the alcohol is the chief form in the plasma, and Glover *et al.* (1947) suggested from their experiments on rats that the vitamin A level in the plasma is more closely related to the amount of the alcohol in the liver than to the ester content. The alcohol is said to be dispersed in the aqueous medium, perhaps carried by proteins, while the esters are in solution in fat droplets; such a difference in state might well be expected to affect the activity of the vitamin on the tissues, but as far as we are aware, studies on the composition and state of vitamin A in the plasma in experimental hypervitaminosis A, with concurrent examination of the pathology, have not been reported.

F. The Mechanism of Action of Vitamin A Excess on the Skeleton

It has been suggested from time to time that the effects of excess of vitamin A is in some way related to the metabolism of other vitamins, but this has not in general been substantiated. The fact that the bone lesions and other manifestations can be produced with pure vitamin A, as already mentioned, rules out the simultaneous presence of large amounts of vitamin D as an essential factor. In spite of the apparent, but probably superficial, resemblance of the bone lesions in hypervitaminosis A to those of scurvy, T. Moore and Wang (1945) and Walker *et al.* (1947) were able to show that vitamin C supplements had no noticeable effects on the development of either these lesions or of hemor-rhages. Light *et al.* (1944) demonstrated that the prothrombin level is low and the clotting time increased in hypervitaminotic rats and that these abnormalities can be largely corrected by addition of vitamin K; the fractures and hemorrhages cannot, however, be prevented in this way according to Walker *et al.* (1947), and dosage with Dicumarol can produce extensive hemorrhages but no bone changes.

The possibility of an indirect action of vitamin A mediated by endo-crine organs has also received consideration. Baumann and Moore (1939) found that young rats given excess of vitamin A together with thyroxine died earlier than rats given vitamin A alone. Wolbach and Maddock (1952) found that excess of vitamin A produced the character-istic bone lesions in hypophysectomized rats that have been described in intact animals. There are no reports of abnormalities in the parathy-roid glands in hypervitaminosis A, and the bone lesions seem to differ in detail from those described in experimental hyperparathyroidism.

Although there is no definite evidence that the effects of vitamin A excess on the skeleton are an indirect result of a primary action on some other tissue, nevertheless, histological and biochemical abnormali-ties in this syndrome are by no means confined to the skeleton; the kidney, liver, and skin, for example, show pathological changes. The effects of vitamin A overdosage in the intact animal are, therefore, no doubt complex. Even though the action of the vitamin might be a direct one on bone tissue, the response of the bone to the vitamin might per-haps be modified by concomitant changes in the cellular environment brought about by the actions of the vitamin elsewhere in the body. Some experiments by Barnicot (1950) in which an attempt was made to restrict the locus of action of the vitamin to bone tissue have some relevance here. Small fragments of crystalline vitamin A acetate were attached to the endocranial surface of pieces of parietal bone cut from the freshly dissected skulls of mice about 1 week old, and the grafts were then thrust into the cerebral hemispheres of littermates. After a period of 1–2 weeks the grafts were examined either by maceration or by histological sectioning *in situ*. The macerated grafts (Fig. 9, see p. 214) showed large perforations where the vitamin was attached, or, in other cases, an area of spongy new bone, which, as could be demon-strated from histological examination (Fig. 16A–D), closed over a per-foration produced in the original grafted bone. Using the technique of supravital staining with neutral red, which, as Barnicot (1947) showed, colors the osteoclasts an intense red, it was possible to demonstrate that after a few days of grafting there were no osteoclasts remaining on the surface of the grafted bone, but after about a week these cells began to

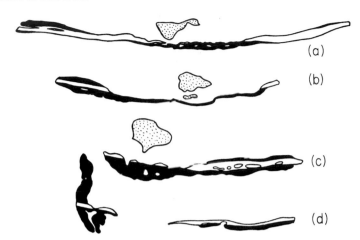

FIG. 16(a–d). Projection drawings of histological sections of intracerebral grafts of pieces of mouse parietal bone bearing implants of vitamin A acetate. The residue of the vitamin is indicated by stippling, the original bone of the graft is white, and newly formed bone black. It will be observed that in all cases the original bone of the graft has been perforated adjacent to the vitamin implant and the hole closed at least partially by new bone. c and d show different levels from the same specimen. In d the original bone is perforated, but in the area shown in c the hole is closed by new bone. (Reproduced from Barnicot, 1950, by courtesy of the editors of the *Journal of Anatomy*, London.)

appear in the immediate vicinity of the vitamin implant. In later stages, as illustrated in the drawing reproduced in Fig. 17, they became extremely numerous.

These experiments suggest rather strongly that the vitamin can exert a direct action on bone tissue leading to enhanced production of osteolasts and increased bone resorbtion. If the implanted vitamin stimulated some organ or tissue remote from the graft site, and resorption was secondary to this, it is not clear why the effect on the grafted bone should be so localized unless the implant also sensitizes the tissue locally to the product of its primary action site. In fact, no sign of generalized hypervitaminosis in the host animals was seen; indeed, it is doubtful whether the amount of implanted vitamin was sufficient to produce it. Since certain other solid materials including carotene crystals, cholesterol crystals, and glass fragments do not cause local resorption it is unlikely that the effect was merely mechanical; nor did the histology of the grafts suggest that necrosis and inflammation were important factors although a local increase in blood supply may perhaps play a part.

Fell and Mellanby (1952), at the start of a long and interesting series

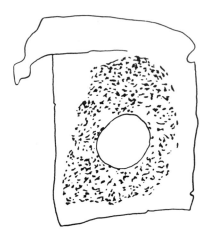

Fɪɢ. 17. Projection drawing of a fragment of parietal bone of a mouse which had been grafted for 14 days to the cerebral hemisphere of a littermate. There is perforation of the bone at the site of implantation of a fragment of vitamin A plus estradiol. The position of osteoclasts, supravitally stained with neutral red on an area of new bone around this perforation is also shown. (Reproduced by courtesy of the editors of the *Journal of Anatomy*, London; Barnicot, 1950.)

of studies using embryonic limb rudiments cultured *in vitro*, wrote, in relation to these graft experiments "a direct action of vitamin A on the bone seems to have been clearly demonstrated" although Fell, reviewing the field some 10 years later, stated that there was no evidence on this point at the time their work started. As Fell and Mellanby (1952) pointed out, the situation in the grafts differed from hypervitaminosis A produced *in vivo* in that the bone was exposed to adjacent crystals of the vitamin rather than to "relatively minute concentrations" present in the bloodstream. In their experiments vitamin A acetate or alcohol was either dissolved in the plasma medium by adding an alcoholic solution or plasma from a hypervitaminotic fowl was used.

The organ culture method has the advantage that it decisively eliminates the possibility that the vitamin acts primarily on some organ or tissue other than those present in the culture and it also allows various biochemical observations to be made. Strictly speaking, it does not exclude the possibility that the vitamin acts by enhancing the response of the bone to some product of other organs or tissues that is present in the plasma medium. The simplification of the experimental system achieved by organ culture may be offset to some extent by the fact that the bone is in a more or less abnormal environment, deprived of its blood supply, so that its responses may deviate from those of the tissue *in vivo*.

Fell and Mellanby (1950, 1952) showed that remarkable changes took place in cartilaginous rudiments from 5 to 6 day chick embryos and in more fully ossified rudiments from late fetal mice when cultured in a vitamin A–enriched medium. In the former the cartilage lost its metachromatic staining and most of the matrix surrounding the cartilage cells ultimately disappeared. In the mouse bones similar dissolution of cartilage occurred and the shaft bone was largely resorbed so that sometimes only a vestige of the original explant remained. They noted that osteoclasts were not especially abundant in the resorbing bones. They also found that plasma from a hypervitaminotic fowl was less effective in producing these dramatic changes than plasma directly enriched by dissolving vitamin in it.

Much of the subsequent work concerns cartilage rather than bone and will therefore be reviewed only briefly. Fell *et al.* (1956) showed that ^{35}S previously incorporated into limb rudiment cartilage was released when vitamin A was added to the culture and further incorporation was inhibited. They suggested that the vitamin caused the liberation of a proteolytic enzyme that attacked cartilage matrix. The increase of acid-soluble nitrogen observed in vitamin A–treated cultures was also suggestive of proteolysis (Dingle *et al.*, 1961). The proteolytic enzyme, papain, produces softening of the ear cartilage when injected into rabbits and this, together with loss of basophilic staining of articular cartilages, can also be produced by massive doses of vitamin A (Thomas *et al.*, 1960). Papain also produces similar changes to vitamin A in limb rudiment cultures (Fell and Thomas, 1960). It had already been shown by de Duve and his colleagues that lysosomal enzymes, including a protease active at low pH, can be released from some tissues by treatment with hypotonic fluids. Similar experiments performed by Lucy *et al.* (1961) on limb rudiments showed that treatment with water followed by incubation at pH 4–5 led to rapid release of hexosamine. An acid protease is liberated when liver "mitochondrial" fractions are treated with vitamin A (Dingle, 1961). Treatment of particulate fractions from cartilage homogenates with the vitamin also leads to release of a protease which has a similar low pH optimum to that released from limb rudiments by vitamin A or hypotonic treatment (Fell and Dingle, 1963). The disruptive effect of certain vitamin A derivatives on cellular membranes is not confined to those of lysosomes; under certain conditions they lyse red cells (Dingle and Lucy, 1962), swell mitochondria (Lucy *et al.*, 1963), and produce blebs on the surface of fibroblasts (Dingle *et al.*, 1962). Dingle and Lucy (1965) attributed these lytic effects to the ability of the vitamin to insert itself into lipid films, noting that the lytic potency of various derivatives roughly parallels their curative power in hypovitaminosis A. Whether these effects of the vitamin at relatively high concentrations tell us much about its normal function is open to question, but these authors suggested that at physiological levels it may be able to *stabilize* membranes because its hydrophobic end can bind to lipids and its polar end to proteins.

Less is known about the biochemistry of bone resorbtion in hypervitaminosis A, but there is some evidence that lysosomal enzymes may also be implicated here. Vaes (1969), in reviewing this subject, stated that bone homogenates are rich in acid proteases and he observed an increase of released lysosomal enzymes in bone cultures treated with parathormone although this hormone does not itself destabilize lysosomes. Observations on living osteoclasts in cultures by Gaillard, Goldhaber, and Hancox (see Hancox, 1965) leave no doubt that these cells can resorb bone, but whether resorption can sometimes occur without them is less certain. Osteoclasts show abundant neutral red granules when supravitally stained (Barnicot, 1947), and it is interesting that such staining is now thought to be characteristic of lysosomes (Allison *et al.*, 1966). Various lysosomal enzymes have been detected in osteoclasts by histochemical staining of sectioned material or whole cells in culture (see Hancox and Boothroyd, 1963). The matrix of calcified bone is said to resist the attack of proteolytic enzymes (Vaes, 1969), and electron microscopy suggests that removal of bone salt and organic matrix in the vicinity of the osteoclast ruffled border goes on more or less simultaneously. Although numerous vacuoles are seen in the cytoplasm of osteoclasts, most electron microscopists have not detected typical dense primary lysosomes. However, Scott (1967) described dense, membrane-limited bodies 0.2–0.5 μ in diameter in the ruffled-border zones of some osteoclasts in the tibiofemoral epiphyses of fetal rats and has seen apparent transitional forms leading to vacuoles via larger, less dense inclusions. She believed that some of the vacuoles, which presumably contain lysosomal enzymes, may discharge to the bone surface by way of the channels of the ruffled border. It is not clear how bone salts are removed from the organic matrix, but microcrystals of bone salt have often been described in the canals of the ruffled border and adjacent vacuoles, and Hancox and Boothroyd (1963) have found collagen fragments in these positions. According to Woods and Nichols (1965) a collagenase, active at pH 6.0 on undenatured bone collagen, is present in the lysosome-containing fraction of bone homogenates. Owen and Shetlar (1968) showed by autoradiography that ingested glucosamine is rapidly taken up by osteoclasts and later appears on the immediately surrounding bone surface. If, as they tentatively suggested, this indicates production of mucoid by osteoclasts, it might connect the effects of vitamin A on bone with the surprising induction of mucus-secreting cells in cultured skin by treatment with the vitamin (Fell and Mellanby, 1952).

There is thus a good deal of circumstantial evidence that lysosomal enzymes may be involved in resorption of both cartilage and bone and that vitamin A may be concerned in their release, but much remains to be discovered about the role of the vitamin in the normal differentiation and activity of bone cells. Very little is known about the biochemistry of vitamin A deficiency at the cellular level. The graft experiments described above show that high local concentrations induce not only bone resorption but also differentiation of numerous osteoclasts, and the curious distribution of these cells in Mellanby's hypovitaminotic dogs remains unexplained.

We conclude by mentioning certain experiments in which the effects of other biologically active substances on the skeletal effects of vitamin A in excess were examined. Selye (1958) found that cortisone exacerbated bone resorption induced by high doses of vitamin A in rats, but Fell and Thomas (1961) reported retardation of cartilage resorption *in vitro*. They suggested that cortisone *in vivo* decreases liver storage of the vitamin thus leading to higher plasma levels. Selye (1957) also found that samatotrophic hormone abolished bone resorption in young rats given high doses of vitamin A. According to Vaes (1969) calcitonin inhibits bone resorption in cultures treated with parathormone but does not affect the release of lysosomal enzymes. He suggested that the action of calcitonin may be specifically on the mechanisms for bone salt removal, whatever that may be. It would be interesting to know whether this is also the case when resorption is induced by vitamin A.

References

Allison, A. C., Magnus, I. A., and Young, M. R. (1966). *Nature (London)* **207**, 874.
Baer, M. J. (1954). *Hum. Biol.* **26**, 80.
Bair, G. (1951). *J. Amer. Med. Ass.* **146**, 1573.
Barnicot, N. A. (1947). *Proc. Roy. Soc., Ser. B* **134**, 467.
Barnicot, N. A. (1950). *J. Anat.* **84**, 374.
Baumann, C. A., and Moore, T. (1939). *Biochem. J.* **33**, ii and 1639.
Blackfan, K. D., and Wolbach, S. B. (1933). *J. Pediat.* **3**, 679.
Bomskov, C., and Sievers, G. (1933). *Z. Gesamte Exp. Med.* **89**, 780.
Bourne, G. H. (1953). *In* "Biochemistry and Physiology of Nutrition" (G. H. Bourne and G. W. Kidder, eds.), Vol. 2, p. 44. Academic Press, New York.
Caffey, J. (1951). *Amer. J. Roentgenol. Radium Ther.* **65**, 12.
Clausen, S. W., Baum, W. S., McCoord, A. B., Rydeen, J. O., and Breese, B. B. (1942). *J. Nutr.* **24**, 1.
Clovell, W. P. (1940). *Laryngoscope* **50**, 632.

Collazo, J. A., and Rodriguez, J. S. (1933). *Klin. Wochenschr.* 12, 1732 and 1768.
Davies, A. W., and Moore, T. (1934). *Biochem. J.* 28, 288.
Dingle, J. T. (1961). *Biochem. J.* 79, 509.
Dingle, J. T., and Lucy, J. A. (1962). *Biochem. J.* 84, 611.
Dingle, J. T., and Lucy, J. A. (1965). *Biol. Rev.* 40, 422.
Dingle, J. T., Lucy, J. A., and Fell, H. B. (1961). *Biochem. J.* 79, 497.
Dingle, J. T., Glauert, A. M., Daniel, M., and Lucy, J. A. (1962). *Biochem. J.* 84, 76P.
Drigalski, W. (1933). *Klin. Wochenschr.* 12, 308.
Fell, H. B., and Dingle, J. T. (1963). *Biochem. J.* 87, 403.
Fell, H. B., and Mellanby, E. (1950). *Brit. Med. J.* 2, 535.
Fell, H. B., and Mellanby, E. (1952). *J. Physiol. (London)* 119, 470.
Fell, H. B., and Thomas, L. (1960). *J. Exp. Med.* 111, 719.
Fell, H. B., and Thomas, L. (1961). *J. Exp. Med.* 114, 343.
Fell, H. B., Mellanby, E., and Pelc, S. B. (1956). *J. Physiol. (London)* 134, 179.
Gerlings, P. G. (1947). *Acta Oto-Laryngol.* 35, 91.
Glover, J., Goodwin, T. W., and Morton, R. A. (1947). *Biochem. J.* 41, 97.
Goodwin, T. W. (1951). *Brit. J. Nutr.* 5, 94.
Gray, E. LeB., Hickman, K. C. D., and Brown, E. F. (1940). *J. Nutr.* 19, 39.
Hancox, N. M. (1965). *In* "Cells and Tissues in Culture" (E. N. Willmer, ed.), Vol. 2, p. 261. Academic Press, New York.
Hancox, N. M., and Boothyroyd, B. (1963). *In* "Mechanisms of Hard Tissue Destruction," Publ. No. 75, p. 497. Amer. Ass. Advance. Sci., Washington, D.C.
Hess, A. F., McCann, G. F., and Pappenheimer, A. M. (1921). *J. Biol. Chem.* 47, 395.
Irving, J. T. (1949). *J. Physiol. (London)* 108, 92.
Josephs, H. W. (1944). *Amer. J. Dis. Child.* 67, 33.
Lacroix, P. (1947). *J. Bone Joint Surg.* 29, 292.
Light, R. F., Alscher, R. P., and Frey, C. N. (1944). *Science* 100, 225.
Lucy, J. A., Dingle, J. T., and Fell, H. B. (1961). *Biochem. J.* 79, 500.
Lucy, J. A., Luscombe, M., and Dingle, J. T. (1963). *Biochem. J.* 89, 419.
Maddock, C. L., Wolbach, S. B., and Maddock, S. (1949). *J. Nutr.* 39, 117.
Mellanby, E. (1944). *Proc. Roy. Soc., Ser. B* 132, 28.
Mellanby, E. (1950). "A Story of Nutritional Research." Williams & Wilkins, Baltimore, Maryland.
Moore, L. A. (1939). *J. Nutr.* 17, 443.
Moore, T., and Wang, Y. L. (1945). *Biochem. J.* 39, 222.
Owen, M., and Shetlar, M. R. (1968). *Nature (London)* 220, 1335.
Pavceck, P. L., Herbst, E. J., and Elvehjem, C. A. (1945). *J. Nutr.* 30, 1.
Perlman, H. B. (1949). *Arch. Otolaryngol.* 50, 20.
Perlman, H. B., and Willard, J. (1941). *Ann. Otol., Rhinol., & Laryngol.* 50, 349.
Rodahl, K. (1949). *Nature (London)* 164, 530.
Rodahl, K. (1950). *Nor. Polarinst., Skr.* 95.
Rodahl, K., and Moore, T. (1943). *Biochem. J.* 37, 166.
Scott, B. L. (1967). *J. Ultrastruct. Res.* 19, 417.
Selye, H. (1957). *J. Endocrinol.* 16, 231.
Selye, H. (1958). *Arthritis Rheum.* 1, 87.
Strauss, K. (1934). *Beitr. Pathol. Anat. Allg. Pathol.* 94, 345.
Sweet, L. K., and K'ank, H. J. (1935). *Amer. J. Dis. Child.* 50, 699.

Takahashi, K., Nakamiya, Z., Kawakami, K., and Kitasato, T. (1925). *Sci. Pap. Inst. Phys. Chem. Res., Tokyo* 3, 81.
Thomas, L., McCluskey, R. T., Potter, J. L., and Weissman, G. (1960). *J. Exp. Med.* 111, 705.
Vaes, G. (1969). *In* "Lysosomes in Biology and Pathology." (J. T. Dingle and H. B. Fell, eds.), Vol. 1, p. 217. North-Holland Publ., Amsterdam.
van Metre, T. E. (1947) *Bull. Johns Hopkins Hosp.* 81, 305.
Vedder, E. B., and Rosenberg, C. (1938). *J. Nutr.* 16, 57.
Wald, G. (1968). *Nature (London)* 219, 800.
Walker, S. E., Eylenberg, E., and Moore, T. (1947). *Biochem. J.* 41, 575.
Wilson, J. R., and Du Bois, R. O. (1923). *Amer. J. Dis. Child.* 26, 431.
Wolbach, S. B. (1946). *Proc. Inst. Med. Chicago* 16, 118.
Wolbach, S. B. (1947). *J. Bone Joint Surg.* 29, 171.
Wolbach, S. B., and Bessey, O. A. (1941). *Arch. Pathol.* 32, 689.
Wolbach, S. B., and Hegsted, D. M. (1952a). *AMA Arch. Pathol.* 54, 13.
Wolbach, S. B., and Hegsted, D. M. (1952b). *AMA Arch. Pathol.* 54, 30.
Wolbach, S. B., and Hegsted, D. M. (1952c). *AMA Arch. Pathol.* 54, 548.
Wolbach, S. B., and Hegsted, D. M. (1953). *AMA Arch. Pathol.* 55, 47.
Wolbach, S. B., and Howe, P. R. (1925). *Proc. Soc. Exp. Biol. Med.* 22, 402.
Wolbach, S. B., and Maddock, C. L. (1951). *Proc. Soc. Exp. Biol. Med.* 77, 835.
Wolbach, S. B., and Maddock, C. L. (1952). *AMA Arch. Pathol.* 53, 273.
Woods, J. F. and Nichols, G., Jr. (1965). *J. Cell Biol.* 26, 747–757.
Ypsilanti, H. (1935). *Klin. Wochenschr.* 14, 90.
Zechmeister, L. (1944). *Chem. Rev.* 34, 267.

CHAPTER 6

Vitamin C and Bone

GEOFFREY H. BOURNE

I. Introduction

The distinguished pathologist, S. Burt Wolbach, had originally agreed to write this chapter in the first edition. Despite the fact that his health was failing and that major surgical interference seemed necessary, he devoted considerable thought to the subject and prepared a table of contents which promised to give us the considered judgment of one who had for 25 years been working on and thinking about the pathology of vitamin C deficiency. His death robbed us of this privilege and the scientific world of a distinguished pathologist. The burden of writing this chapter has fallen on my shoulders and I have tried to follow the line which Dr. Wolbach might have taken; my efforts, however, will inevitably seem but a feeble glim by comparison with the light that would have been shed by the master.

II. Vitamin C Deficiency and Intercellular Substances in General

A. COLLAGEN AND WOUNDS

In 1748, Richard Walter, chaplain to Lord Anson's expedition round the world (1740–1744), described how old wounds broke open under the influence of scurvy:

> At other times the whole body, but more especially the legs, were subject to ulcers of the worst kind, attended with rotten bones, and such a luxuriance of fungous flesh, as yielded to no remedy. But a most extraordinary circumstance, and what would be scarcely credible upon any single evidence, is that the scars of wounds which had for many years healed, were forced open again by this violent distemper: of this, there was a remarkable instance in one of the invalids upon the *Centurion* who had been wounded about fifty years before at the battle of Boyne (1690); for although he was cured soon after, and had continued well for a great number of years past, yet on his being attacked by the scurvy, his wounds, in the progress of his disease, broke out afresh, and appeared as if they had never been healed. Nay, what is still more astonishing, the callous of the broken bone, which had been completely formed for a long time, was found to be hereby dissolved, and the fracture seemed as if it had been consolidated.

This account constitutes the earliest record of the effects of scurvy on wounds and since the tensile strength of wounds is a function of the fascial scar, it becomes the first indication that vitamin C is associated with the maintenance of collagen. Lind, in 1753, referred to a letter from Mr. Ives describing a seaman on *H. M. S. Dragon* who had a "shattering of the humerus from a Spanish musket ball," the healing of which was delayed by the onset of scurvy.

Many other references exist in the older literature which show not only that healing of wounds was delayed but also that they were likely to break open again in scurvy (see, for example, Smart, 1888; Eve, 1888).

That vitamin C was essential for the maintenance of collagen was suggested by the work of Höjer (1923–1924), and more recently Hunt (1941) showed a reversion of newly formed collagen in a wound to an argyrophilic precollagenous state when his animals were made scorbutic. Pirani and Levenson (1953) showed that ascorbic acid was necessary for the maintenance of scar tissue many weeks old which had formed during the healing of experimental wounds. Although there are relatively few references to the necessity of vitamin C for the maintenance of formed collagen there are many references to the effect of vitamin C deficiency on delaying the healing of wounds, thus indicating an inhibition of collagen production and/or maturation.

Most of the early literature already quoted makes reference to this and there is a record that even during the 1914–1918 war Turkish soldiers suffered severely from scurvy and that in those who developed the disease both skin and flesh wounds and fractures healed poorly.

Höjer showed in 1923–1924 that in experimental guinea pig tuberculosis there was deficient scar production by the lung tissues resulting from the inability to produce collagen. Ishido (1923) and later Saitta (1929) showed that there was considerable delay in the healing of wounds in scorbutic animals. Lauber (1933) found that application of vitamin C to skin wounds in mice stimulated healing but that injections of vitamin C into normal guinea pigs had no effect on the speed at which wounds healed (see also Proto, 1936). This is not surprising since the guinea pigs were already receiving their optimum dose of vitamin C, and it has been shown (Bourne, 1942b) that there is an optimum requirement of vitamin C for healing wounds. It may be possible that the increased local concentration of the vitamin as a result of its direct application to the lesion in animals such as mice (which synthesize their own vitamin C) may have enabled the repair process to proceed faster than if the injured tissues had been dependent upon the slower diffusion from the blood. However, rabbits are also able to synthesize their own vitamin C, and it is possibly surprising therefore that Mann and Pullinger (1940) were unable to find that local applications of vitamin C had any stimulatory effect on the regeneration of a cornea which had been damaged with mustard gas. If an increased local concentration of vitamin C was important in securing rapid regeneration one would have thought that an avascular tissue such as the cornea would have been ideal for demonstrating such an effect. The positive result obtained by Saitta with mice might therefore have been owing to lack of adequate statistical means of measuring regeneration. Lauber and Rosenfeld (1938) showed that if animals on a low vitamin C intake are wounded most of the organs and tissues lose their vitamin C, which appears to become mobilized in the injured region. Thus, there seems to be some local concentration of the vitamin in a lesion, but presumably under normal circumstances an optimum concentration is secured fairly rapidly. Bartlett *et al.* (1942) found in fact that the tensile strength of a scar depended directly upon its vitamin C content; e.g., scars with 7.65 mg of vitamin C per 100 gm of tissue broke at 258 mm Hg and those having 0.31 mg vitamin C per 100 gm tissue burst at 127 mm Hg.

Wolbach (1953) has pointed out that the rate of production of intercellular material has a quantitative relationship to the amout of ascorbic acid administered. The first quantitative experiment which demonstrated this was described by Lanman and Ingalls (1937), who carried out direct measurements of the force required to break wounds in normal and scorbutic animals. The wounds were made in the abdominal wall, and measurements of their strength was obtained by distending the abdomen with air and noting the pressure on a mercury manometer at which the wounds burst. Similar observations were made on wounds in the stomach wall. The results are given in the accompanying tabulation. Similar results were obtained on the stomachs of guinea pigs by

	Bursting pressure	
Wounds	2 mg vitamin C	0.5 mg vitamin C
Abdominal	160 mm Hg	65 mm Hg
Gastric	70 mm Hg	30 mm Hg

Taffel and Harvey (1938), Hunt (1941), and Hartzell and Stone (1942). Wolfer and Hoebel (1940) demonstrated that patients in whom the plasma vitamin C was lowest showed the slowest healing of surgical wounds. Wolfer *et al.* (1947), working with human volunteers, concluded that up to 50% reduction of tensile strength in a wound could be produced by a diet deficient in vitamin C. Crandon *et al.* (1940) recorded their results on experimental human scurvy and showed that only after a subject had been on a diet completely deficient in vitamin C for about 6 months, and after the plasma vitamin C had been nil for over 2 months, did a wound in the back refuse to heal. The subject, however, was adult; a very different result may have been obtained with a child. In growing guinea pigs, for example, it was shown (Bourne, 1944a) that the curve of tensile strength of skin wounds against plasma vitamin C ran roughly parallel (see Fig. 1). It was further shown that there was a close correlation between tensile strength of these wounds and the intake of vitamin C by the animal (see Table I).

This work also showed that in the animals receiving the least amount of vitamin C there was a greater amount of reticular (precollagen) fibers than in those receiving the greatest amount, and this was correlated with the tensile strength of the wounds. Carney (1946) was

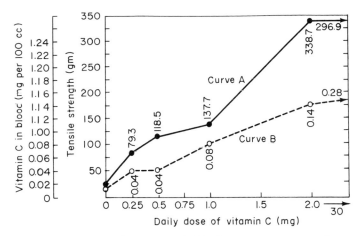

FIG. 1. Curves showing relationship of blood vitamin C to tensile strength of wounds in guinea pigs. Curve A: Tensile strength of wounds in 52 guinea pigs on graded doses of vitamin C after healing for 1 week. Curve B: Blood vitamin C in 14 quinea pigs on varying doses of vitamin C (see Bourne, 1944a).

not able to find a relationship between wound healing and the level of vitamin C in the plasma in military patients; however, he too was dealing with adults.

The relationship between wound healing and vitamin C intake is now amply confirmed; see, for example, the more recent work of Campbell

TABLE I
TENSILE STRENGTH IN GRAMS OF WOUNDS IN GUINEA PIGS
GIVEN GRADED DOSES OF VITAMIN C
Each figure is the average tensile strength of two wounds

	Dose of vitamin C per day (mg)				
None	0.25	0.5	1.0	2.0	30
0 gms.	58 gms.	156 gms.	111 gms.	343 gms.	255 gms.
0	56	86	143	331	255
46	65	220	231	185	270
21	91	150	120	480	310
55	125	123	95	400	394
0	101	123	150	295	313
21	34	62	96	320	281
34	120	40	135	316	—
50	64	206	158	378	—
Means $\begin{cases} 25.3 \\ \pm\ 7.4 \end{cases}$	79.3 $\pm\ 10.4$	118.5 $\pm\ 18.0$	137.7 $\pm\ 13.9$	338.7 $\pm\ 26.8$	296.9 $\pm\ 18.5$

et al. (1950), Campbell and Ferguson (1950), Galloway *et al.* (1948), and Pirani *et al.* (1952). Hines *et al.* (1944) have shown that the vitamin is essential for the healing of nerves.

That this failure of wounds to heal normally results primarily from failure of collagen production is also unequivocal. The relationship between vitamin C and collagen production is demonstrated by the work of various authors; for example, Jeney and Törö (1936) found that if vitamin C is added to the culture medium in which fibroblasts were being grown, fibers were produced more rapidly. Mazoué (1937) injected kieslguhr intraperitoneally into a guinea pig and demonstrated a close association between the dose of vitamin C and the time of the first appearance of fibroblasts and fibers; he also showed that vitamin C deficiency had a profound effect on the organization of a clot produced by severing the limb muscles of guinea pigs. Querido and Gaillard (1939) demonstrated the relationship between the vitamin and the production of collagen fibers by culturing osteogenetic cells from the chick in three types of plasma: (1) from scorbutic guinea pigs, (2) from scorbutic guinea pigs with crystalline vitamin C added, and (3) from scorbutic guinea pigs which had been treated with large doses of vitamin C for a few days before the experiment. Hardly any fibers were formed by the cells in the first plasma, but in the second and third, fibers were formed as rapidly as in the normal plasma. The cells in the scorbutic plasma showed fatty degeneration. However, Hass and McDonald (1940) found that vitamin C did not promote the formation of fibers in guinea pig tissue cultures. Hunt (1941), Bourne (1942b), and Danielli *et al.* (1946) also showed that there was a delay in the change from precollagen to mature collagen in scorbutic guinea pigs. The latter authors also showed a lack of phosphatase in wounds in scorbutic guinea pigs, a finding which has been confirmed by Bunting and White (1948). The present author (1943) found also a deficiency of phosphatase in healing bones, but this appeared to be due not so much to the fact that there was less phosphatase in the osteoid that did form but that less osteoid was formed. That which was present appeared to contain as much as normal osteoid. It is of interest that Danielli and his co-workers found that in the healing of wounds the precollagen fibers formed (as in healing bone injuries) contained phosphatase and that as they matured into collagen the phosphatase disappeared.

Although the relationship between collagen production and vitamin C seems to be well established, the relationship between the maintenance of the collagen fiber (as distinct from the intercellular substance) is perhaps not so certain in view of the fact that Neuberger *et al.* (1951) have shown that, at least in the rat, once collagen is formed its metabolic turnover is virtually negligible. It is of interest, too, that Ham and Elliott (1938) have claimed that the basic defect in scurvy is a failure to produce new fibers, not a weakening or destruction of those already formed. This suggestion is supported by the work of Elster (1950), Robertson (1950), and Burns *et al.* (1951). This may explain why the development of scurvy is much more rapid in the growing animal than in the adult. Wolbach (1953) has drawn attention to the necessity that "Biochemists, interested in quantitative studies of collagen under conditions of dietary deficiency or in the estimation of collagen turnover by the use of heavy nitrogen or amino acids containing radioactive carbon, should not fail to take into account the growth rate of their experimental animals."

B. GROUND SUBSTANCE

Although vitamin C deficiency is known to affect collagen production there is no certainty as to how this is done. Any explanation is affected by the fact that the method of formation of collagen fibers is in dispute. Wolbach and Howe (1926) claimed that collagen fibers were produced in the intercellular ground substance by a sort of jellying process and that in scurvy it was this which was affected, whereas the cells remained more or less normal. This view has been supported by a number of other workers including Dalldorf (1939). However, others including Höjer (1923–1924), Fish and Harris (1934), and Ham and Elliott (1938) considered that it is the cells which are primarily affected. Other authors, e.g., Follis (1948), claimed that the gelation theory is not proved. Evidence is accumulating that in fact, as Margaret Lewis claimed in 1917, the collagen fiber is secreted in the cell and excreted to the exterior. It may be of interest that Barnett and Bourne (1942) found that many mesenchyme cells in a 5-day-old chick embryo contained numerous vitamin C granules (demonstrated by the acid silver nitrate technique). The presence of these granules may have been related to the production of fibers. It is of interest, too, that mesenchyme cells in certain sites become chondroblastic and the first morphological indication that they are about to do this is the withdrawal of their processes and the appearance of a "mucoid matrix," the resulting tissue being called *precartilage.* Before this happened an increased deposit of vitamin C appeared, mainly in the processes of the cells. A similar process was observed, not only in the early embryo but also later when some cartilage was already formed and was undergoing accretionary growth. Such cartilage showed a well-defined outer zone of mesenchyme, which was precartilage; both layers contained ascorbic acid, and the amount diminished with increasing distance from the surface. Perhaps this accumulation of ascorbic acid is associated with the formation of intercellular matrix of ground substance. It may be significant that the majority of differentiated cartilage cells showed little or no reaction. In the earlier stages although most of the vitamin C granules were present in the cells some granules could be seen in the ground substance of the precartilage. Although there was not much evidence that cartilage was affected in scurvy, Wolbach and Maddock (1952) had recently produced proof that it is. This was particularly apparent in the epiphyseal cartilage plates of the long bones of young guinea pigs; it is not so obvious in costal cartilages which grow more slowly.

In scurvy, Wolbach and Maddock found cartilage cells failed to produce matrix, developed an abnormal appearance, and became shrunken and irregular; the nuclei stained very deeply with basic dyes; and the cells were separated from each other by small quantities of material which did not give the normal staining reaction for matrix. Reddi and Norström (1954) have shown, using radioactive sulfur, that the incorporation of sulfate into chondroitin sulfate is reduced to about one-third in scurvy. This had also been demonstrated autoradiographically in the present author's laboratory by Miss C. R. Hill (see Fig. 2, A and B). Friberg and Ringertz (1954) found reduction of uptake of radioactive sulfur in scurvy all over the body but not particularly in cartilage. It is of interest, too, that Follis (1951) has shown that in cartilage cells in scorbutic guinea pigs there is no cytochrome oxidase, no mucopolysaccharide, and a reduction in ribonucleic acid and glycogen.

Gersh and Catchpole (1949) have shown that fibroblasts contain a glycoprotein to which a CHO radical is attached. This, they believed, may be the precursor of the ground substance. They speculated that the fibroblast might secrete a glycoprotein of high molecular weight which would then become precipitated in the extracellular fluid. Con-

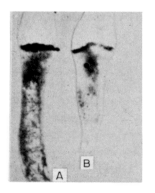

FIG. 2. (A) Autoradiograph of costochondral junction of normal guinea pig showing incorporation of radiosulfur (^{35}S) into cartilage (below) and at junction. (B) Autoradiograph of costochondral junction of scorbutic guinea pig showing greatly reduced uptake of radiosulfur in cartilage and at junction. (from preparations by Miss C. R. Hill made in the author's laboratory.)

tinued precipitation would result in fiber formation which would eventually crystallize into the highly organized cross-striated elements which compose mature collagen. This is fundamentally a modified view of the gelation theory of Wolbach, but whether such precipitations occur or not this substance presumably represents the nonfibrillar ground substance of connective tissue which must be a product of cell secretion, and which is believed to be affected by vitamin C deficiency.

In healing wounds of scorbutic guinea pigs, Penney and Balfour (1949) found that a considerable amount of metachromatic substance (acid mucopolysaccharide) was produced. An increased concentration of periodic acid Schiff (PAS) positive material was also found associated with the edges of the trabeculae in costochondral junctions (Hill and Bourne, 1954) (see Figs. 3 and 4) although there was a decrease of this material in the inner parts of the trabeculae. Increased mucopolysaccharides were also demonstrated in scurvy by Bunting and White (1948). Thus, one effect of vitamin C deficiency appears to be an increase of intercellular material, but this material is abnormal in nature according to Bradfield and Kodicek (1951). It appeared to be nonsulfated and not capable of removal by amylase or hyaluronidase.

Wolbach (1953) has drawn attention to the fact that the first material

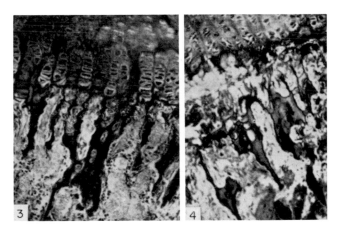

Fig. 3. Periodic acid Schiff reaction in costochondral junction of normal guinea pig. Note even distribution of reaction through developing trabeculae and in cartilage matrix.

Fig. 4. Periodic acid Schiff reaction in costochondral junction of scorbutic guinea pig. Note general reduction of reaction but greatly increased intensity along the edges of developing trabeculae.

(Figures 3 and 4 are from preparations by Miss C. R. Hill made in the author's laboratory.)

which has staining properties similar to collagen appears as a homogeneous substance surrounding the fibroblast and its processes and that fibers subsequently appear in this material. However, as Wolbach mentioned, these first-formed fibers are argentophilic and do not have the staining properties of collagen. The fact that this amorphous material has a similar reaction to collagen is therefore not evidence that it represents the first stage of the cycle of collagen production. It seems more likely to represent matrix, perhaps eventually associated with the mature fibers but not necessarily forming an integral part of its structure. Wolbach, in referring to the glycoprotein granules of fibroblasts described by Gersh and Catchpole, noted that the vacuoles which apparently contain these granules were described by him in 1933. He suggested that the extracellular liquid, frequently described in different parts of the body in both experimental and clinical scurvy, may result from the failure of polymerization of this glycoprotein after excretion from the cells and that normally it becomes polymerized to form part of the connective tissue matrix.

The tendency to hemorrhage in scurvy has suggested some alteration in the permeability of the capillary vessels, and this indicates some alteration in the intercellular cement substance binding the endothelial cells together. In this respect one should mention that Chambers and Cameron (1943) found that vitamin C was not necessary in tissue culture of epithelial cells to enable the cells to cohere into sheets. Findlay (1921) observed "diapedesis" of red cells between the endothelial cells of the capillaries of scorbutic guinea pigs (see also the findings of Hess, 1920), but it has been found that various dyes passed through the capillary walls of scorbutic animals no faster than through those of normal animals (see Elster and Schack, 1950). Göthlin *et al.* (1937), however, have produced substantial evidence based on human experiments that the capillary resistance was lowered in scurvy and could be restored with crystalline vitamin C, but Lazarus *et al.* (1948) demonstrated that many scorbutic patients show no signs of increased capillary fragility. Wolbach and Bessey (1942) stated that the capillary bleedings in scurvy may have resulted either from the changes in the cement substance binding the endothelial cells together or in the collagen fibrils supporting the capillary. They pointed out that new capillary formation was prevented by a severe deficiency of vitamin C.

In interpreting the effects of vitamin C deficiency we are hindered by the absence of the knowledge as to what biochemical function the vitamin serves in the body. King (1950) has shown biochemically, and Hill and Bourne (1954) histochemically, that there is a decrease in activity of oxidative enzymes, e.g., cytochrome oxidase and succinic dehydrogenase. Furthermore, King showed a decrease in phosphatase and esterase activities and a decreased ability to metabolize tyrosine and phenylalanine. These reactions suggest, as King has stressed, that there is a general lowering of normal cellular metabolic activities in scurvy and none of these decreased reactions appears to be associated specifically with the failure of formation of intercellular substances. One can only assume that since the secretion of these substances is a normal metabolic activity of these cells the lowered metabolism of the cells in scurvy results in lowered production of matrix. According to Lloyd and Sinclair (1953) ascorbic acid or its oxidation products may play a part in the removal of polysaccharides in the final stages of collagen formation, or they may have a catalytic function in the organization of cross-linkages such as —S—S— bonds between the protein chains of collagen. Lloyd and Sinclair also suggested that ascorbic acid and its oxidation products may be associated with the oxidation of organic sulfur to sulfate in the production of chondroitin sulfate. Support for this is seen in the work of Reddi and Nörstrom (1954). According to Barrenscheen and Valyi-Nagy (1948) there may be also an association between ascorbic acid and the oxidation of methionine sulfate.

More recently, it has been established that there are two major metabolic defects which occur in connective tissue and cartilage in scurvy. A number of authors have now confirmed that there is a defect in chondroitin fulfate production; thus, a significant decrease of this material is found in mature connective tissue and cartilage. Decreased uptake of radioactive sulfur (^{35}S-sulfate) in scorbutic animals has been described by a number of authors (Friberg and Ringertz, 1954; Reddi and Norström, 1954; Kodicek, 1965). Studies with ^{14}C glucose have also demonstrated a decreased uptake of this compound in scorbutic animals, and Antoniwicz and Kodicek (1964) have shown that vitamin C deficiency causes a gross decrease of incorporation of this radioactive glucose into galactosamine in cartilage and in granulation tissue. Since galactosamine is an important constituent of chondroitin sulfate, the decrease of this material in vitamin C deficiency can be explained by the block in the formation of galactosamine. Kodicek (1965) has also drawn attention to the increased destruction of preformed galactosaminoglycans.

Kodicek and his colleagues believed, that the block in galactosamine formation results from an impairment of the UDP-4-epimerase reaction (Kalckar and Maxwell, 1958). According to Kodicek, this step "catalyses" the conversion of UDP-acetyl-galactosamine by an oxido-reduction mechanism. An active UDP-N-acetylpyrophosphorylase has been found in granulation tissue by Guha *et al.* (1962). Kodicek believed that if this enzyme is impaired in scurvy, the amounts of mucopolysaccharides containing glucosamine would be reduced.

Kodicek has published a scheme which summarizes the steps involved in the biosynthesis of hexosamine (see Scheme I).

Bates *et al.* (1969) showed that in granulation tissue of healing tendonectomy wounds in guinea pigs, vitamin C deficiency caused a drop in galactosamine content without affecting the glucosamine content. Fractionation of the digested granulation tissue gave three fractions: (1) glycopeptide, (2) hyaluronic acid, and (3) a sulfated glycosaminoglycan mixture of which half behaved like dermatan sulfate. In vitamin C deficiency there was a drop in the glycosaminoglycan fraction which explained why there was a decrease on galactosamine. There was also a drop in the amount of hyaluronic acid but a slight rise in the glycopeptide fraction. These changes may have resulted in part from changes in the endoplasmic reticulum and various cell organelles (see Ross, 1968). It has also been suggested that these biochemical changes are secondary to hormonal changes produced by the vitamin deficiency (see Kitabchi, 1967; Sulimovici and Boyd, 1968). Other authors have suggested these changes result from liberation of hydrolytic enzymes, e.g., polysaccharidases (Messina *et al.*, 1968). Bates *et al.* suggested that the absence of fresh collagen fibers in vitamin C deficiency results in a failure to bind these intercellular substances in place.

A second change in connective tissue in scorbutic animals which is now well documented is the failure of hydroxylation of proline to hy-

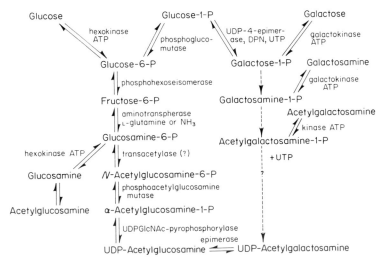

Scheme 1. Biosynthesis of hexosamine (Kodicek, 1965).

droxyproline (see Fig. 5). Chvapil and Huryck (1959) and Breslow and Lukens (1960) showed this was true *in vitro,* and a number of authors including Gould (1961), Gross (1959), Ross and Benditt (1964) showed that it was true in scorbutic tissues *in vivo.* D. S. Jackson (1958) and Green and Lowthern (1959) believed that the process of hydroxylation of proline occurs early in the biosynthesis of collagen and before the complete collagen chain is formed. The process is also believed to have occurred during proline activation on sRNA. Peterkofsky and Udenfriend (1963), according to Kodicek (1965) (see Fig. 6), "conclude from their studies with the cell-free system from the chick embryo that the hydroxylation of proline may occur beyond the terminal stage of biosynthesis of a proline polypeptide on polysomal RNA, namely when the final polypeptide esterified through its terminal hydroxyl group to the last sRNA remaining attached to the messenger RNA if formed."

It appears that vitamin C affects the hydroxylation of proline locally. The fact that vitamin C is concentrated in the tissues of healing wounds supports this possibility (Cmuchalova and Chvapil, 1963).

There has also been some discussion as to whether vitamin C affects the formation of intramolecular bonds in collagen (Gould and Manner, 1962).

How vitamin C facilitates hydroxylation of proline is not known.

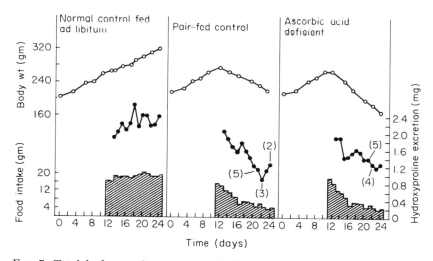

Fig. 5. Total hydroxyproline excretion, body weight, and food intake of normal, pair-fed, and scorbutic guinea pigs. Results are expressed as the mean of individual determinations for each group. The numbers in parentheses refer to the number of animals surviving within the group from the original of six: (○) body weight and (●) hydroxyproline excretion (from Barnes *et al.,* 1969).

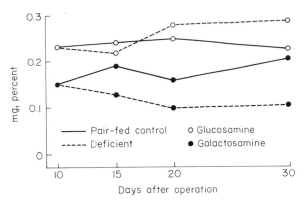

Fig. 6. Effect of scurvy on individual hexosamines of 10-day-old normal granulation tissue from tendonectomized guinea pigs (from Kodicek, 1965).

Kodicek (1965) pointed out that this process has been shown to require molecular oxygen with the production of free hydroxyl radicals. This type of reaction according to Kodicek is one of an "oxygenase" type which attaches molecular oxygen to a variety of substances in the body. *In vitro* ascorbic acid can produce hydroxylation of proline without enzymic activity, and Buhler and Mason (1961) have decided that vitamin C does not support enzymic hydroxylation. Kodiccek (1965) was attracted by the possibility, suggested by a number of authors, that vitamin C, *in vivo*, provides free hydroxyl radical as monodehydroascorbic acid.

Summing up the possibilities, Kodicek said:

> According to the electron microscope studies of Ross and Benditt (1961), ascorbic acid deficiency causes intracellular changes mainly in the micro-somes and endoplasmic reticulum and this could result in alteration of protein synthesis. The studies of Staudinger et al. (1961) on microsomal electron transport and hydroxylation reactions in the presence of ascorbic acid are the most consistent approach to elucidate the mode of action of the vitamin; they have isolated a NADH-monodehydroascorbic acid transhydrogenase, a flavoprotein which catalyses proton transfer from NADH to the ascorbic acid radical to form reduced ascorbic acid. In this manner, ascorbic acid would be involved indirectly in the electron transport chain . . . Recently Mapson (1964) suggested that the ascorbate system might act as an electron donor and acceptor in the photosynthetic process in plants.

Figure 7 shows changes in mucopolysaccharides in normal and scorbutic rats.

The question also arises as to whether the changed mucopolysaccharide component of granulation tissue affects the formation of collagen.

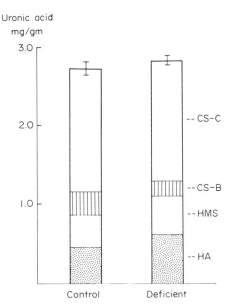

FIG. 7. Acid mucopolysaccharides of normal and scorbutic guinea pig aortas indicating the relative proportions of hyaluronic acid (HA), heparitin monosulfate (HMS), and chondroitin sulfate C (CS-C) (Gore *et al.*, 1965).

Bradfield and Kodicek, in 1951, showed that in scorbutic skin wounds the collagen fibers were thick and cornified in a chaotic fashion, and Bourne (1956) and others have shown that the nature of the collagen in such wounds appeared to be different in that it stained like reticulin and not like mature collagen. In a wound in a normal animal, the collagen fibers are slender, and although they interlace there is a general pattern of their arrangement parallel with the skin surface. Perhaps this first-formed collagen, which is rapidly matured into mature collagen in normal animals, contains nonhydroxylated collagen. It appears to contain less sulfur than normal collagen. Barnes *et al.* (1969) concluded that the formation of elastin hydroxyproline was dependent upon vitamin C and that in scurvy elastin which is formed and retained is deficient in hydroxyproline. Barnes *et al.* (1969) and others have shown an increase in excretion of amino nitrogen in the urine in scorbutic guinea pigs. This has also been observed in scorbutic infants (Janxis and Huisman, 1954) and in monkeys (Banerjee, 1962). The latter author also found an increase in the excretion of ammonia in scorbutic monkeys, and Barnes *et al.* confirmed this in scorbutic guinea pigs.

It is obvious that we have advanced some distance in our understanding of the role which vitamin C plays in connective tissue metabolism, but there is still much to be understood.

C. CORTISONE AND WOUND HEALING

Since 1928 it has been known that the adrenal gland contains a considerable amount of vitamin C, usually estimated at about 10 times that found in any other organ. Similar high concentrations are, however, found in the anterior pituitary gland, the corpus luteum, and the interstitial cells of the testes. Because of the association of vitamin C with the adrenal cortex it is of interest that cortisone injections delay or suppress wound healing. This was first described by Ragan et al. (1949). They found that in the course of treating patients with various complaints there was a delay in the healing of previously incised wounds and an inhibition of the growth of granulation tissue in open wounds. They confirmed this with experimental wounds in rabbits (Ragan et al., 1949, 1950; Plotz et al. 1950). In these animals histological study of the wounds showed that there was a suppression of fibroblast migration and proliferation; new capillary vessels did not form, and there was less ground substance than normal. A decrease in skin thickness was also noted. In addition, the authors found a suppression of callus formation of a broken bone by cortisone. Similar results were obtained by the use of ACTH. Ragan's work was repeated and confirmed by Bangham (1951). Spain et al. (1950a,b) repeated the work in mice, and Plotz et al. (1950) found delay in the healing of incised wounds of both skin and stomach as well as with fractures. Howes et al. (1950) also showed that the bursting strength of sutured wounds was reduced in cortisone-treated rats and that fracture healing was delayed; in addition, they noted that cortisone delayed the absorption of extravasated blood. Further work confirming the failure of wound healing and of collagen production in cortisone-treated human beings and animals was published by Baxter et al. (1951), Aldrich et al. (1951), and Magarey and Gough (1952). It is also of interest that Tauberhaus and Amromin (1950) found that deoxycorticosterone acetate stimulated fibroblasts and fibrous tissue development (supported by Selye, 1949; Pirani et al., 1951; Bourne et al., 1952) and that cortisone exerted a suppressive effect. This suggested a balance of cortical hormones controlling fibroblast activity and fiber production. Baker and Whitaker (1950) and Castor and Baker (1950) found that hog adrenal extract applied locally had a striking inhibitory effect on the closing of experimental wounds in animals and that when cortisone, or compound F, was applied a similar result was obtained.

Baldridge *et al.* (1951) and Steen (1951), however, found no effect of cortisone on fibroblast proliferation and migration. Nevertheless, in embryos cortisone was found to disturb growth in chick, mouse, and rat (Karnovsky *et al.*, 1951a,b). Follis (1951) found that the growth of long bones was retarded by cortisone; in fact, he found the growing ends of such bones to be composed of spindles of calcified cartilaginous matrix enclosed in bone.

The effects of cortisone on wound healing were virtually identical with those produced by scurvy. This led both the present author (Bourne, 1952) and Wolbach and Maddock (1952) to endeavor to prevent the effects of cortisone on connective tissue by treatment with vitamin C. The present author worked with experimental wounds in rabbits and guinea pigs and studied the effects of cortisone and vitamin C upon their tensile strength and their histological nature.

In control rabbits the average tensile strength of three wounds on the left flank of each of five rabbits was 340 gm; in the same rabbits injected with cortisone daily for a week the mean of three wounds on the right flank of each was 192 gm. The tensile strength of these wounds was therefore only about half that of the controls.

The similarity between the effects of cortisone and scurvy had impressed other authors and was commented upon by Plotz *et al.* (1950) and Spain *et al.* (1950a,b). The first of these groups of authors were so impressed by this similarity that they considered the possibility of cortisone inducing a scurvylike condition in the connective tissue. Accordingly, they made determinations of the vitamin C levels in animals treated with cortisone but found them to be normal. They also tried flooding patients with vitamin C who were receiving either cortisone or ACTH, but this had no effect on the action of the hormones. This is of interest since ACTH causes a pronounced loss of vitamin C from the adrenal cortex.

To study this problem further the present author used a second series of rabbits: control incisions on the left flank gave a mean tensile strength of 237 gm; then each animal was given daily injections of cortisone together with 1 gm of sodium ascorbate injected parenterally at the same time. The mean tensile strength of wounds on the right flank was then found to be 134 gm, still only a little more than half the tensile strength of the controls. It was obvious therefore that cortisone did not exert its effect on healing wounds by depriving them of vitamin C. Histologically, scars of the cortisone-treated animals showed less fibrous tissue and there were few fibroblasts and other tissues present. There were also unabsorbed blood clots. These characteristics were the same as those found in scurvy. In animals treated with vitamin C as well as cortisone the wounds showed exactly the same changes without any signs of mitigation.

It is of interest that Schaffenberg *et al.* (1950) put forward the theory that vitamin C deficiency (in view of the association of the vitamin with the adrenal cortex) might lead to inadequate production of glucocorticoids. This is supported by the fact (Persson, 1953) that adrenalectomy aggravates the effects of scurvy. This seems a strange denial of the work of the various authors which has just been discussed. However, Schaffenberg *et al.* (1950) and Hyman *et al.* (1950) found that both cortisone and ACTH ameliorated some of the effects of scurvy. As against this Clayton and Prunty (1951) found that cortisone did not affect the weight loss in scorbutic guinea pigs, and Upton and Coon (1951) and Bourne (1952) found that it had no beneficial effects on wound healing in such animals. It may be of interest at this point to mention that cortisone in general seems to retard wound healing in those species of animals which synthesize their own vitamin C.

Wolbach and Maddock in their investigation into the problem asked three questions:

(1) Will cortisone administered after the development of the lesions of scurvy produce a demonstrable histological effect?

(2) Will the daily concurrent administration of cortisone modify the progress of events in guinea pigs fed a diet deficient in vitamin C?

(3) Will cortisone modify the reparative sequences resulting from ascorbic acid treatment of scorbutic guinea pigs?

These questions, they stated, were all decisively answered in the negative after examining a number of organs and tissues including epiphyseal cartilage, bone, adrenal, and other soft tissues.

Persson (1953) has made a detailed study of the changes in scurvy and compared them with those produced by cortisone. The summary of his results is reproduced below.

(1) An increased amount of ground substance mucopolysaccharides is found in scurvy; the concentration of hexosamine within the skin is significantly increased in comparison with normal animals.

(2) The ground substance complex is present in an abnormal state of organization in scurvy showing an increased solubility in water and a significantly lowered resistance toward penetrating agents; the dermal spread of Evans blue is increased similar to the velocity of flow of Ringer's solution through isolated muscle fascia.

(3) The water binding capacity of the skin is increased in scurvy.

(4) In repair after wounds in scurvy a depolymerized water-soluble

ground substance is found within the granulation tissue. This ground substance does not show any metachromatic potency but reacts with Schiff's reagent after periodic acid and with Hale's colloidal iron. The fibroblasts contain large amounts of Schiff-reactive material.

(5) Adrenalectomy aggravates the symptoms of scurvy and seems to inhibit the cellular activity in granulation tissue.

(6) Cortisone induces a marked gelation of the matrix. The dermal spreading of Evans blue shows a tendency to be depressed; the amount of hexosamine in the skin decreases and the dermal content of water is lowered as compared to untreated scorbutic animals. The histochemical properties of the ground substance change at treatment with cortisone in scurvy, the matrix becomes metachromatic and its reactivity to the periodic acid Schiff staining seems to be diminished.

(7) Local treatment of skin wounds with ascorbic acid and dehydroascorbic acid are effective when the treatment is extended over several days.

From these results it is obvious that the changes brought about by cortisone treatment are not directly comparable with those resulting from scurvy.

It seems fairly certain that, as Persson pointed out, the ground substance is present in scurvy in a disaggregated and depolymerized state and shows no metachromatic activity although it gives a positive reaction with the periodic acid Schiff technique for polysaccharides. It is impossible to say whether this ground substance is secreted by the fibroblasts in this depolymerized state or whether it is subjected to depolymerization after secretion possibly because of excess activity of hyaluronidase. Persson referred to the work of Bensley (1934) who characterized all healing processes by the three stages of (1) edema, (2) gelation, and (3) fiber production. Bensley and Persson pointed out that in scurvy the process stops at the first stage, namely, edema. In cortisone-treated animals, however, it stops at the second stage, i.e., gelation. The setting of the intercellular matrix is believed by some workers to be associated with the production of chondroitin sulfuric acid, but there is evidence that cortisone inhibits the formation of this substance. In fact, Layton (1951) claimed that the hormone prevents the incorporation of labeled inorganic sulfate *in vivo* or *in vitro* into chondroitin sulfate in connective tissue ground substance. However, the gelling is probably not a property dependent entirely upon chondroitin or mucoitin sulfate and is undoubtedly also concerned with the state and amount of the hyaluronic acid present.

It therefore appears to be soundly established that vitamin C deficiency is associated with profound changes in connective tissue, and since the principal elements of connective tissue are also present in bone it might be expected that bone would also be affected. There is ample evidence also for this.

III. Bone

A. Vitamin C in Chick Embryo

In the chick embryo, mesenchyme that is to form bone contains vitamin C distributed in the cells in the same way as in precartilage. When the differentiation into osteoblasts begins the cells lose their vitamin C; the early osteoblasts themselves generally containing few granules. In well-developed bone, such as is seen in the femur 2 days after hatching, a few cells are heavily impregnated. The deposit is always granular and diffuse (Barnett and Bourne, 1942). Klein (1938) using $AuCl_3$ instead of $AgNO_3$ for the demonstration of ascorbic acid had observed a similar impregnation in periosteal mesenchyme in pig embryos; he found that the osteoblasts also give a strong reaction, either local or diffuse, both when on the surface and when embedded in the calcified matrix. In regions where the collagenous (osteogenic) fibers have appeared, extracellular granules of what appears to be vitamin C are present. These granules can often be observed to be arranged in rows along the collagen fibers. Very fine granules are also present, rather unevenly distributed, in freshly calcified bone laminae. In the development of cartilage bone, whether endochondral or perichondral, the osteoblasts do not differ from those of membrane bone. The special phenomenon associated with this process is the appearance of a deposit in the cartilaginous matrix around the hypertrophied cartilage cells; the latter do not contain vitamin C. There is a possibility that in this case the granules may be of bone salt. Before cartilage cells enlarge and degenerate they align themselves in a characteristic fashion; at this stage they may contain ascorbic acid in small amounts, generally localized at one pole of the nucleus. This association of the differentiation of the osteoblast with the disappearance (the using up?) of the vitamin C they contain is of interest in view of the claim by MacLean *et al.* (1939) that in young scorbutic guinea pigs the differentiaton of mesenchymal cells to osteoblasts is impaired in scurvy.

It is of interest that in most developing cartilage groups of strongly vitamin C—positive cartilage cells occur, particularly in the regions of active cell division (Fig. 8). Prior to cell division the vitamin C was

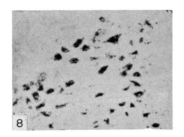

FIG. 8. Group of cartilage cells in 12-day chick embryo stained to demonstrate vitamin C. They show a strong positive reaction (see Barnett and Bourne, 1942).

found to be collected around the nucleus, which was consequently obscured; when the spindle elongated it, too, was surrounded by granules containing the vitamin. In what appeared to be the telophase the reaction was confined to the regions of the two daughter nuclei. It is of interest that other dividing cells in the chick embryo do not seem to contain this high concentration of vitamin C. Cartilage cells seem to be unique in accumulating the vitamin before division: As a rule in animal cells the presence of vitamin C is not a correlate of cellular proliferation (Barnett and Bourne, 1942).

B. SCURVY AND BONE REPAIR—HISTORICAL

The association of scurvy with the failure of injured bone to undergo repair has been well known for some two-hundred years. It is however, a little difficult to accept, in the account by Richard Walter (1748) of Lord Anson's voyage around the world, the claim that the callus in the leg of an old soldier which had been broken at the battle of the Boyne 50 years before, softened and refractured.

Mead, in 1762, quoted the case of a sailor who had suffered from a fractured clavicle which had apparently healed normally and which broke again 4 months later when the sailor was suffering from scurvy. Six months after this when the sailor had been on a diet of green vegetables for some time the fracture reunited.

Marrigues (1783), J. Bell (1788), Callisen (1798), and Budd (1840) all found softening of the callus of old fractures of bones in scurvy, sometimes with a separation of the ends of the bones. Hammick (1830) reported a number of cases of spontaneous refracture of bones and pointed out that it was impossible to secure the uniting of a fracture as long as the patient had scurvy. Dr. Lonton (quoted in the *Medical and Surgical History of the British Army which served in Turkey and the Crimea*, 1858) described the case of a grenadier aged 23 who broke his humerus while carrying a log across some frozen snow. After he had been put in hospital, old ulcers on his leg opened up and his gums became spongy. The callus which formed at the site of the fracture in the humerus was unusually small (suggesting a reduced inflammatory reaction to injury). Only when this man was placed on a nonscorbuto-genic diet did his fracture unite and his ulcers heal.

Moore (1859) has recorded two cases of fractures of the forearm in which healing was prevented because the patients also had scurvy. Moore stated that this disease has a "powerful effect in retarding the consolidation of fractures."

Even during the First World War, Lobmayer (1918) claimed that Turkish soldiers suffered severely from scurvy and that in those who developed the disease both skin and flesh wounds and fractures healed poorly. In many cases the fractures showed not the slightest sign of formation of a callus even after several months. In confirmation of the fact that it was lack of the antiscorbutic substance which was responsible for this failure of fractures to unite, he quoted two cases who suffered from pseudoarthrosis of the humerus and who recovered rapidly and completely as soon as they were put on a diet which was rich in antiscor-butic material.

Since these original clinical observations, various authors have called attention to their importance in the treatment of fractures (notably Bier, 1923, 1925; Kappis, 1927).

Experimental work with animals has supported these clinical observa-tions. It might be of interest at this point to mention various refracture experiments which have been carried out in order to test the old and oft-repeated clinical observations that an old fracture would soften and break again when a person developed scurvy. The first of these experi-ments was carried out by Israel and Frankel (1926) and Israel (1925, 1926). They claimed to confirm the clinical observations on human scurvy by their experiments on guinea pigs. Roegholt (1932) has also supported this fact. Hertz (1936), however, believed that their experi-ments were not critically carried out and that what really occurred was a new fracture resulting from the fragility of bones which ordinarily accompanies scurvy. Murray and Kodicek (1949a), when repeating Israel and Frankel's experiments, were unable to support them.

The earliest experimental observations on the importance of vitamin C in the healing of bone was that of Shinya (1922). He concluded that when bones from scorbutic guinea pigs are transplanted into normal animals they do not take. He attempted also to transplant sound bones into scorbutic animals, but the latter died of scurvy before results could be obtained.

Ferraris and Lewi (1923) found that in scorbutic animals there was not only a delay in the reformation of bone after a fracture but also there appeared to be inhibition of the normal process of the removal of cellular debris, e.g., the hematoma which formed as a result of the fracture persisted for a very long time.

Watanabe, in 1924, sawed furrows in the skulls of guinea pigs suffering from acute scurvy and as each animal died he examined the injury histologically. He found that the scorbutic animal showed practically no power of bone regeneration Wolbach and Howe (1925, 1926) investigated the effect of vitamin C deficiency on the regeneration of bones in small saw cuts made in the femora of guinea pigs. In the scorbutic animals there was complete lack of formation of osteoid trabeculae, and although there was some fibrous organization of the clot resulting from the injury there was no penetration into it of capillaries and blood vessels.

Schilozew (1928) repeated the work of many other authors, including that of Watanabe and of Israel and Frankel. His findings were in agreement with theirs. He also showed that a diet containing adequate vitamin C resulted in the formation of massive well-ossified calluses and found that if he added plenty of fresh vegetables to the diets of patients suffering from fractures the healing was accelerated. Similar results, derived from wounds made in the heads of scorbutic animals were obtained by Jeney and Korpàssy (1934).

Hanke (1935, 1936) found that a vitamin C–free diet retarded fracture healing not only in guinea pigs but also in rabbits, which are thought not to require this vitamin in their diet. Lauber (1936) and Taubor *et al.* (1937) stated that once the normal requirements of a rabbit were satisfied extra vitamin C had no further effect on the rate of regeneration of injured bone. It is difficult to appreciate that a rabbit has a normal dietary requirement for vitamin C if it synthesizes the vitamin. Giangrasso (1939a,b) and Giangrasso and Gangitano (1939) were also able to secure more rapid regeneration of fractured bones in rabbits by giving vitamin C. These facts might possibly be explained by assuming that the healing of a fractured bone calls for more vitamin C than the animal is able to manufacture for itself. It has been shown (Bourne, 1942b) that in a relatively small injury of the bone in rats, which also synthesize vitamin C (e.g., a 1-mm hole bored in the femur) the administration of vitamin C has no effect on the healing process. It should be noted, however, that when calcium ascorbate was injected subcutaneously into rats the amount of bone healing was statistically increased over that of animals injected with calcium gluconate. However, this may be associated with the availability of the calcium in calcium ascorbate rather than with the effect of the ascorbate fraction (see later).

These experiments were also repeated with rabbits in which the calcium ascorbate was injected intravenously in the marginal ear vein. A similar increased rate of bone healing was observed.

One of the most detailed of the earlier investigations of the effect of vitamin C in bone healing was that of Hertz (1936). He studied the formation of callus in a fractured fibula of a guinea pig, choosing this bone because the tibia acted as a splint. He found delayed absorption of the fracture hematoma, deficient production of osteoid trabeculae, and increased necrosis of the broken ends.

Lexer (1939a,b) also found a failure of fracture healing in scorbutic guinea pigs. He studied the process in a fractured femur by means of X-rays. The failure to heal in scorbutic animals was ascribed by Lexer to collapse of blood vessels and failure of proper blood supply to develop around the fracture. Subsequent histological examination showed that, according to the degree of vitamin C deficiency (starting on the day of the fracture), there was a regression of the callus and excess formation of connective tissue. In animals on a normal diet, or with extra vitamin C, there was a rich blood supply at the fracture site and a good callus formation. The majority of the previous papers had stressed deficient fiber or osteoid production in scorbutic animals, Lexer is the only one to lay special stress on the deficiency of blood supply in causing failure of healing of the tissues.

In the experimental work just recorded the results were obtained by depriving animals of foods containing vitamin C and claiming that the results obtained were owing to deficiency of this vitamin. Supplements of vitamin C were administered as natural foods and, in fact, Mazoué, writing even as late as 1939, used lemon juice as his source of vitamin C. The present author (1942b) used graded doses of synthetic crystalline vitamin C. Wolbach (1953) (see Figs. 9A–F, pp. 256 and 257) has described and figured the changes taking place in regenerating connective tissue, in cartilage, and in bone in scorbutic guinea pigs.

C. Quantitative Estimation of Bone Repair in Scurvy

A quantitative estimate of the rate of bone healing has been devised (Bourne, 1942a and b) for measuring the amount of repair taking place in a period of 1 week in a 1-mm hole bored in the femur. Transverse sections were made through the femur in the region of the hole. The outline of the femur and the trabeculae in the section passing through the center of the hole were projected onto paper and drawn. Then the area representing the hole was cut out and weighed as were the trabeculae. Division of the second by the first figure gave an index of density of bone formation, and if the final figure was multiplied by 100, whole numbers were obtained. The result was described as a trabecular index. This technique was applied to the femurs of guinea pigs placed on a scorbutic diet supplemented by 0, 0.25, 0.5, 1.0, or 4.0 mg of vitamin

Vitamin C (mg)	Trabecular index ($\times$ 100)
0.00	7.73 ± 2.25
0.25	6.70 ± 2.30
0.50	9.74 ± 2.48
1.00	19.41 ± 3.53
2.00	23.73 ± 6.75
4.00	18.09 ± 4.48

C daily. The results obtained are given in the accompanying tabulation. It is obvious that the critical level for vitamin C in healing of bone injury lies somewhere between 0.5 and 1.0 mg [see Fig. 10(A–E) p. 258].

In 1936, Boyle *et al.* investigated the rate of dentine formation in the persistently growing incisor teeth of guinea pigs. By administering alizarin to the animals, which stains the dentin pink as it is formed, they were able to measure the amount of dentin formed in response to the administration of various amounts of vitamin C. Their results have been graphed and the curve compared with that obtained by the present author for bone regeneration. It can be seen that the two sets of results give virtually identical curves (Fig. 11 p. 259).

The effects of complete deficiency of vitamin C on bone injury obtained in this work were similar to those obtained by other workers (e.g., Wolbach and Howe, 1926; Hertz, 1936). Hertz pointed out that in a completely scorbutic animal following bone injury there was no periosteal hyperemia, that in general it is difficult for a scorbutic animal to produce an inflammatory reaction in response to injury, and that in the absence of such a reaction the normal process of healing could not be induced. The enlargement of the cambial layer of the periosteum is, of course, an essential stage in the reaction. Hertz, like Watanabe, noticed a delayed absorption of the hematoma at the fracture site in scorbutic animals. The same phenomenon has been observed by the present author (1942b). For example, in guinea pigs receiving no vitamin C and in those receiving only 0.25 mg of the vitamin, by the end of the experimental period the whole of the connective tissue supporting the muscles associated with the femur was permeated with blood which had not been absorbed even as long as 7 days after the injury. It appeared that this blood had not clotted very readily and had continued

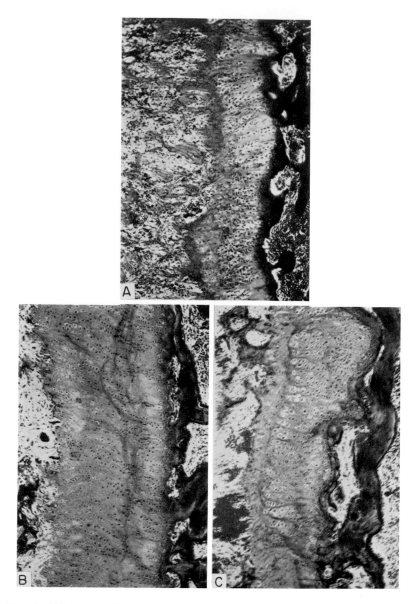

Fig. 9. (A) Proximal epiphyseal cartilage of tibia. Scorbutic guinea pig showing failure of matrix formation. Mallory's connective-tissue stain. (B) Repair after 72 hours following ascorbic acid administration. Proximal epiphyseal cartilage tibia. (C) Repair after 96 hours, proximal epiphyseal cartilage, tibia, guinea pig. To show approximately normal cartilage cells and matrix.

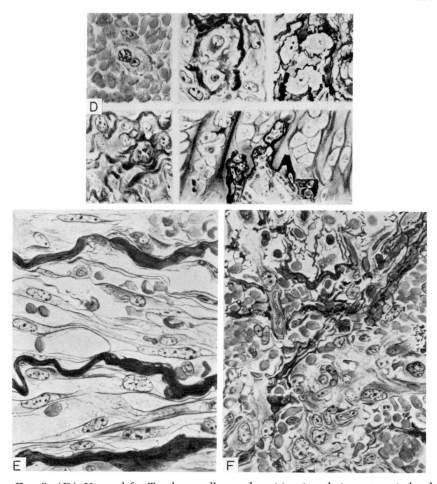

FIG. 9. (D) Upper left. To show collagen deposition in relation to an isolated cell deep within a ·blood clot. Repair after 72 hours following excision of muscle. Middle upper. Same preparation to show collagen deposition of cells which have penetrated fibrin strands. Repair after 72 hours. Upper right. A corresponding field, reticulum stain, repair of a blood clot after 72 hours. Lower left. Repair of a blood clot after 96 hours. To show collagen deposition in a group of fibroblasts which have not yet assumed their normal morphology. Lower right. Resumption of deposition of matrix in endochondral bone formation. Reticulum stain. Recovery period of 40 hours. (E) Fibroblasts in relation to fibrin strands in organization of a blood clot in absolute scorbutus. Note prominence of fibroglia fibrils and cytoplasmic vacuoles in fibroblasts. No stainable collagen or argyrophile fibrils present. Guinea pig operated on the twenty-third day of deficient diet, killed on the thirty-third day. (F) To illustrate collagen formed in organization deep within a blood clot, following 42 hours of ascorbic acid therapy. Note the homogeneous appearance of the collagen. (From Wolbach, 1953, by permission of the British Journal of Nutrition and Proceedings of the Nutrition Society.)

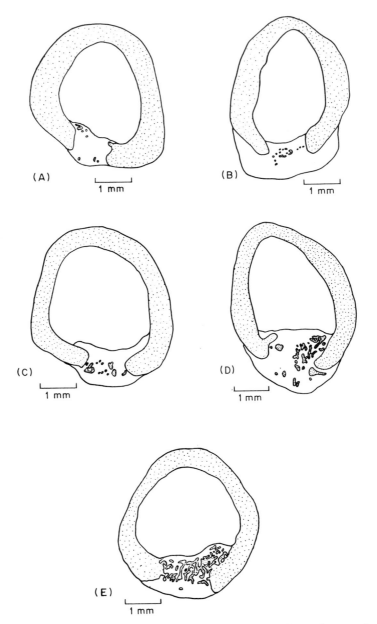

FIG. 10. Projection drawings of sections through healing holes of femurs of guinea pigs on graded doses of vitamin C. One week after injury. The drawings show the development of bony trabeculae in the area of injury to be greater as the dose of vitamin C increases. (A) No vitamin C, (B) 0.25 mg vitamin C daily, (C) 0.5 mg vitamin C daily, (D) 1.0 mg vitamin C daily, and (E) 2.0 mg vitamin C daily (see Bourne, 1942b).

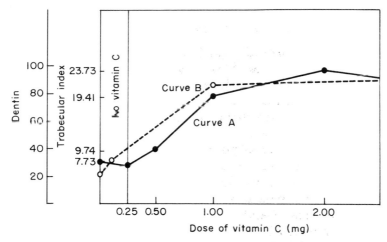

FIG. 11. Curves showing rate of formation of dentin compared with rate of formation of bony repair tissue in healing holes in femurs of guinea pigs on graded doses of vitamin C. Curve A shows rate of formation of trabeculae. Curve B shows rate of formation of dentin. The two curves are seen to be similar.

to ooze from the hole for some time after the operation. Finally, it had extended through practically the whole of the soft tissues of the upper part of the leg. The connective tissue (as has been found by other workers) was edematous and had a soft jellylike appearance. Animals receiving 0.5 mg of vitamin C showed a small hematoma at the site of injury, but in animals receiving 1, 2, or 4 mg it had disappeared by the time the animals were killed.

There is no agreement (as already shown) that extra vitamin C given to animals which normally synthesize their own supplies of this vitamin accelerates healing processes in bone. Halasz and Marx (1932) found that by administering amounts of orange juice much greater than that needed to prevent guinea pigs from getting scurvy they obtained no acceleration of the normal time of fracture healing. None of the authors working in this field subjected their results to statistical analysis or indeed used methods which lent themselves to such an analysis, although Hanke (1935), who used rabbits, published some rather convincing X-ray photographs. The present author, using rats and the technique for estimating bone regeneration already described and subjecting the results to statistical analysis, was unable to find any significant difference between controls and vitamin C–treated animals.

The weight of evidence suggests there is an optimum level of vitamin C intake for bone regeneration and there is no detectable advantage in administering more than this amount.

D. Vitamin C and the Phosphatase Reaction

Although techniques are, and have been for some time, available for demonstrating phosphatase in decalcified sections of bone (see this volume, Chapter 2), the present author preferred to study the effect of vitamin C on the phosphatase reaction in healing bone injury by undecalcified sections of 1 mm drill holes in the skull and of costochondral junctions.

In such preparations it was found (Bourne, 1948) that one of the effects of injury to the bone is to stimulate the absorption or synthesis of phosphatase by the periosteal cells. Also, 24 hours after injury a large number of phosphatase-positive cells were found to be present in the blood clot (a similar result was found by Danielli *et al.*, 1946, in skin wounds). The phosphatase in such cells appeared to be present mainly in the nucleus and the cells appeared to be mainly polymorph leukocytes. Further experiments using trypan blue showed that there was simultaneously a large number of macrophages in the injured area, but they showed no signs of phosphatase activity. After 3 days the numbers of both these types of cell were greatly reduced but phosphatase-positive fibroblasts and fibers were present. Later, these cells and fibers lost their phosphatase and a second cycle of phosphatase production developed with the appearance of calcified trabeculae (see this volume, Chapter 2).

In the injured areas in the scorbutic animals there were fewer of any kind of cell. However, such cells as were present, mainly fibroblasts, appeared to contain as much phosphatase (histochemically) as those present in the normal animal. Although the deficiency delayed the migration of these cells into the injured area it did not completely inhibit them, and by 4 days there were an many present (and with a phosphatase reaction apparently equal to normal) as could be found in 24 hours in the normal animal. However, in the scorbutic animal no fibers could be seen. The vitamin C deficiency therefore delays cell migration to the injury area (polymorphs, macrophages, and fibroblasts), does not affect profoundly the synthesis of phosphatase by the fibroblasts, but tends to prevent completely (if it is severe enough) the formation of phosphatase-impregnated fibers.

Experiments in which Gomori phosphatase preparations were first made on whole femurs containing a healing hole, and which were subsequently decalcified and sectioned, showed a reduced amount of phosphatase-positive trabeculae compared with the normal control (Figs. 12 and 13). Also, there was less phosphatase activity in the periosteum of the scorbutic femur (Bourne, 1943); see also Figs. 14 and 15.

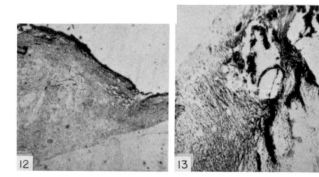

Fig. 12. Phosphatase preparation of repair tissue in hole bored in femur of scorbutic guinea pig. One week after operation. Virtually no phosphatase is present in this area with the exception of a line of activity on the surface of the repair tissue (see Bourne, 1942a).

Fig. 13. Phosphatase preparation repair tissue in hole bored in femur of normal guinea pig. One week after operation. Note phosphatase-positive fibers and a number of phosphatase-positive trabeculae (see Bourne, 1942a).

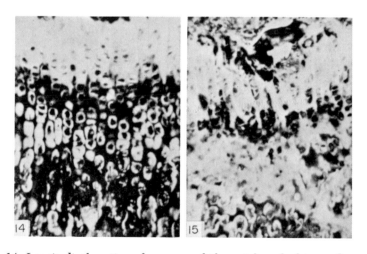

Fig. 14. Longitudinal section of an area of the epiphyseal plate at the proximal end of the tibia of a control guinea pig. Phosphatase is present in the columnar cells and hypertrophic cells. Less activity occurs in the zone of calcification. The dark gray appearance of the trabeculae in the metaphysis results from bone salts which were not completely removed in this section.

Fig. 15. Scorbutic animal. Area comparable to that of 5. Some indication of columnar arrangement of cells is present. The cells contain the enzyme but the amount is less than in the controls. (Figures 14 and 15 and legends are reproduced by permission of Drs. Zorzoli and E. M. Nadel, and the Journal of Histochemistry and Cytochemistry.)

If alizarin is added to Gomori's substrate mixture for demonstrating alkaline phosphatase it forms a "lake" with calcium ions and when these are deposited owing to the activity of phosphatase they produce a pink-stained calcium phosphate. If a formalin-fixed whole guinea pig femur and an alcohol-fixed one are incubated in such a mixture the alizarin stains the recently formed bone salt on the surface of the bones a light pink but in the alcohol-fixed bone (in which the phosphatase is still active) there is intense red staining in regions of greatest phosphatase activity. Femurs from scorbutic guinea pigs showed greatly reduced acitivity, indicating a decrease in phosphatase activity in this condition (Bourne, 1942b).

Sections of costochondral junctions also showed a histochemical reduction of phosphatase activity in scorbutic guinea pigs (Figs. 16 and 17). The activity was reduced in periosteum, in both fibrous and cellular parts, in the osteoblasts at the junction and in the osteocytes in the trabeculae. There was also a reduction in phosphatase activity in the endosteum. At the junction in normal animals there was a line of intense phosphatase activity which was continuous at the periphery with the periosteum. In this line the enzyme appeared both extra- and intracellular. The line was greatly reduced in width in scorbutic animals (Bourne, 1943). It is of interest that Gould and Schwachman (1942) and Zorzoli and Nadel (1950) have shown reduction of bone phosphatase in scurvy.

Van Wersch (1954) has recorded the results of an extensive investigation into chemical, histochemical, and X-ray changes in experimental scurvy in guinea pigs. After 3–4 weeks on a scorbutic diet he found

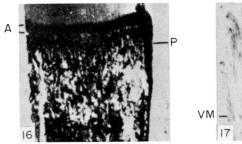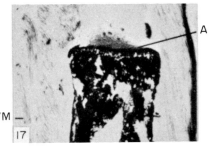

Fig. 16. Phosphatase preparation of undecalcified section of costochondral junction of normal guinea pig. Moderately dark reaction given by cartilage is artifact. Note thick line of phosphatase activity at A which is continuous on right with phosphatase-positive periosteum (P). (Note: periosteum has been cut away on the left side of the shaft.) See Bourne (1943).

Fig. 17. Phosphatase preparation of undecalcified section of costochondral junction of scorbutic guinea pig. Note great reduction of line of phosphatase (A) at junction (see Bourne, 1943).

histochemically a decrease of phosphatase activity in bones, particularly in osteoblasts and in soft tissues such as the kidney. He confirmed this biochemically by showing that the alkaline phosphatase activity of bone and kidney was reduced to about one-fifth of the normal. However, in hemopoietic islands in the bone marrow he found that there was an accumulation of phosphatase-positive cells. In addition, he found histochemically by the use of the periodic acid Schiff method and by chemical analysis that there was an accumulation of glycogen in scorbutic bones; in the histochemical preparations it was noted that there was considerable accumulation of glycogen in the osteocytes and that there was also an increase in extracellular glycogen. Also, in the marrow there was an accumulation of granulocytes loaded with glycogen.

Although van Wesch found a general increase in PAS-positive substances, in addition to glycogen he recorded a decrease in toluidine blue metachromasia, suggesting a loss of chondroitin or mucoitin sulfate.

E. Vitamin C and Calcification

Vitamin C obviously plays an important part in the production of an inflammatory reaction to injury of bone—in the organization of the blood clot resulting therefrom and in the formation of the ground substance of trabeculae. It remains to be considered whether it plays any part in the process of calcification, particularly in view of its apparent association with phosphatase production, either directly or through its association with phosphatase activity. Calcium has been found to be deposited in various tissues in scurvy, but it is deposited in an amorphous form. This is probably a result of the absence of an adequate fibrous matrix. Fish and Harris (1934) have pointed out that in scurvy calcium salts may be deposited in teeth but that there was no matrix available for their reception. It is of interest, however, that as long ago as 1934 Schmidt suggested that when collagen fibers are first formed they adsorb precipitated inorganic salts, and he has pointed out that such fibers possess the ability to orientate particles precipitated in their presence.

The calcium balance appears to be disturbed in scurvy (see Hess's summary of the work of Baumann and Howard, 1917). This has been shown also for scurvy in adult human beings (Lust and Klocman, 1912; Moll, 1919), infantile scurvy (Moll, 1919), and monkey scurvy (Howard and Ingvaldsen, 1917). Lust and Klocman found a positive calcium balance in the scurvy stage and a negative balance in the healing stage. Bahrt and Edelstein (1913) found a diminished calcium content of the bones of a scorbutic infant, but Kapp and Schetty (1937) found the mineral content of bones remained normal in scurvy. Höjer (1923–1924) stated that his histological observations gave no reason to suppose that the calcium metabolism is primarily disarranged in scurvy. He stated that dying tissue generally has a greater affinity for calcium and that this "explains" the calcification of late scurvy.

Humphreys and Zilva (1931) found that calcium and phosphorus retention by guinea pigs was lowered in scurvy but only in the last stages when the whole metabolism was affected. Matricardi (1938) found that blood phosphate fell in scurvy, and Lucké and Wolf (1938) claimed that extra vitamin C administered to an animal led to a greater retention of calcium and phosphorus. If one adrenal of an animal was removed there was an upset of the calcium-phosphorus balance which was restored by the administration of vitamin C (Lucké and Heckman, 1938).

Lanford (1939) claimed that orange juice added to the diet of rats caused increased calcium retention. Against this observation Henry and Kon (1939) found that the addition of 2 mg daily of vitamin C to rats had no influence on the retention of calcium. Ruskin (1938) and Ruskin and Jonnard (1938a,b) held that there was an intimate association between vitamin C and calcium, believing that calcium was absorbed from the intestine as calcium ascorbate. This compound they found to be adsorbed onto the blood proteins much more strongly than other salts of calcium.

If, in fact, calcium is absorbed from the intestine as ascorbate and if this ascorbate is more efficiently adsorbed onto the blood proteins than other salts of calcium, one might expect that by artificially increasing the amount of calcium ascorbate available it might be possible to secure a higher conentration of ionic calcium in the blood [since McLean and Hastings (1934, 1935) have shown that $Ca^{2+} + protein^-/Ca$ proteinate $= K$]. It is possible that such a higher ionic calcium (see Logan, 1940) might stimulate the formation of bone in an injured area.

The present author (Bourne, 1942a) found that, in fact, subcutaneous injection of calcium ascorbate produced statistically more bone in drill holes in the femora of rats than animals receiving normal saline, or equivalent amounts of vitamin C, or equivalent amounts of calcium as calcium glucono-galacto-gluconate, or equivalent amounts of vitamin C and calcium glucono-galacto-gluconate injected together. In fact, the last of these appeared to depress the rate of bone formation. It was also shown that calcium ascorbate did not affect the earlier healing processes at 3 and 4 days, and an effect could only be demonstrated when active formation of osteoid trabeculae was taking place. Further investigation was carried out on rabbits by injecting the calcium ascorbate into the marginal veins of the ears. Increased bone formation over the calcium glucono-galacto-gluconate–injected animals was obtained (Fig. 18, A and B). Further confirmation was also obtained from experiments on guinea pigs, and in these animals the calcium ascorbate was found to be superior also to calcium lactate in stimulating bone regeneration.

Possibly, if more bone is formed by injecting calcium as the ascorbate, this substance may cause an increase in the calcium ion concentration in the serum, a result which is difficult to achieve by feeding. According to Shohl (1939), calcium is present in serum in a concentration of only 10.0–10.5 mg/100 ml of serum and that unless an animal has been on a calcium-deficient diet the ingestion of calcium salts produces only a minute rise in serum calcium. This rise is so small that for some time it was thought not to be significant. Whether calcium ascorbate does cause a rise in ionic calcium in the blood can, of course, only be determined for certain by direct estimation. On the other hand, G. H. Bell *et al.* (1941) stated that a daily consumption by growing rats of dietary calcium up to 0.36 gm of calcium per 100 gm dry weight of food, increased the weight, the calcium content, the bending and twisting strength, and the thickness of the cortices of their femora.

The promotion of bone formation by calcium ascorbate even if one

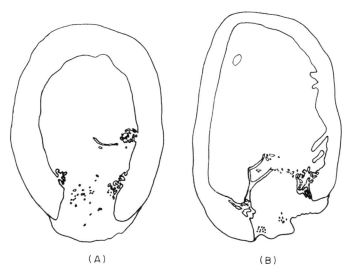

(A)   (B)

Fɪɢ. 18. (A) Projection drawing of section through the femur of a rabbit 1 week after drilling a hole and daily injection of calcium glucono-galacto-gluconate. Formation of trabeculae just beginning. (B) Projection drawing of section through the femur of a rabbit 1 week after drilling a hole and daily injections of calcium ascorbate. Note great increase in formation of bony trabeculae.

assumes that it works by increasing the ionic calcium is not easy to explain. The calcium cannot be deposited unless there is an organic matrix to receive it and the results described imply, therefore, that calcium ascorbate, either by increasing the ionic calcium or by some other means, stimulates the more rapid formation of bone matrix even in animals saturated with vitamin C.

If there is failure of matrix formation, calcification is not likely to take place except for the type of calcification represented by the amorphous deposits of calcium which sometimes occur in acute scurvy. In the long bones of animals bone salt is constantly being deposited on the outside and withdrawn from the inside. The brittleness and thinning of the cortex of long bones in scurvy seems likely to result from the process of resorption of bone continued during scurvy while the process of deposition of bone on the outside ceases. This would explain why Kapp and Schetty (1937) found the mineral content of the bones of scorbutic guinea pigs to be normal. That bone salt deposition does cease in scurvy is shown by the work of Salter and Aub (1931); see also Figs. 19 and 20. These authors found that in normal animals injections of sodium alizarin sulfate stained the long bones of young guinea pigs a bright pink. In scorbutic animals the bones were unstained. In the normal animals the trabeculae in the cancellous tissue of the ends of the long bones were also stained (this indicates that bone salt is being deposited in this region). Externally, the heads of the bones near the epiphysis stained more intensely than the shaft. None of these parts stained in the scorbutic animal.

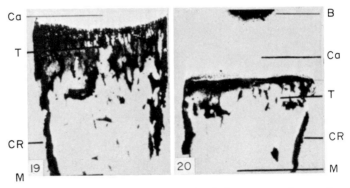

Fig. 19. Von Kossa preparation of costochondral junction of normal guinea pig to show number of trabeculae. Ca, cartilage; T, trabeculae; CR, cortex of bone; M, marrow. See Bourne (1943).

Fig. 20. Von Kossa preparation of costochondral junction of ascorbic guinea pig to show greatly reduced number of trabeculae. B, deposit of cartilaginous bone salt in portion of rib. See Bourne (1943).

If vitamin C promotes the absorption of calcium from gut, then presumably the greater the amount of vitamin C given by mouth the greater the amount of calcium absorbed and available for deposition on bone. On the other hand, if no vitamin C is given by mouth and the animal receives all its vitamin C by injection, minimal absorption of calcium should occur and less calcification of bones should take place—assuming, of course, that more calcium absorbed will result in more calcification. However, we cannot neglect the possibility that in a state of emergency calcium will be taken from the trabeculae and laid down on the surface of the bones. If, however, we use alizarin to stain freshly deposited bone salt the trabeculae would be unstained should this occur and the superficial part of the shaft stained. But another source of calcium is the inner surface of the shaft, and alizarin experiments would not show whether or not calcium was being removed from this region.

In experiments described by the present author (Bourne, 1943) vitamin C was administered by mouth or by injection to guinea pigs, and the animals were also injected with alizarin; the staining of the bones obtained was compared with another group of animals injected with equivalent amounts of calcium ascorbate. The results obtained were not entirely unequivocal but indicated that there might be more bone laid down in animals receiving vitamin C by mouth or injected as ascorbate than in animals receiving vitamin C by injection.

Despite the work of Salter and Aub (1931) already mentioned, Boyle (1938) and Boyle *et al.* (1940) stated that the process of calcification continues in the incisor teeth of guinea pigs even when they have been for some time on a scorbutic diet; but Friberg and Ringertz (1954) found a lowered uptake of radiophosphorus in bone in scurvy. Wolbach and Bessey (1942) stated that it was a generally accepted fact that vitamin C played no part in the process of calcification. The present author (Bourne, 1943) using $1:2:5:8:$tetrahydroxyanthraquinone (alizarin Bordeaux) and alizarin itself (dihydroxyanthroquinone) was able to stain recently formed bone *in vivo* and showed that the degree of staining (and therefore the amount of calcification) varied directly with the amount of vitamin C in the diet. This suggests that the vitamin does play a part in the process of calcification. However, calcification in normal animals does not take place in the absence of the appropriate matrix to receive the mineral salts; thus, this result may still only mean that vitamin C deficiency affected the matrix formation.

Further investigations were made on the effect of vitamin C on the calcification of bone regeneating in a 1-mm hole in the guinea pig femur. Alizarin staining again was greatest in the repair tissue in the holes in the animals receiving the largest amount of vitamin C (5 mg). Further experiments showed that this difference did not result from progressive differences in calcification but from variation in the amount of osteoid trabeculae present. In other words, if the amount of vitamin C given to the animals permitted any trabeculae to form at all then these trabeculae were as heavily calcified, as far as can be shown, by the technique used, as those formed in an animal receiving optimum amounts of the vitamin.

The result to be deduced from this work is therefore that the significance of vitamin C in bone formation and bone healing lies in its ability to promote the growth of the matrix.

It is of interest that vitamin P and sodium citrate had no effect in promoting bone healing or in increasing the alizarin staining of normal growing bones. On the other hand, an interesting result was obtained by the present author (1949) by administering certain sugars and other substances to guinea pigs on a scorbutic diet.

The substances used were D-arabinose, D-glucose, D-mannose, sorbitol, sorbose, ketogulonic acid, L-rhamnose, rhamnolactone, sodium D-isoascorbate, and galactouronic acid. Animals receiving rhamnose and rhamnolactone gave almost as intense as *in vivo* stain in the skeleton with alizarin as those receiving ascorbic acid. The animals receiving the other substances showed little or no staining. This work suggests that rhamnose and rhamnolactone can permit matrix formation in the absence of vitamin C. Collagen and presumably ossein appear to be made of long chain protein molecules with carbohydrate and probably vitamin C linkages. If the latter is correct then the deficiency of collagen in scurvy results, at least in part, from the absence of sufficient vitamin C to maintain these linkages. It would appear that rhamnose and rhamnolactone might be able to replace vitamin C in this respect. However, the fact that McManus and Saunders (1950) found that collagen is attacked by a polygalacturonidase suggests that galacturonic acid may be involved in these intrafibrillar linkages in the collagen fiber, in which case it is surprising that this acid did not have the same effect as rhamnose. Although the possibility exists that the carbohydrate in ossein may be different from that of collagen, galactose and galactosamine have been separated from ossein.

F. Histological Changes in Scorbutic Bones and Teeth

In intact bones characteristic changes develop in scurvy. In human scurvy the epiphyses in young persons were often found to be separated from the shafts of the bones (Aschoff and Koch, 1919; Hess, 1920) and beading of the ribs may occur both in scorbutic infants and monkeys (Hart and Lessing, 1913).

Histologically, in scorbutic human bones one of the most obvious signs was subperiosteal hemorrhage. Marked thinning of the cortex of the bone (which was also brittle) was also present and the marrow had become yellowish and developed a gelatinous consistency (Gerüst-mark). It is of interest that in experimental animal scurvy the Gerüstmark does not form in an artificially immobilized limb (Follis, 1951). At the junction of bone and cartilage in the heads of bones or at costochondral junctions the line becomes wavy instead of straight. At the junction a Trümmerfeld zone develops in which irregular and unorientated trabeculae are scattered, and in which irregularly shaped and scattered cells are also present. Cell and bone detritus is also present. According to Hess, "the picture is that of weakened bone having been crushed by the pressure of the more compact cartilage." The cells which are present are mainly spindle or stellate connective tissue cells with relatively few osteoblasts. Those which are present in association with the reduced trabeculae become spindle-shaped and shriveled. It is of interest that there is no increase of osteoclasts associated with those trabeculae or with the walls of the medullary cavity so that the rarefaction observed does not obviously result from increased osteoclastic activity Hess, in fact, suggested that the thinning of the trabeculae results from the combination of normal bone resorption and the failure of normal bone regeneration. Aschoff and Koch showed that the cells of the framework "marrow" (Gerüstmark) are normally able to make bone trabeculae but that in scurvy there is a lack of the material required to build the osteoid; however, since the cells presumably make this material it is difficult to follow their reasoning.

Follis (1948), describing bone changes in scurvy, based his report on a study of the experimentally induced disease in guinea pigs and on a hundred cases of human scurvy. As the scorbutic state developed, he found that the cartilage cells of the epiphyseal plate continued to multiply and orientate themselves and calcium salts continued to be deposited between the rows; however, beyond that point trouble occurred: The osteoblasts failed to lay down osteoid, and the calcified matrix was not absorbed. The result was an accumulation of calcified matrix under the cartilaginous plate of the epiphysis which continued to grow rapidly. Park described this arrangement as a "scorbutic lattice." Breaking the spindles of bone in the matrix produced the "crushing" effect described by Hess. Finally, constant fracturing of the spicules resulted in the building up of an area completely lacking in orientation which is the Trümmerfeld zone of the earlier authors.

Follis (1948), however, showed that if he immobilized one leg by placing it in a plaster cast thus protecting it from normal stresses and strains, it did not exhibit the characteristic changes of scurvy while the opposite leg did. The absence of fractures, hemorrhage, pink-staining material, and fibroblastic proliferation from such a femur, i.e., the absence of a Trümmerfeld zone, indicated that these were all secondary to the stresses and strains and that the fundamental lesion caused by the deficiency was simply an unabsorbed calcified lattice and absence of osteoid formation.

Although a good deal of experimental work has been carried out on the effects of acute deficiency of vitamin C on experimental animals, only Murray and Kodicek (1949a,b,c) appear to have studied the effects of prolonged partial deficiencies. In guinea pigs subjected to such treatment they found that stiffness of the knee joint was a characteristic early symptom and that this resulted from degeneration and edematous changes in muscles and the formation of hyperplastic connective tissue at and around the joint. Later, the shafts of some of the long bones showed a considerable amount of spongy subperiosteal bone. Associated with this was a typical osteoporosis. It was of interest that this osteoporosis was restricted to the old bone of the shaft; the new bone which formed simultaneously showed no signs of it. Höjer had also shown in 1924 (1923–1924) that in scurvy it was possible to obtain osteoporosis of the jaw bone simultaneously with the production of spongy bone on the surface. The diaphyseal thickenings of scurvy had also been demonstrated by Mouriquand and his colleagues by radiographical means (1937, 1940a,b; Mouriquand and Dauvergne, 1938).

Kodicek (1965) found rheumatoid-like joint lesions in guinea pigs with chronic vitamin C deficiency. He found swelling of the knee joints which eventually became ankylosed. Such changes in acute scurvy often follow hemorrhages, but this was not the case in the lesions Kodicek described; they were directly comparable with those of human rheumatoid arthritis. The synovial membrane was hyperplastic, the joint was packed with hyperplastic connective tissue, and the joint capsule was thickened. All these changes combined to immobilize the joint. Fibrin was deposited on the joint surfaces and synovial membranes. Foci of lymphatic cells were present in the synovial villi. Eventually, the articular surfaces were destroyed. The adrenals of these deficient animals were greatly enlarged ansd showed damage in the zona fasciculata. These joint changes have been described by Peric-Golia *et al.* (1960) as being secondary in nature and resulting from the primary damage to the adrenals produced by the vitamin C deficiency.

Murray and Kodicek (1949 a, b, and c) stated that a process of absorption of the old subperiosteal bone preceded the production of new subperiosteal bone. In the space so formed between the periosteum and the shaft of the bone a diffuse mesenchyme-like tissue developed and in this appeared a number of stellate osteoblasts which bore many resemblances to fibroblasts. These cells deposited a granular bone which subsequently became covered with a fibrillar bone. If the bone was fractured the amount of periosteal bone formed was greatly increased. The summary of the changes found by these authors in a fractured bone (fibula) in the chronically scorbutic guinea pigs is as follows. There was more absorption from the broken ends of the bones, no cartilage formed (unlike the normals), and the subperiosteal bone (a small amount of which forms in all fractured bones some distance back from the injury, "distant periosteal reaction") increased enormously and formed a great thickening which extended the whole length of the diaphysis. Eventually this newly formed subperiosteal bone moved toward the fracture and in some cases covered it. The callus formed inside, however, was never complete and remained of light trabecular construction.

As already mentioned there are characteristic changes in the teeth as well as in bone of guinea pigs on a scorbutic diet. The teeth which are particularly susceptible to such changes are the persistently growing incisors.

L. Jackson and Moore (1916) and Zilva and Wells (1919) were the first to show that when guinea pigs are placed on a scorbutic diet they suffer from characteristic changes in the incisor teeth. Howe (1920, 1921, 1923) was able to produce alveolar resorption, spongy gums, irregularities in the teeth, and even caries with a scorbutic diet. Histological studies of scorbutic teeth were made by Höjer and Westin (1925), Toverud (1923), and Key and Elphick (1931); and in 1934 Fish and Harris published a very detailed work on this subject. They found that in full scurvy the odontoblasts lost their fibrils and died. Even in subscurvy the odontoblasts degenerated before their normal time, casting off their fibrils in the process. The normal process of scar formation in the pulp was also interfered with. The ameloblasts were also affected, although rather later in the disease than the odontoblasts. In subscurvy some enamel continued to be formed by in full scurvy there was a complete failure of formation—the ameloblasts either disappeared altogether or became completely keratinized. Normal cementum was also found to be absent in scorbutic teeth, being replaced by an amorphous deposit of calcific scar tissue which enclosed occasional cementoblasts.

Harris and Fish concluded that deficiency of vitamin C in guinea pig diets affected the viability of all cells associated with the laying down of the three hard tissue components of teeth. This was associated with general degeneration of the connective tissue of the dental pulp and congestion of its vessels. Other changes present in the teeth were obviously secondary to the degeneration of the cells. Particularly was this so in the case of the dentin where any changes in this tissue naturally followed the degeneration of the odontoblastic fibrils. One of the results of this process was the deposition of calcific scar tissue, which had been described by a number of earlier workers as "pulp bone," inferring that the odontoblasts changed to osteoblasts and produced bone instead of dentin. There is no real evidence in the literature that such a meta-plasia of the odontoblasts occurs and the explanation is much more likely to be, as Fish and Harris asserted, that the so-called pulp bone is simply calcific scar tissue. Other workers on this problem include Wolbach and Howe (1926), Dalldorf and Zall (1930), Wolbach (1933), Boyle *et al.* (1936, 1940); Glasunow (1937), Boyle (1938), Ham and Elliott (1938), Dalldorf (1939), and McLean *et al.* (1939). All have established the essential nature of vitamin C for the development of incisor teeth in guinea pigs and in particular that it is necessary for the production of predentin, which can be regarded as the equivalent in the tooth of the osteoid of bone. Boyle *et al.* (1936) claimed that vitamin C was not essential for the calcification of teeth and Wolbach and Howe that the pulp became shrunken, completely detached from the dentin, and appeared to float in a fluid material. It seems that this latter appearance may have resulted from an artifact. Wolbach and Bessey (1942) claimed that the prompt appearance of bone matrix and of dentin when vitamin C was administered to a scorbutic animal sug-gested "that the failure of cells to produce an intercellular matrix in scorbutus is the result of the absence of an agent common to all support-ing tissues which is responsible for the setting, fibrillation, or jelling of a product which would otherwise remain liquid."

G. Conclusions

Follis (1951), in summing up the effect of vitamin C deficiency, said:
"It would seem best to designate scurvy as that part of the overall picture of ascorbic acid deficiency which is characterized by a failure of certain specialized cells, i.e., fibroblasts, osteoblasts and odontoblasts to promote the deposition of their respective fibrous proteins: collagen, osteoid and dentin."

That the effects of the disease primarily result from the failure of specific cells is also borne out by Follis' observations that osteocytes, osteoblasts, and the cells of the Gerüstmark showed a lowered oxidative activity (Nadi reaction for cytochrome oxidase). Administration of the vitamin brought about simultaneous return to normal of cytochrome oxidase activity and of fiber production. The Gerüstmark cells also showed very little PAS-positive material (see Figs. 3 and 4 for altered distribution of PAS-positive material in scorbutic trabeculae). When the scurvy was cured the spindle-shaped cells of this tissue changed into a plumper shape and their cytoplasm became metachromatic and gave a stronger PAS reaction. A return of basophilia in these cells and in osteoblasts and osteocytes was shown to result from ribonucleic acid, which in the scorbutic condition had been depressed.

We are faced with the established fact, enunciated by Wolbach some twenty years ago, that there is a failure of the production of intercellular materials in scurvy. Although a relationship has been shown between vitamin C and tyrosine metabolism, the most important effects of vitamin C deficiency seem to be the defect in chondroitin sulfate formation resulting, in part, from the failure of galactosamine synthesis, and the decrease in the formation of hydroxyproline, an essential constituent of collagen. In addition, we have the information that the respiratory activity of most cells in the body (Hill and Bourne, 1954; King, 1950), particularly those associated with the connective tissues (Follis, 1951), is depressed in scurvy, which might itself explain the decrease in synthetic activity of these cells. Although there appears to be loss of phosphatase activity in scorbutic bones, this seems to mainly result from decrease of phosphatase-impregnated matrix. Histochemically, the matrix-producing cells appear to give as intense a histochemical reaction for phosphatase as the normal, and any matrix that is produced seems to contain at least a near normal amount of phosphatase (however, see King's results). It appears to be the synthesis of both fibers and structureless matrix which are inhibited by lack of vitamin C, and the decreased incorporation of radioactive sulfur into chondroitin sulfate appears to be an indication of one type of breakdown in the synthetic mechanism. It is of interest that a decreased synthesis of chondroitin sulfate also occurs under the influence of cortisone, and in this case it seems unlikely to result from decreased respiratory activity of the cells since it has been shown (Malaty and Bourne, 1953) that coritsone appears to increase the respiratory activity of the cells of many organs. Further work on these lines, however, should ultimately reveal the complete secret of the role of vitamin C in the maintenance and repair of the connective tissues.

References

Aldrich, E. M., Carter, J. P., and Lehman, E. P. (1951). *Ann. Surg.* **133**, 783.

Antoniwicz, I., and Kodicek, E. (1964). *Med. Eur. Biochem. Ass.* p. 61 (Proc.).

Aschoff, L., and Koch, W. (1919). "Skorbut: Eine pathologische Studie." Fischer, Jena.

Bahrt, H., and Edelstein, F. (1913). *Z. Kinderheilk.* **9**, 415.

Baker, B. L., and Whittaker, W. L. (1950). *Endocrinology* **46**, 544.

Baldridge, G. D., Kligman, A. L., Lipnik, M. J., and Pillsbury, D. M. (1951). *AMA Arch. Pathol.* **51**, 593.

Banerjee, S. (1962). *Nat. Abstr. Rev.* **32**, 783.

Bangham, A. D. (1951). *Brit. J. Exp. Pathol.* **32**, 77.

Barnes, M. J., Constable, B. J., and Kodicek, E. (1969). *Biochem. J.* **113**, 387.

Barnes, M. J., Constable, B. J., and Kodicek, E. (1969). *Biochim. Biophys. Acta* **184**, 358.

Barnett, S. A., and Bourne, G. H. (1942). *Quart. J. Microsc. Sci.* **83**, 259.

Barrenscheen, H. K., and Valyi-Nagy, T. (1948). *Hoppe-Seyler's Z. Physiol. Chem.* **283**, 91.

Bartlett, M. K., Jones, C. M., and Ryan, A. E. (1942). *N. Engl. J. Med.* **226**, 469.

Bates, C. J., Levine, C. I., and Kodicek, E. (1969). *Biochem. J.* **113**, 783.

Baumann, L., and Howard, C. P. (1917). *Amer. J. Med. Sci.* **153**, 650.

Baxter, H., Schiller, C., and Whiteside, J. H. (1951). *Plast. Reconstr. Surg.* **7**, 85.

Bell, G. H., Cuthbertson, D. P., and Orr, J. (1941). *J. Physiol.* (*London*) **100**, 299.

Bell, J. (1788). "A System of Surgery," Vol. 6. Crowther, London.

Bensley, S. H. (1934). *Anat. Rec.* **60**, 93.

Bier, A. (1923). *Arch. Klin. Chir.* **127**, 1.

Bier, A. (1925). *Arch. Klin. Chir.* **138**, 107.

Bourne, G. H. (1942a). *Quart. J. Exp. Physiol.* **31**, 319.

Bourne, G. H. (1942b). *J. Physiol.* (*London*) **101**, 327.

Bourne, G. H. (1943). *J. Physiol.* (*London*) **102**, 319.

Bourne, G. H. (1944a). *Lancet* **1**, 688.

Bourne, G. H. (1944b). *Proc. Roy. Soc. Med.* **37**, 275.

Bourne, G. H. (1948). *J. Anat.* **82**, 208.

Bourne, G. H. (1949). *Brit. J. Nutr.* **3**, xi.

Bourne, G. H. (1952). *Int. Z. Vitaminforsch.* **24**, 318.

Bourne, G. H., ed. (1956). "The Biochemistry and Physiology of Bone," 1st ed. Academic Press, New York.

Bourne, G. H. (1960). Unpublished data.

Bourne, G. H., Parkes, M. W., and Wrigley, F. (1952). *Z. Rheumaforsch.* **11**, 17.

Boyle, P. E. (1938). *Amer. J. Pathol.* **14**, 843.

Boyle, P. E., Wolbach, S. B., and Bessey, O. A. (1936). *J. Dent. Res.* **15**, 331.

Boyle, P. E., Bessey, O. A., and Howe, R. R. (1940). *Arch. Pathol.* **30**, 90.

Bradfield, J. R. G., and Kodicek, E. (1951). *Biochem. J.* **49**, xvii.

Breslow, R., and Lukens, L. N. (1960). *J. Biol. Chem.* **235**, 292.

Budd, A. (1840). Quoted by Hertz (1936).

Buhler, D. R., and Mason, H. S. (1961). *Arch. Biochem. Biophys.* **92**, 424.

Bunting, H., and White, R. F. (1948). *Arch. Pathol.* **49**, 500.

Burns, J. J., Burch, H. B., and King, C. G. (1951). *J. Biol. Chem.* **191**, 501.

Callisen, H. (1798). Quoted by Hertz (1936).

Campbell, F. W., and Ferguson, I. D. (1950). *Brit. J. Ophthalmol.* 34, 329.

Campbell, F. W., Ferguson, I. D., and Garry, R. C. (1950). *Brit. J. Nutr.* 4, 32.

Carney, H. M. (1946). *Ann. Surg.* 123, 1111.

Castor, C. W., and Baker, B. L. (1950). *Endocrinology* 47, 234.

Chambers, R., and Cameron, G. (1943). *Amer. J. Physiol.* 139, 21.

Chvapil, M., and Huryck, J. (1959). *Int. Rev. Connect. Tissue Res.* 4, 67.

Clayton, B. E., and Prunty, F. T. G. (1951). *Brit. Med. J.* 2, 927.

Cmuchalova, B., and Chvapil, M. (1963). *Prokovni Lekar.* 15, 30.

Crandon, T. H., Lund, C. C., and Dill, D. B. (1940). *N. Engl. J. Med.* 223, 353.

Dalldorf, G. (1939). *J. Amer. Med. Ass.* 111, 1376.

Dalldorf, G., and Zall, C. (1930). *J. Exp. Med.* 52, 57.

Danielli, J. F., Fell, H. B., and Kodicek, E. (1946). *Brit. J. Exp. Pathol.* 26, 367.

Elster, S. K. (1950). *J. Biol. Chem.* 186, 105.

Elster, S. K., and Schack, J. A. (1950). *Amer. J. Physiol.* 161, 283.

Eve, W. (1888). *In* "Medical and Surgical History of the War of the Rebellion." U. S. Govt. Printing Office, Washington, D. C.

Ferraris, C., and Lewi, M. (1923). Quoted by Hertz (1936)

Findlay, G. M. (1921). *J. Pathol. Bacteriol.* 24, 446.

Fish, E. W., and Harris, L. J. (1934). *Phil. Trans. Roy. Soc. London, Ser. B* 223, 489.

Follis, R. H. (1948). "The Pathology of Nutritional Diseases." Blackwell, Oxford.

Follis, R. H. (1951). *Bull. Johns Hopkins Hosp.* 89, 9.

Friberg, U., and Ringertz, N. R. (1954). *Exp. Cell Res.* 6, 527.

Galloway, N. M., Garry, R. C., and Hitchin, A. D. (1948). *Brit. J. Nutr.* 2, 228.

Gersh, I., and Catchpole, H. R. (1949). *Amer. J. Anat.* 85, 457.

Giangrasso, G. (1939a). *Boll. Soc. Ital. Biol. Sper.* 14, 522.

Giangrasso, G. (1939b). *Boll. Soc. Ital. Biol. Sper.* 14, 525.

Giangrasso, G., and Gangitano, C. (1939). *Boll. Soc. Ital. Biol. Sper.* 14, 531.

Glasunow, M. (1937). *Virchows Arch. Pathol. Anat. Physiol.* 299, 120.

Göthlin, G. F., Frisell, E., and Rundquist, N. (1937). *Acta Med. Scand.* 92, 1.

Gore, I., Tanaka, Y., Fujinami, T., and Goodman, M. L. (1965). *J. Nutr.* 87, 311.

Gould, B. S. (1961). *Ann. N. Y. Acad. Sci.* 92, 168.

Gould, B. S., and Manner, O. (1962). *In* "Collagen," p. 311. Wiley (Interscience), New York.

Gould, B. S., and Schwachman, H. (1942). *Amer. J. Physiol.* 135, 489.

Green, N. M., and Lowthern, D. A. (1959). *Biochem. J.* 71, 55.

Gross, J. (1959). *J. Exp. Med.* 109, 557.

Guha, A., Pattabiraman, T. N., and Backhawat, B. K. (1962). *In* "Collagen," p. 405. Wiley (Interscience), New York.

Halasz, G., and Marx, J. (1932). *Arch. Klin. Chir.* 169, 121.

Ham, A. W., and Elliott, H. C. (1938). *Amer. J. Pathol.* 14, 323.

Hammick, S. L. (1830). "Practical Remarks on Computations, Fractures and Strictures of the Urethra." Published privately, London.

Hanke, H. (1935). *Z. Chir.* 245, 530.

Hanke, H. (1936). *Klin. Wochenschr.* 15, 1121.

Hart, C., and Lessing, O. (1913). "Der Skorbut der kleinern Kinder." Enke, Stuttgart.

Hartzell, J. B., and Stone, W. E. (1942). *Surg., Gynecol. Obstet.* **75**, 1.
Hass, G. M., and McDonald, F. (1940). *Amer. J. Pathol.* **16**, 525.
Henry, K. M., and Kon, S. K. (1939). *Biochem. J.* **33**, 1652.
Hertz, J. (1936). "Studies on the Healing of Fractures." Oxford Univ. Press, London and New York.
Hess, A. F. (1920). "Scurvy Past and Present." Lippincott, Philadelphia, Pennsylvania.
Hill, C. R., and Bourne, G. H. (1954). *Brit. J. Nutr.* **13**, 116.
Hines, H. M., Lazere, B., Thompson, J. D., and Cretzmeyer, C. H. (1944). *J. Nutr.* **27**, 303.
Höjer, J. A. (1923–1924). *Acta Paediat. (Stockholm)*, Suppl. 3.
Höjer, J. A., and Westin, A. (1925). *Dent. Cosmos* **67**, 1.
Howard, C. P., and Ingvaldsen, T. (1917). *Bull. Johns Hopkins Hosp.* **28**, 221.
Howe, P. R. (1920). *Dent. Cosmos* **62**, 586.
Howe, P. R. (1921). *Dent. Cosmos* **63**, 1086.
Howe, P. R. (1923). *J. Amer. Dent. Ass.* **10**, 201.
Howes, E. L., Plotz, C. M., Blunt, J. W., and Ragan, C. (1950). *Surgery* **28**, 177.
Humphreys, F. E., and Zilva, S. S. (1931). *Biochem. J.* **25**, 579.
Hunt, A. H. (1941). *Brit. J. Surg.* **28**, 436.
Hyman, G. A. C., Ragan, C., and Turner, J. C. (1950). *Proc. Soc. Exp. Biol. Med.* **75**, 470.
Ishido, B. (1923). *Virchow's Arch. Pathol. Anat. Physiol.* **240**, 241.
Israel, A. (1925). *Arch. Klin. Chir.* **138**, 105.
Israel, A. (1926). *Arch. Klin. Chir.* **142**, 145.
Israel, A., and Frankel, R. (1926). *Klin. Wochenschr.* **5**, 94.
Jackson, D. S. (1958). *N. Engl. J. Med.* **259**, 814.
Jackson, L., and Moore, J. J. (1916). *J. Infec. Dis.* **19**, 478.
Janxis, J. H. P., and Huisman, T. H. J. (1954). *Pediatrics* **14**, 238.
Jeney, A., and Korpàssy, B. (1934). *Z. Chir.* **61**, 2836.
Jeney, A., and Törö, E. (1936). *Virchow's Arch. Pathol. Anat. Physiol.* **298**, 87.
Kalckar, H. M., and Maxwell, E. S. (1958). *Physiol. Rev.* **38**, 77.
Kapp, H., and Schetty, A. (1937). *Biochem. Z.* **290**, 58.
Kappis, H. (1927). *Deut. Med. Wochenschr.* **53**, 1734.
Karnofsky, D. A., Ridgway, L. P., and Stock, C. C. (1951a). *Fed. Proc., Fed. Amer. Soc. Exp. Biol.* **10**, 204.
Karnofsky, D. A., Ridgway, L. P., and Patterson, P. A. (1951b). **48**, 596.
Key, K. M., and Elphick, G. K. (1931). *Biochem. J.* **25**, 888.
King, C. G. (1950). *J. Amer. Med. Ass.* **142**, 563.
Kitabchi, A. E. (1967). *Nature(London)* **215**, 1385.
Klein, L. (1938). *Anat. Anz.* **87**, 14.
Kodicek, E. (1965). *In* "Structure and Function of Connective and Skeletal Tissue" (S. Fitton Jackson *et al.*, eds.), p. 307. Butterworths, London.
Lanford, C. S. (1939). *J. Biol. Chem.* **130**, 87.
Lanman, T. H., and Ingalls, T. H. (1937). *Amer. J. Surg.* **105**, 616.
Lauber, H. J. (1933). *Beitr. Klin. Med.* **158**, 293.
Lauber, H. J. (1936). *Beitr. Klin. Med.* **161**, 565.
Lauber, H. J., and Rosenfeld, W. (1938). *Klin. Wochenschr.* **17**, 1587.
Lauber, H. J., Nafziger, H., and Bersin, T. (1937). *Klin. Wochenschr.* **16**, 1313.
Layton, L. L. (1951). *Proc. Soc. Exp. Biol. Med.* **76**, 596.
Lazarus, S., Munro, H. N., and Bell, G. H. (1948). *Clin. Sci.* **7**, 175.

Lewis, M. R. (1917). *Carnegie Inst. Contrib. Embryol.* 6, 45.

Lexer, E. W. (1939a). *Klin. Wochenschr.* 18, 208.

Lexer, E. W. (1939b). *Arch. Klin. Chir.* 195, 611.

Lind, J. (1753). "Treatise on Scurvy." Millar, London.

Linton, C. (1858). See Medical and Surgical History of the British Army which served in Turkey and the Crimea (1858).

Lloyd, B. B., and Sinclair, H. M. (1953). *In* "Biochemistry and Physiology of Nutrition" (G. H. Bourne and G. W. Kidder, eds.), Vol. 1, p. 370. Academic Press, New York.

Lobmayer, G. (1918). *Arch. Klin. Chir.* 18, 208.

Logan, M. A. (1940). *Physiol. Rev.* 20, 522.

Lucké, H., and Heckman, E. (1938). *Naunyn-Schmiedebergs Arch. Exp. Pathol. Pharmakol.* 189, 87.

Lucké, H., and Wolf, J. (1938). *Naunyn-Schmiedebergs Arch. Exp. Pathol. Pharmakol.* 189, 628.

Lust, F., and Klocman, L. (1912). *Jahrb. Kinderheilk.* 75, 663.

MacLean, D. L., Sheppart, M., and McHenry, E. W. (1939). *Brit. J. Exp. Pathol.* 20, 451.

McLean, F. C., and Hastings, A. B. (1934). *J. Biol. Chem.* 107, 337.

McLean, F. C., and Hastings, A. B. (1935). *J. Biol. Chem.* 108, 285.

McManus, J. F. A., and Saunders, J. C. (1950). *Science* 111, 204.

Magarey, F. R., and Gough, J. (1952). *Brit. J. Exp. Pathol.* 33, 76.

Malaty, H. A., and Bourne, G. H. (1953). *J. Physiol. (London)* 122, 178.

Mann, I., and Pullinger, B. D. (1940). *Brit. J. Ophthalmol.* 15, 444.

Mapson, L. W. (1964). *Phytochemistry* 3, 429.

Marrigues, A. (1783). Quoted by Hertz (1936).

Matricardi, M. (1938). *Riv. Clin. Pediat.* 36, 351.

Mazoué, H. (1937). *Arch. Anat. Microsc.* 33, 129.

Mazoué, H. (1939). *Arch. Anat. Microsc.* 35, 91.

Mead, R. (1702). "Medical Works." London.

Medical and Surgical History of the British Army which served in Turkey and the Crimea. (1858). Official Account presented to Parliament, Session 3rd December 1857–2nd August 1858. Accounts and Papers, Vol. 38, Part II.

Messina, A., Girlando, M., and Brucchen, A. (1968). *Int. Z. Vitaminforsch.* 38, 409.

Moll, L. (1919). *Mitt. Ges. Inn. Med. Wien.* 18, 29.

Moore, W. G. (1859). *Brit. Med. J.* 1, 443.

Mouriquand, G., and Dauvergne, M. (1938). *Presse Med.* 46, 1081.

Mouriquand, G., Tête, H., Wenger, G., and Viennois, P. (1937). *C. R. Acad. Sci.* 204, 921.

Mouriquand, G., Dauvergne, M., and Edel, V. (1940a). *Presse Med.* 48, 268.

Mouriquand, G., Tête, H., and Edel, V. (1940b). *C. R. Acad. Sci., Ser. D* 210, 515.

Murray, P. D. F., and Kodicek, E. (1949a). *J. Anat.* 83, 158.

Murray, P. D. F., and Kodicek, E. (1949b). *J. Anat.* 83, 205.

Murray, P. D. F., and Kodicek, E. (1949c). *J. Anat.* 83, 285.

Neuberger, A., Perrone, J. C., and Slack, H. G. B. (1951). *Biochem. J.* 49, 199.

Penney, J. R., and Balfour, B. M. (1949). *J. Pathol. Bacteriol.* 61, 171.

Peric-Golia, L., Eik-Nes, K., and Jones, R. S. (1960). *Endocrinology* 66, 48.

Persson, B. H. (1953). "Studies on Connective Tissue Ground Substance." Almqvist & Wiksell, Stockholm.

Peterkovsky, B., and Udenfriend, S. (1963). *J. Biol. Chem.* **238**, 3966.

Pirani, C. L., and Levenson, S. M. (1953). *Proc. Soc. Exp. Biol. Med.* **82**, 95.

Pirani, C. L., Stepto, R. C., and Sutherland, K. J. (1951). *J. Exp. Med.* **93**, 217.

Pirani, C. L., Stepto, R. C., and Conzolazio, C. F. (1952). *Fed. Proc., Fed. Amer. Soc. Exp. Biol.* **11**, 423.

Plotz, C. M., Blunt, J. W., Lattes, R., and Ragan, C. (1950). *Ann. Rheum. Dis.* **9**, 399.

Proto, M. (1936). *Ann. Ital. Chir.* **15**, 37.

Querido, A., and Gaillard, P. J. (1939). *Acta Brevia Neer. Physiol., Pharmacol., Microbiol.* **9**, 70.

Ragan, C., Howes, E. L., Plotz, C. M., Meyer, K., and Blunt, J. W. (1949). *Proc. Soc. Exp. Biol. Med.* **12**, 718.

Ragan, C., Howes, E. L., Plotz, C. M., Meyer, K., Blunt, J. W., and Lattes, R. (1950). *Bull. N.Y. Acad. Med.* [2] **26**, 251.

Reddi, K. K., and Norström, A. (1954). *Nature (London)* **173**, 1232.

Robertson, W. van B. (1950). *J. Biol. Chem.* **187**, 673.

Roegholt, A. (1932). *Arch. Klin. Chir.* **168**, 783.

Ross, R. (1968). *Biol. Rev.* **43**, 51.

Ross, R., and Benditt, E. P. (1961). *J. Biophys. Biochem. Cytol.* **11**, 677.

Ross, R., and Benditt, E. P. (1964). *Fed. Proc., Fed. Amer. Soc. Exp. Biol.* **23**, 41.

Ruskin, S. L. (1938). *Amer. J. Dig. Dis.* **5**, 408.

Ruskin, S. L., and Jonnard, R. (1938a). *C. R. Soc. Biol.* **128**, 266.

Ruskin, S. L., and Jonnard, R. (1938b). *Amer. J. Dig. Dis.* **5**, 676.

Saitta, S. (1929). *Scritti Biol. Castaldi* **4**, 301.

Salter, W. T., and Aub, J. C. (1931). *Arch. Pathol.* **11**, 380.

Schaffenberg, C., Masson, G. M. C., and Corcoran, A. C. (1950). *Proc. Soc. Exp. Biol. Med.* **74**, 358.

Schilozew, S. P. (1928). *Arch. Klin. Chir.* **209**, 320.

Schmidt, W. J. (1934). *Handb. Biol. Arbeitsmeth.* **5**, 435.

Selye, H. (1949). *Brit. Med. J.* **2**, 1129.

Shinya, D. H. (1922). Quoted by Hertz (1936).

Shohl, R. J. (1939). "Mineral Metabolism." Van Nostrand-Reinhold, Princeton, New Jersey.

Smart, C. (1888). *In* "Medical and Surgical History of the War of the Rebellion," Vol. 1, Part 3. U. S. Govt. Printing Office, Washington, D. C.

Spain, D. M., Molomut, N., and Haber, A. (1950a). *Amer. J. Pathol.* **26**, 710.

Spain, D. M., Molomut, N., and Haber, A. (1950b). *Science* **112**, 335.

Staudinger, H. J., Kirsch, K., and Leonhauser, S. (1961). *Ann. N.Y. Acad. Sci.* **92**, 195.

Steen, A. G. (1951). *Brit. J. Ophthalmol.* **35**, 741.

Sulimovici, S., and Boyd, G. S. (1968). *Eur. J. Biochem.* **3**, 332.

Taffel, M., and Harvey, S. C. (1938). *Proc. Soc. Exp. Biol. Med.* **38**, 518.

Tauberhaus, M., and Amromin, G. D. (1950). *J. Lab. Clin. Med.* **36**, 7.

Toverud, K. (1923). *J. Biol. Chem.* **58**, 583.

Upton, A. C., and Coon, W. W. (1951). *Proc. Soc. Exp. Biol. Med.* **77**, 153.

van Wersch, H. J. (1954). "Scurvy as a Skeletal Disease." Dekker & van de Vegt, Utrecht.

Walter, R. (1748). "A Voyage 'round the World." Knapton, London.

Watanabe, T. (1924). *Virchows Arch. Pathol. Anat. Physiol.* **251**, 281.

Wolbach, S. B. (1933). *Amer. J. Pathol., Suppl.* 9, 689.

Wolbach, S. B. (1947). *J. Bone Joint Surg.* 29, 171.

Wolbach, S. B. (1953). *Brit. J. Nutr.* 12, 247.

Wolbach, S. B., and Bessey, O. A. (1942). *Physiol. Rev.* 22, 233.

Wolbach, S. B., and Howe, P. R. (1925). *Proc. Soc. Exp. Biol. Med.* 22, 400.

Wolbach, S. B., and Howe, P. R. (1926) *Arch. Pathol.* 1, 1

Wolbach, S. B., and Maddock, C. L. (1952). *AMA Arch. Pathol.* 53, 54.

Wolfer, J. A., and Hoebel, F. C. (1940). *Surg., Gynecol. Obstet.* 69, 745.

Wolfer, J. A., Farmer, C. J., Carroll, W. W., and Marshardt, O. (1947). *Surg., Gynecol. Obstet.* 84, 1.

Zilva, S. S., and Wells, A. (1919). *Proc. Roy. Soc. Ser. B* 90, 505.

Zorzoli, A., and Nadel, E. M. (1950). *J. Nat. Cancer Inst.* 6, 1366.

CHAPTER 7

Vitamin D and Bone*

ROBERT J. COUSINS† AND HECTOR F. DELUCA

* Work from the author's (H.F.D.) laboratory reported herein was supported by a grant from the U. S. Public Health Service, No. AMO-5800-10 and a contract from the U. S. Atomic Energy Commission, No. AT(11-1)-1668.
† U. S. Public Health Service Postdoctoral Fellow No. 5F02AM41810-02.

I. Introduction

There is now a vast body of experimental data compiled over the last fifty years which supports the idea that the major, if not sole, role of vitamin D in the prevention of bone disease is the elevation of plasma calcium and phosphate to levels sufficiently high to effect the normal mineralization of bone. Vitamin D affects these levels by at least two distinct mechanisms. First, it stimulates the active absorption of dietary calcium and secondarily phosphate by the small intestine. Second, it induces the mobilization of mineral from bone. Whether the vitamin is involved in osteoblastic calcification directly or in renal handling of calcium and phosphate remains unknown at the present time. In any case, the processes of bone mobilization and intestinal absorption working in concert with other homeostatic mechanisms supersaturate the plasma with calcium and phosphate which in turn allow the mineralization of bone to proceed at a normal rate. The action of vitamin D on bone at this point, therefore, must be viewed from its overall effect on plasma calcium.

II. Historical Review—Chemistry and Methods

A. Dawn of the Vitamin Era

The disease rickets, generally recognized as a disease of civilization, was first chronicled in the seventeenth century by Whistler (1645) and

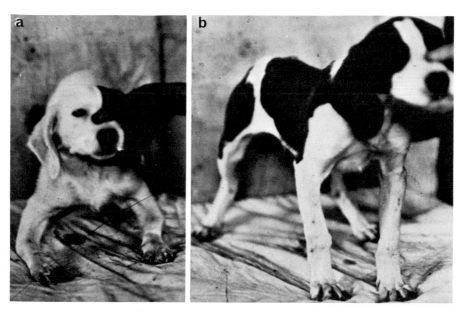

FIG. 1. Gross morphologic changes in rickets: (a) rachitic dog and (b) normal dog.

Glisson (1650). Numerous investigators thereafter implicated the disease with an improper or inadequate diet since the disease could readily be cured by administering cod-liver oil. These early observations have been carefully reviewed elsewhere (Harris, 1956; Fourman *et al.*, 1968).

Hopkins (1912) and Funk (1912) proposed that the absence of a specific dietary factor was responsible for producing rickets. This hypothesis was substantiated when Sir Edward Mellanby (1919a,b) provided the first clear-cut experimental data on rickets, producing the disease in dogs by excluding either cod-liver oil or butter from the diets of these animals (Fig. 1). Years before, McCollum and Davis (1913) and Osborne and Mendel (1913a,b) independently established the existence of fat-soluble vitamin A in cod-liver oil which led Mellanby to incorrectly attribute the antirachitic activity of cod-liver oil to this substance. Proof that vitamin A and the "antirachitic factor" were two distinct substances was finally provided by McCollum and co-workers (1922b) who demonstrated that vitamin A activity (anti-xerophthalmia) is destroyed in cod-liver oil by heat and aeration while the antirachitic activity remains. The newly established antirachitic factor was named *vitamin D* (McCollum *et al.*, 1922c).

B. VITAMIN D AND ULTRAVIOLET RADIATION

Nearly ten years before the discovery of vitamin D, Steenbock and Hart (1913) reported that lactating goats when housed outdoors maintained positive calcium balance while similar animals maintained indoors did not. This observation and the suggestion by Palm (1890) that rickets was most prevalent in the temperate zones where sunlight is limited remained enigmatic until Huldschinsky (1919) demonstrated rickets in children could be cured by exposure to irradiation from a mercury vapor "sun" lamp. Then, five years later, Steenbock and Black (1924) and independently Hess and Weinstock (1924) made the brilliant discovery that ultraviolet irradiation of either the animal or its diet was equally as effective as cod-liver oil in curing rickets. This culminated in the commercial process of irradiating milk to induce vitamin D activity (Steenbock, 1924). This process, which has now been replaced by the direct addition of vitamin D to milk, essentially eliminated rickets as a pediatric health problem in the areas of the world where the practice was adopted.

C. IDENTIFICATION OF VITAMIN D

The antirachitic factor induced in diets by ultraviolet (UV) irradiation received widespread attention following the discoveries of Steenbock and of Hess. Hess and associates (1925), Steenbock and Black (1925), and Rosenheim and Webster (1925) independently demonstrated that the heterogeneous steroid component of the unsaponifiable fraction of cod-liver oil contained a pro-vitamin D. Numerous steroid preparations were then screened for pro-vitamin D activity. One such sterol possessing pro-vitamin activity was ergosterol, a compound derived from fungi. Finally, years later, vitamin D_2, which was then considered to be "the" vitamin D, was isolated in pure form from irradiation products of ergosterol and its structure identified by Askew *et al.* (1930) and Windaus and co-workers (1932) and named *ergocalciferol*. Waddell (1934) made the important observation that the vitamin D derived from UV-activated cod-liver oil (i.e., cholesterol analogs) differed biologically from that derived from ergosterol. The isolation and identification of vitamin D_3 followed shortly thereafter. Named *cholecalciferol*, vitamin D_3 was obtained and identified from irradiated 7-dehydrocholesterol by Windaus and associates (Windaus *et al.*, 1936; Schenk, 1937). The structures of vitamins D_2, D_3, and D_4 shown in Fig. 2 are drawn in the conformation forms determined by Crowfoot and Dunitz (1948) from their X-ray defraction studies.

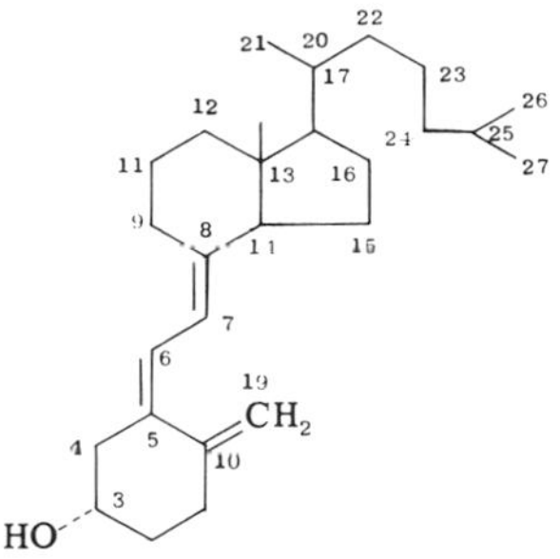

Vitamin D₃
Cholecalciferol
Rat assay   40 IU/μg

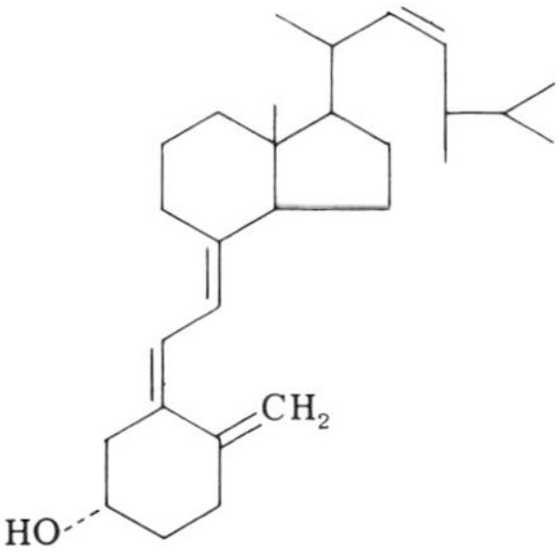

Vitamin D₂
Ergocalciferol
40 IU/μg

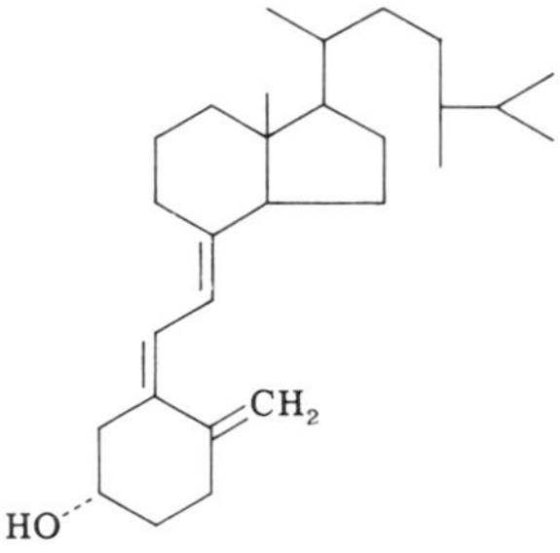

Vitamin D₄
22, 23-Dihydro-
ergocalciferol
Rat assay   20-30 IU/μg

FIG. 2. Structures of the common dietary D vitamins.

The conformation of the ring structure of all biologically active vitamin D compounds known to date with the notable exception of the dihydrotachysterols is the same. A modification of the side chain, however, markedly alters the ability to cure rickets. Various side chain analogs of vitamin D and their respective antirachitic activities are shown in Fig. 3. The reasons for this structure–activity relationship are not well understood, but data to be presented later in this review provide some clues to this phenomenon.

Recently, DeLuca and co-workers (Blunt *et al.*, 1968a; Suda *et al.*, 1969) have isolated and identified the 25-hydroxy derivatives of vitamins D_2 and D_3 which appear to be the metabolically active forms of these substances at the organ level. These compounds and similar analogs will be discussed in detail in the following sections. The experimental

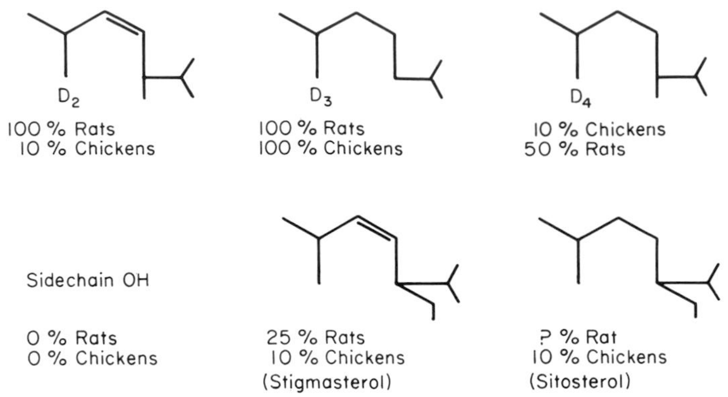

FIG. 3. Side chain modifications of vitamin D_3 and the respective biological activities in rats and chicks.

and clinical applications of these new compounds have triggered a resurgence of research in the area of the role of vitamin D in maintaining calcium homeostasis.

The chemistry of the D vitamins is too vast a subject to be covered in this chapter, and only the more salient work will be mentioned. Excellent reviews and monographs are available on this and related subjects (Sebrell and Harris, 1954; Fieser and Fieser, 1959; DeLuca, 1970a).

D. Assay of Vitamin D Compounds

1. Biological Assay Methods

The most widely accepted assay methods involve the measurement either directly or indirectly of the increased ash content of bone following administration of vitamin D or one of its biologically active analogs. The production of rickets to a moderate but reproducible degree is a prerequisite in the rat "line test" assay. This method originally developed by McCollum and co-workers (1922a) quantitates the deposition of calcium salts in the calcification zone (epiphyseal plate) of the rat tibia or radius. After 18 to 21 days on a standard rachitogenic diet, the bone ash content has dropped from 50–60% to 25–35% on a dry fat-free basis. The animals are then dosed with the test compound (in oil) and after a 7-day test period the tibia or radius is removed, split, and stained with silver nitrate solution. The highly stained calcified zones can then be compared to line test standards (Fig. 4) (U. S. Pharmacopoeia, 1955; Oser, 1965). This method is sensitive to the submicrogram level; however, its lack of precision limits its use.

A method based on maintenance of normal calcification in chicks has

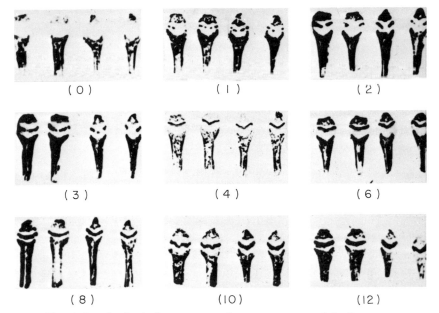

Fɪɢ. 4. Standard calcification scores for interpretation of the line test.

been developed; however, its use as an assay is limited to products intended for this species (Association of Official Analytical Chemists, 1966). Recently, Schachter and co-workers (1961) have based a bioassy on the *in vitro* uptake of ^{45}Ca by rat intestinal slices, but the method has not received widespread use.

2. Chemical Assay Method

A colorimetric assay procedure has been developed and is the official U.S.P. method for vitamin D (U. S. Pharmacopoeia, 1965). Samples must first be saponified and then extracted with hexane. After interfering substances such as sterols, vitamin A, and carotenes are removed by chromatography on siliceous earth, a color complex between the vitamin D and antimony trichloride both in ethylene dichloride is measured at 500 nm exactly 45 seconds after the two solutions are combined. The vitamin D content is determined by comparison to standards treated in an identical fashion. This method unfortunately is only sensitive to 250 μg (10,000 IU) and fails to differentiate between biologically active analogs (Oser, 1965; DeLuca, 1970a). Its use is limited to the assay of vitamin D in pharmaceuticals and prepared animal feed concentrates. Oser (1965) has reviewed the numerous spectrophotometric methods for vitamin D analysis.

Gas-liquid chromatographic methods have been proposed by Avioli and Lee (1966), Murry *et al.* (1966), and Edlund *et al.* (1970). These methods are much more convenient and are far more sensitive than spectrophotometric procedures plus having the advantage of being able to separate vitamins D_2 and D_3. Recently, Nair and deLeon (1968) have obtained limited success in detecting nanogram quantities of vitamins D_2 and D_3 using high temperature electron capture coupled with gas-liquid chromaotgraphy.

3. Radioactive Vitamin D Preparations

The most significant metabolic studies concerning the effect of vitamin D on bone and other targets of its action have involved the use of radioactively labeled vitamin D preparations, which are now available commercially as radiochemically pure compounds of high specific activity. These [14]C- and ^{3}H-labeled materials, when used in conjunction with liquid scintillation analysis, provide high assay sensitivity allowing the use of physiological doses (e.g., 0.25 μg of vitamin D_3 per rat or chick) in whole animal experiments.

III. Metabolic Bone Disease and Vitamin D

A. TYPES OF BONE DISEASE

Metabolic diseases of bone can, according to Fourman *et al.* (1968), be divided into three major types. The first is the lack of bone matrix as occurs, for example, in the disease osteoporosis. The second is the inability of normally synthesized matrix to calcify as occurs in rickets and osteomalacia, analogous diseases in growing and adult animals, respectively. The third is an abnormally high rate of bone resorption most often resulting from hyperparathyroidism. Vitamin D deficiency and excess are primarily involved in the second and third categories, respectively.

B. RICKETS

Rickets and osteomalacia from an etiological viewpoint are the same disease in the young and adult, respectively. That is to say, they are both the direct result of hypovitaminosis D. The biochemical lesion responsible in both diseases is a failure of the calcification process to keep abreast of the synthesis of calcifiable organic bone matrix.

1. Morphologic Changes in Rickets

Grossly the rachitic animal is characterized by soft, twisted, bowed and generally misshapen long bones. The endochondral or joint regions of the bone shafts become enlarged and eventually a crippling dislocation of the epiphysis results (Figs. 1 and 5). These gross morphological changes are the result of the failure of extracellular calcification; hence, the hypertrophic cartilage cells fail to mature. As the immature cartilage cells accumulate the epiphyseal plate widens, and eventually large amounts of osteoid tissue appear at the base of the epiphyseal plate (Fourman *et al.*, 1968).

Intramembranous bone formation as well as periosteal and endosteal lesions are also associated with rickets. The deficiency of calcium and phosphate at the calcification sites resulting from hypovitaminosis D concomitant with normal osteoblastic activity yields secreted but uncalcified organic matrix in these areas. Osteoid tissue accumulates as uncalcified seams in the diaphyseal regions of the long bones (DeLuca, 1970b).

Prolonged vitamin D deficiency rickets is terminal. The primary reason appears to be a combination of complications induced by a flattening of the intramembranous bones of the skull and a collapse of the chest cavity seriously impairing normal body processes (DeLuca, 1970a). Tetany occurs only in advanced rickets since in early stages of the disease the parathyroid glands stimulate bone resorption thus releasing enough mineral to maintain calcium in body fluids. However, eventually this calcium reserve is exhausted, and in addition the bone becomes resistant to parathyroid hormone and tetany develops. Terminal respiratory spasm owing to tetany results unless intravenous calcium or vitamin D is administered.

2. Physiological Basis of Rickets

Originally it was suggested that vitamin D functions directly on the calcification of bone since rachitic bone has been shown to have one-half the ash content (on a dry, fat-free basis) of normal bone (Steenbock and Herting, 1955). However, Howland and Kramer (1921) found that the $[Ca^{2+}] \times [HPO_4^{2-}]$ product of rachitic blood was below normal as well. Shipley *et al.* (1925, 1926) demonstrated that the metabolic defect in rickets was probably a failure of sufficient calcium and phosphate supply at calcification sites. They found that rachitic bone is able to calcify normally *in vitro* when incubated in blood serum from normal animals or in an inorganic salt solution approximating a normal blood electrolyte composition, while blood from rachitic animals had no calcifying ability *in vitro*. Neuman and Neuman (1958) demonstrated that

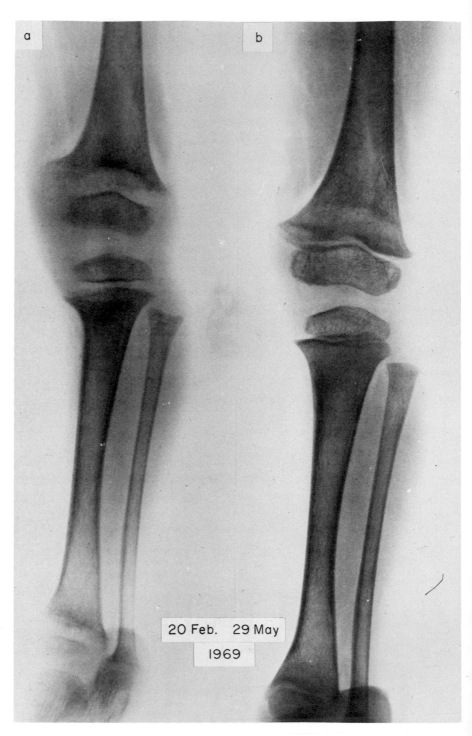

FIG. 5. Radiographs of a knee joint of a 2-year-old rachitic girl treated with 25-HCC: (a) before treatment, and (b) 14 weeks after receiving 2600 IU/day. Courtesy of Dr. S. Balsan.

blood normally is supersaturated with bone forming minerals, but in rickets the serum is undersaturated (Neuman, 1958). The collagen fibrils serve to catalyze the crystallization of the bone mineral as hydroxyapatite. This suggests that the metabolic lesion in rickets is the failure in supply of calcium (Ca^{2+}) and phosphate (HPO_4^{2-}) to the calcification sites. Whether there is a direct effect of vitamin D on osteoblastic-mediated calcification remains however a possibility unsupposed by adequate experimental data.

3. Production of Rickets and Vitamin D Deficiency

Rickets is easily produced in most domestic animals with the notable exception of rats by omitting vitamin D from the diet and preventing exposure to sunlight or other forms of ultraviolet radiation. Under experimental conditions continuous exposure to fluorescent light, which emits sufficient ultraviolet radiation to induce antirachitic activity, should be eliminated in favor of incandescent illumination. In the case of chickens rickets is sometimes difficult to produce when incubators are heated even with incandescent lights.

Care in the choice of diets must also be emphasized, both to avoid vitamin D deficiency as a public health problem as well as the production of this deficiency. With the widespread fortification of foods for human consumption (particularly milk and milk by-products) in the more highly developed countries, hypovitaminosis D is extremely rare. The vitamin D content of natural foods has the most limited distribution of all the vitamins; hence, in the underdeveloped countries as well as those areas where governmental legislation has limited vitamin D fortification, rickets is still a common pediatric health problem.

Animal diets vary greatly in vitamin D content, particularly those ingredients that have been prepared with limited exposure to sunlight. Therefore, fortification of commercial animal feeds has become a standard practice in agriculture (Maynard and Loosli, 1962). For experimental purposes in animal experiments the use of purified diets fed from the time of weaning cannot be overemphasized. These diets have been discussed and evaluated in detail (Steenbock and Herting, 1955). They yield well-defined and rapidly conducted experiments of high precision.

Rickets is clearly a disturbance of calcium and phosphorus metabolism, and the mineral as well as the vitamin D content of the diet is important. Seed grains and their by-products are essentially devoid of the vitamin and rations of oatmeal and corn were used in preparing rachitogenic diets, particularly in the early years. The phosphate in these preparations is primarily in the phytate form which has only limited biological availability. This unavailability of phosphorus produces a low phosphate–high calcium diet. This calcium-to-phosphorus imbalance coupled with a vitamin D-deficient ration is necessary to produce in rats the bone lesions that are characteristic of rickets. A normal calcium-phosphate ratio produces bone lesions but not to the extent of those found in rickets in this species. In all domestic animals of economic importance rickets with accompanying retarded growth rate and low serum calcium is produced by eliminating vitamin D from the diet regardless of the calcium and phosphate content (DeLuca, 1970a). The effect of varying the calcium and phosphate levels in diets of rats has been described in detail (Steenbock and Herting, 1955). It must be emphasized that true rickets in rats can only be obtained by means of a high calcium–low phosphorus, vitamin D-deficient diet. If the diet contains adequate calcium and phosphorus, bone lesions do occur (Baylink *et al.*, 1970) as well as with low calcium diets and are associated with a hypocalcemia. Morphologically however, the bone lesions are not true rickets.

4. Detection of Rickets and Vitamin D Deficiency

As has been mentioned previously rickets is accompanied by a 50% reduction in bone ash which can be used for terminal diagnosis of rickets. Similarly silver nitrate staining of tibia, radius, and ulna as employed in the line test (Fig. 4) method of vitamin D assay can be used to detect the disease.

Of great value clinically are serum calcium, phosphorus, and alkaline phosphatase determinations. In rickets serum alkaline phosphatase is markedly elevated while serum phosphorus and/or serum calcium are depressed. It should be borne in mind however that other disease conditions, e.g., neoplastic growth in the liver, also elevate the synthesis or activity of this enzyme in the blood; hence, serum alkaline phosphatase is usually not a singularly definitive diagnostic criterion. Most widely used however is X-ray examination of the long bones. The characteristic epiphyseal cartilage enlargement is usually well defined in active rickets and is a supplemental diagnostic tool for some species (Thomas *et al.*, 1954).

C. Osteomalacia

Osteomalacia is a disease most generally found in adults and is characterized by a failure of calcification of either existing bone matrix which has become decalcified or new matrix. It differs from rickets inasmuch as little new bone growth is occurring. The bone acting as a buffer for extracellular calcium supply is often drawn upon to supply calcium to maintain the $[Ca^{2+}] \times [HPO_4^{2-}]$ product in the blood. During pregnancy and particularly during lactation the drain of metabolic calcium is very high (McLean and Urist, 1968). If sufficient vitamin D is not available to supply this needed calcium through increased absorption of dietary calcium and possibly by increased renal reabsorption, then severe hypocalcemia is observed. The net result is that the blood becomes undersaturated with respect to calcium and the matrix fails to recalcify (DeLuca, 1970b).

While the disease rarely progresses to the same gross morphological changes as seen in rachitic children, osteomalacia is still a public health problem where insufficient vitamin D is provided. In complicating disease conditions such as steatorrhea (Guyton, 1966) insoluble calcium soaps are formed and both vitamin D and dietary calcium are poorly absorbed thus advancing the disease. Azotemic chronic renal failure is also often associated with osteomalacia, perhaps the result of a type of metabolic vitamin D deficiency.

D. VITAMIN D-RESISTANT RICKETS

Health surveys reveal that rickets and osteomalacia are no longer serious health problems in areas where the vitamin D intake is adequate either through adequate nutrition and food fortification or routine consumption of vitamin tablets. Hence, attention has recently focused on the less common metabolic bone diseases associated in some way with vitamin D.

Vitamin D-resistant rickets (VDRR) first described by Albright *et al.* (1937) is probably best described as a hereditary disease (or a series of closely related syndromes, Fanconi, 1956) characterized by rachitic or osteomalacic bone lesions which are resistant to normal vitamin D therapy. In addition, a marked and consistent dysfunction of the renal tubules occurs resulting in a depressed net reabsorption of inorganic phosphate and concomitant hypophosphatemia. The low blood phosphate level in turn disturbs the normal balance of $[Ca^{2+}]$ and $[HPO_4^{2-}]$ necessary for optimal bone calcification. Decreased absorption of dietary calcium is also a common finding in this malady (Avioli *et al.*, 1967b). These workers observed an abnormal metabolism of ^{3}H-labeled vitamin D in patients with VDRR. Specifically, these individuals exhibit a decrease in the plasma fractional turnover rate of $[^3H]$-vitamin D_3 as well as a decrease in the conversion of the vitamin to polar metabolites including 25-hydroxycholecalciferol (25-HCC). Adult relatives with familial hypophosphatemia, but without rachitic symptoms themselves, appear to have similar though less severe alterations in vitamin D metabolism. This may correspond to the less severe pathological changes associated with hypophosphatemia.

The familial nature of VDRR inheritance has been fairly well documented as a sex-linked dominant trait (Graham *et al.*, 1959), although the pathogenisis is disputed. Undoubtedly, some of the lesions associated with VDRR familial hypophosphatemia result from secondary hyperparathyroidism (DeLuca, 1970a). While the serum calcium level does not fall appreciably, poor calcium absorption triggers the release of parathyroid hormone (PTH), which promotes bone resorption and therefore maintenance of the serum calcium level. The increased PTH activity would also exert its action on the kidney and decrease reabsorption of phosphate thus accounting for the hypophosphatemia.

The most likely explanation for VDRR and familial hypophosphatemia is thus an impaired ability of the intestine to absorb dietary calcium which could be the result of a genetic defect that could occur at any of several levels. DeLuca (1970b) has suggested that the defect lies not in the metabolism of vitamin D itself but in its active metabolite 25-HCC at the hepatic or the target tissue level where an abnormal rather than a functional metabolite is formed. Goldstein *et al.* (1968) has proposed that the affinity of a vitamin D "receptor" is altered in those afflicted with VDRR. Evidence for a vitamin D receptor in the intestinal mucosal cell has been demonstrated (Stohs and DeLuca, 1967; Haussler and Norman, 1969; Chen *et al.*, 1970) and will be discussed later.

E. RENAL OSTEODYSTROPHY

Chronic renal disease gives rise to bone lesions which are resistant to therapeutic doses of vitamin D. Avioli *et al.* (1968), in a detailed study of the metabolism of [^{3}H]-vitamin D_3 in normal and uremic patients, found a twofold increase in fractional turnover of the vitamin in plasma, an abnormal accumulation of polar metabolites in the plasma, and an increased urinary excretion of these polar metabolites. These workers suggested that an acquired defect in the metabolism and excretion of vitamin D in patients with renal disease precludes its ability to function normally at target sites, particularly the intestine. This, in turn, alters normal mineral metabolism since calcium is drawn from the bone reserves and leads to the osteodystrophic condition. The exact pathogenisis of the altered vitamin D metabolism is, however, not known at present (DeLuca and Avioli, 1970).

Recently, Fraser and Kodicek (1970) followed by Gray *et al.* (1971)

have shown that the metabolically active form of vitamin D for intestinal calcium transport is formed in renal tissue. It is therefore attractive to speculate that in this disease there is a defective calcium absorption which results from a metabolic "vitamin D"-deficient intestine. The hypocalcemia which results brings about an excessive PTH secretion and thus osteodystrophy. When the specific vitamin D metabolite becomes available, it should be possible to prevent renal osteodystrophy by supplying the specific active form of vitamin D for the intestine.

F. Bone Disease and Vitamin D Therapy

A number of disease conditions affecting bone are benefited by vitamin D administration although the exact role the vitamin plays in these conditions is not clear. The use of vitamin D compounds to treat these disease states has until recently been rather straightforward. However, the synthesis of newly identified biologically active metabolites of vitamin D has provided the clinician with new therapeutic agents to treat bone diseases.

Classically, rickets has been treated with vitamin D_3 with generally successful results. Recently, 25-HCC has been shown to be a very useful agent for the treatment of this disease (Balsan, 1970a). Figure 5 shows the radiographs of a 2-year-old rachitic child previous to and 6 weeks after being treated with 2600 IU of 25-HCC per day. The reduction of metaphyseal size and vast improvement in calcification are evident. In a limited number of cases, 25-HCC has been a successful treatment of osteomalacic patients found resistant to unmodified vitamin D (Hioco et al., 1970). Surprisingly, however, in VDRR the effectiveness of 25-HCC in controlling this disease has been inconsistent (Balsan, 1970b; Earp et al., 1970). However, recent evidence (Seely and DeLuca, 1970) suggests that 10,000–20,000 IU of 25-HCC per day is a highly successful treatment of the disease.

Hypoparathyroidism and concomitant hypocalcemia is usually treated clinically with dihydrotachysterol (DHT). This drug possesses a potent bone mineral mobilizing property at high doses but only a limited ability to stimulate intestinal calcium absorption. Harrison et al. (1967) found DHT to be only one-fifth as effective as vitamins D_2 and D_3 in elevating serum calcium levels in hypocalcemic vitamin D-deficient rats. In hypoparathyroid rats, DHT at high doses is ten times as active in restoring calcium levels to normal. This preferential action on bone makes DHT a unique replacement for PTH in hypoparathyroid patients. Serum calcium changes induced by DHT are more rapid and of shorter duration, hence precluding serious protracted hypercalcemia resulting from hypervitaminosis D (Potts and Deftos, 1969). Dihydrotachysterol may require a 25-hydroxylation before it is biologically active since 25-OHDHT$_3$, which has recently been synthesized and isolated in pure form (Suda *et al.*, 1970d), has a higher biological activity and acts more rapidly on a weight basis than unmodified DHT$_3$ (Suda *et al.*, 1970a). This drug may also be useful clinically in treating hypoparathyroidism.

Idiopathic and acquired postoperative hypoparathyroidism in many instances is accompanied by resistance to vitamin D. Recently, Pak *et al.* (1970) demonstrated that 25-HCC was effective in elevating serum calcium levels in two of three cases. In still other cases, 25-HCC is the most effective compound yet known in the treatment of hypoparathyroidism.

Azotemic chronic renal disease is associated with altered vitamin D metabolism, the nature of which was not clear until very recently (Avioli *et al.*, 1968). DeLuca and Avioli (1970) have found 25-HCC to be one-hundred times more effective than vitamin D in stimulating calcium absorption in uremic rats. These results suggest that 25-HCC could prove to be a useful therapeutic agent in treating the osteodystrophy often associated with chronic renal disease. However, most likely the new metabolite of vitamin D believed to be the metabolically active form in intestine will be the agent of choice in this disease since its production is likely very low in chronic renal disease.

Parturient paresis (milk fever), a disease affecting lactating dairy cows and ewes, is characterized by acute hypocalcemia commencing within 72 hours after parturition (Siegmund, 1961). The exact cause appears to be an abnormally large need for calcium for milk production which in turn places a tremendous drain on reserves of calcium. Massive doses of vitamin D (10–30 million units daily) several days prior to parturition is an effective prophylactic measure; however, toxicity is observed as abnormal calcification if treatment is prolonged. Feeding a high phosphorus–low calcium diet during late pregnancy is somewhat helpful, suggesting the disease results from an inability of the parathyroid glands to meet the calcium needs through increased bone resorption (Maynard and Loosli, 1962). In the past the disease was best treated by intravenous administration of calcium. The use of 25-HCC prophylactically shows great promise in that it is more active than its unhydroxylated parent and is more readily excreted, thus decreasing the chances of toxic reactions (Bringe *et al.*, 1970).

The metabolism and mode of action of vitamin D will be discussed in later sections, but it should be clear that as the exact metabolic picture is delineated and the specific metabolites and analogs are identified and synthesized, these compounds will usher in a new chapter in the use of vitamin D and its analogs as therapeutic agents for bone disorders.

IV. Physiological Basis of Vitamin D Action

A. VITAMIN D AND BONE CALCIFICATION

The calcification promoting properties of vitamin D have been discussed in the section on rickets. It should be emphasized that the overall effect of the vitamin is to maintain calcification. The work of Shipley *et al.* (1926) established that calcification of rachitic bone could proceed *in vitro* only when adequate concentrations of minerals were supplied to the bone via the blood. Neuman and Neuman (1958) then demonstrated that the blood serum must be supersaturated with the essentials of bone mineral if calcification is to occur. Recently, Canas *et al.* (1969) obtained evidence that an early effect of vitamin D on rachitic bone is to stimulate bone collagen synthesis thus providing new organic matrix for calcification. However, a direct involvement of vitamin D in the calcification process *in situ* has yet to be demonstrated experimentally.

B. VITAMIN D AND CALCIUM ABSORPTION

The best-known physiological effect of vitamin D is to increase calcium absorption from the intestine. This phenomenon was first recognized by Orr *et al.* (1923). They correctly concluded from the examination of clinical cases of rickets that vitamin D must be involved in intestinal absorption of calcium. Their observation remained largely unknown until Nicolaysen and co-workers (Nicolaysen, 1937; Nicolaysen and Eeg-Larsen, 1953) established on a firm experimental basis that vitamin D increases intestinal absorption of calcium and secondarily phosphate from the intestinal lumen. This classic work has been confirmed many times using many elegant techniques, reviewed in detail in a book edited by Wasserman (1963). The exact mechanism of increased intestinal absorption of calcium remained relatively obscure until the work of Schachter and Rosen (1959) revealed that the calcium is transported against a concentration gradient in the small intestine. Continued work in his laboratory (Schachter, 1963) and elsewhere (Harrison and Harrison, 1960, 1961; Martin and DeLuca, 1969a) showed this process to be an active one involving the transfer primarily of calcium against an electrochemical potential gradient. Schachter and his colleagues have concluded that vitamin D is involved both in the entrance process of calcium across the brush border membranes of intestinal absorption cells and the exit of calcium from the absorption cells into the extracellular fluid. Harrison and Harrison (1960) have concluded that vitamin D is involved in the nonactive portion of the transport process, whereas Martin and DeLuca (1969b) have demonstrated that the exit of calcium from the intestinal epithelial cells involves extracellular sodium. They have further demonstrated that vitamin D is involved in the initial entrance of calcium from the lumen across the brush border surface (Martin and DeLuca, 1969a). The mechanism is not entirely understood nor agreed upon by current research workers in the field. Clearly, much work remains to be done to delineate the molecular mechanism of calcium transfer across the epithelial cells of intestine.

A very large step toward understanding the molecular mechanism of intestinal calcium transport was taken when very recently Wasserman and his associates demonstrated the existence of and isolated in pure form a calcium binding protein found in the intestine following vitamin D administration (Wasserman and Taylor, 1966; Wasserman *et al.*, 1968). Using fluorescent antibodies to this protein it was demonstrated in large concentrations at the brush border surface of the intestine and appeared to be secreted by the goblet cells (Wasserman, 1971). Wasserman and his colleagues have accumulated massive amounts of evidence suggesting that the calcium binding protein is of fundamental importance of the vitamin D-stimulated intestinal calcium transport.

Recently, Martin *et al.* (1969) and Melancon and DeLuca (1970) have demonstrated the existence of a calcium-dependent adenosinetriphosphatase in the brush borders of intestine from rats given vitamin D. This system was found to be present only following vitamin D administration and is considered to play an important role in the energy-linked transfer of calcium across brush border surface. Exactly how the calcium binding protein of Wasserman and his colleagues and the calcium-dependent adenosinetriphosphatase fit together as an intestinal calcium transport system stimulated by vitamin D remains an obscure point. Undoubtedly both are involved and it seems likely that the calcium binding protein is the specific one made in response to vitamin D and that it together with certain fractions of the brush border membrane constitute a calcium-dependent ATPase or a transport system which utilizes ATP to "pay for" the transfer of calcium from outside the lumen into the intestinal epithelial cell.

Of great physiological interest is the fact that animals fed a low calcium diet have great ability to absorb calcium from the intestine, whereas those animals fed high calcium diets have much less ability to carry out intestinal calcium absorption. Nicolaysen and Eeg-Larsen

(1953) and Malm (1963) have found that man deprived of calcium for long periods of time will maintain a high intestinal absorption rate until such time as the bones are saturated. Nicolaysen postulated the existence of an endogenous factor which serves as the messenger from bone to the intestine instructing it in regard to the level of intestinal calcium absorption. Although this factor is of obvious interest it is yet to be placed on a firm experimental basis.

The form in which calcium from the diet is presented to the intestine affects absorption. Simultaneous ingestion of phosphates, phytic acid, and oxalic acid present in some grains tie up the available calcium as insoluble salts which are not absorbed by the intestine. Lengemann et al. (1959) showed that lactose has beneficial effects on ^{45}Ca absorption. These factors and others have been reviewed in detail (Bronner, 1964).

C. Vitamin D and Bone Mineral Mobilization

Hypervitaminosis D has for a long time been known to mobilize bone with a concomitant hypercalcemic effect (Nicolaysen and Eeg-Larsen, 1953). Harris and co-workers (Harris, 1956) in early work reported that excess vitamin D brought about a greatly increased absorption of calcium and the formation of highly calcified new bone as well as hypercalcemia. The assumption that increased calcium absorption by the gut is responsible for the hypercalcemia is, however, incorrect since Carlsson and Lindquist (1955) showed calcium absorption increases as an asymptotic function of dose. Carlsson (1952) and Bauer et al. (1955) demonstrated conclusively that physiological doses of vitamin D induce a mobilization of bone mineral into the blood thus elevating the serum calcium level. They showed experimentally that when rats are placed on a diet with only a negligible calcium content the vitamin is still able to induce a marked increase in serum calcium. This increased calcium could not be accounted for by increased calcium absorption and hence must have come from the large calcium reserves in bone (Nicolaysen and Eeg-Larsen, 1956). Moreover, it was subsequently established that bone mobilization induced by parathyroid hormone requires the presence of vitamin D (Harrison et al., 1958; Rasmussen et al., 1963), thus establishing a direct involvement of vitamin D in bone resorption.

Recently, Baylink and co-workers (1970) have placed some bone changes associated with vitamin D deficiency on a firm quantitative histological basis. Using tetracycline labeling and pair-fed control animals they were able to measure the following parameters as influenced by hypovitaminosis D: the rates of total bone formation, total matrix formation, periosteal and endosteal apposition, periosteal mineralization rates, and the linear rate of endosteal bone resorption. They concluded that the major bone changes associated with vitamin D deficiency were: (a) a decrease in osteoblastic matrix formation, (b) an inhibition of osteoid mineralization and (c) an increase in osteoclastic bone resorption. They suggested that since vitamin D-deficient rats are hypocalcemic, while concomitantly bone resorption is greater than normal, the deficiency renders them unable to compensate by increased intestinal calcium absorption. The important point is brought out that vitamin D-deficient hypocalcemic rats absorb appreciable but suboptimal amounts of calcium, while vitamin D-adequate rats on a zero calcium diet do not become as hypocalcemic probably as a result of increased bone resorption. They suggested the lack of PTH action in hypovitaminotic D animals is responsible for a defect in osteoclastic resorption found in this deficiency syndrome which nevertheless promotes secondary hyperparathyroidism. The hypocalcemia or secondary hyperparathyroidism causes the reduced rate of bone matrix formation and mineralization.

D. Vitamin D and the Kidney

Vitamin D has been shown to enhance the reabsorption of inorganic phosphate by the kidney (Harrison and Harrison, 1941). It has been suggested (DeLuca, 1967) that this phenomenon is a consequence of secondary hyperparathyroidism induced by hypocalcemia in vitamin D deficiency. Parathyroid hormone promotes phosphate diuresis, an effect of the hormone which is not dependent on the presence of vitamin D (Arnaud et al., 1966). Gran (1960) reported that vitamin D also increases the renal reabsorption of calcium; however, 99% of the filtered calcium is reabsorbed even in deficient animals. This effect of the vitamin, if true, probably is of minor quantitative significance.

Recently, Fraser and Kodicek (1970) have provided evidence that the kidney is a regulator of functional vitamin D metabolism and the small amount of calcium in the kidney could play an important regulatory function, however.

E. Vitamin D, Parathyroid Hormone, and Calcitonin Interactions

Harrison et al. (1958; Harrison and Harrison, 1964) were the first to observe that PTH is unable to increase serum calcium in vitamin D-deficient animals. Rasmussen et al. (1963) further documented this effect and also found the serum phosphate lowering ability of the hormone was independent of vitamin D. More recently, Arnaud and associates (1966) have also found PTH-induced phosphate diuresis is independent of vitamin D. Pechet and co-workers (1967) have demonstrated that bone resorption induced by PTH, as indicated by elevated urinary hydroxyproline excretion rates, is similarly dependent on vitamin D.

Calcitonin (CT), in contrast to PTH, lowers serum calcium and phosphate levels by a process independent of vitamin D (Morii and DeLuca, 1967). This independence was also observed in simultaneous infusion experiments (Pechet *et al.*, 1967). DeLuca *et al.* (1968) proposed a model to explain existing data on vitamin D, PTH, and CT interactions. They suggested vitamin D induces the formation of a calcium mobilizing system of bone while PTH and CT increase and decrease, respectively, the permeability of the basement membrane of bone cells to calcium. The mechanism of action of vitamin D on bone at the molecular level will be discussed in detail in a following section.

F. Overall Physiological Action of Vitamin D

Two main targets of vitamin D action have clearly been established, i.e., small intestine and bone (Fig. 6). The action of the vitamin then is to promote active absorption of calcium and secondarily phosphorus by the intestine and mobilization of these minerals from bone. Both effects aid in maintaining the calcium and phosphate concentration of the plasma at supersaturated levels with regard to bone mineral which in turn is necessary for normal calcification of bone. Possible renal effects of vitamin D as well as direct effects on osteoblastic calcification must remain an open question.

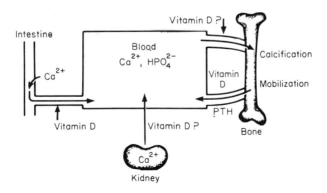

Fig. 6. Physiological actions of vitamin D.

V. Metabolism of Vitamin D

A. EXPERIMENTAL TECHNIQUES

Until recently, the detailed study of vitamin D metabolism progressed rather slowly owing to the lack of sensitive enough methods for the detection of physiological concentrations of vitamin D and its metabolites. The preparation of isotopically labeled vitamin D, the development of powerful chromatographic methods of isolation and physical methods of identification have provided the tools for rapid progress in this area.

1. Radioactive Vitamin D

Preparation of the first labeled vitamin D was carried out by Kodicek (1955). In the intervening years labeled preparations have been made by a variety of methods, biosynthetic and chemical. DeLuca (1967) has reviewed these methods in detail elsewhere. These materials, when used in conjunction with liquid scintillation spectrometry, provide a high degree of sensitivity and allow experiments to be carried out with physiological doses (e.g., 0.25 μg or less of vitamin D_3 per rat) in whole animal experiments. This sensitivity is also especially important in subcellular and in autoradiography experiments which may contribute to the elucidation of the molecular mechanism of vitamin D action.

2. Extraction and Separation Methods

A modification of the Folch chloroform-methanol extraction procedure (Folch *et al.*, 1957) developed by Bligh and Dyer (1959) has received nearly universal acceptance as the method of choice for extraction of vitamin D and its metabolites from bone as well as the soft tissues (Lund and DeLuca, 1966; Cousins *et al.*, 1970b).

Silicic acid column chromatography has until recently provided the main analytical tool for separation of vitamin D (peak III) metabolites. High resolution can easily be obtained by utilizing subtle exponential gradient elution and careful choice of solvent mixtures used as eluents. The resolution obtainable with this type of separation system is illustrated with the chromatographic profiles shown in Fig. 7. For example, peak IV of this plasma extract, which appears as one metabolite (lower profile), is resolvable into eight metabolites (upper profile) by simply altering the elution system (Ponchon and DeLuca, 1969b). Recently, it has become clear that the polar metabolites are extremely important in the overall mode of action of vitamin D. A new chromatographic

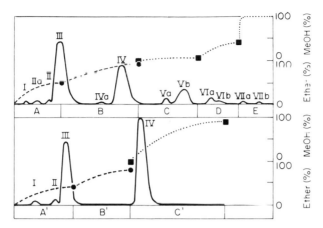

Fig. 7. Chromatography of plasma 24 hours after intravenous injection of 10 IU [1,2-³H]-vitamin D_3 to vitamin D-deficient rats. Resolution of the polar metabolites of vitamin D on silicic acid columns obtained with a modified elution system (upper profile) compared to the original system (lower profile); (——) radioactivity; (- - -) ether in Skelly B; (. . .) methanol in ether.

system using Sephadex LH-20 has been developed (Holick and DeLuca, 1971a), in light of the importance of these metabolites, which definitively separates metabolites of the peak V region on silicic acid into four distinct metabolites, two of which have been identified (Suda *et al.,* 1970b,c).

B. ABSORPTION AND TRANSPORT OF VITAMIN D

Kodicek (1959) and Norman and DeLuca (1963), using radioactive preparations, found that dietary vitamin D in oil is absorbed primarily in the ileum of the small intestine. Bile has been shown to be required for the vitamin D absorption process by Greaves and Schmidt (1933) and Heymann (1937) and more recently by Schachter *et al.* (1964). Schachter and co-workers, in their extensive studies using ligated loops of small intestine, found vitamin D in alcohol and propylene glycol is absorbed principally in the jejunum as is cholesterol. DeLuca (1967), attempting to clarify the point, suggested that the carrier vehicle used accounts for the varying results and that the vitamin may be absorbed in both the jejunum and the ileum.

The once-absorbed vitamin is then transported to the systemic circulation via the thoracic duct of the lymphatic system initially associated with chylomicrons (Schachter *et al.,* 1964). High and low density lipoproteins are also involved in the lymphatic transport to a limited extent.

Once in the circulation, the vitamin is transported initially by the serum lipoproteins. Intravenously administered vitamin D is similarly associated with lipoproteins initially. Rikkers and DeLuca (1967) have demonstrated that with time the task of vitamin D transport is increasingly shifted from the lipoproteins to a protein migrating as an α-globulin on disc gel electrophoresis. Furthermore, this transfer is time-related rather than dose-related. Vitamins D_2 and D_4 have a lower *in vivo* binding affinity for the α-globulin than does vitamin D_3 suggesting that the side chain composition is critical for optimal binding (Rikkers *et al.*, 1969). This dependence on side chain conformation led them to suggest the liver, which has been shown to rapidly take up vitamin D (Neville and DeLuca, 1966) and convert it into an "active" form through an alteration in the side chain (Blunt *et al.*, 1968a), is involved in the lipoprotein to α-globulin transfer.

C. Tissue Distribution of Vitamin D

The fate of circulating vitamin D has been nearly universally studied in vitamin D-deficient animals administered a pulse of isotopically labeled vitamin. Early work in this area involved the use of abnormally large doses of vitamin D preparations of low specific activity. We now have evidence (Holick and DeLuca, 1970) that dose-related aberrant metabolism exists in the hypervitaminotic D animal; therefore, only those more salient experiments employing physiological doses will be discussed.

Norman and DeLuca (1963) and Kodicek and Thompson (1965) both found appreciable amounts of radioactivity in the bones and livers of vitamin D-deficient rats following [³H]-vitamin D_3. Neville and DeLuca (1966) reported that 4 hours after intravenous administration of 10 IU of [³H]-vitamin D_3 virtually all organs have taken up radioactivity (Table I). Expressing these data on a relative incorporation basis (i.e., disintegrations/min/100 mg dry weight) the targets where vitamin D exerts its action, i.e., the intestinal mucosa and bone cells, accumulate the largest concentration of ³H from the labeled vitamin. Moreover this distribution does not change appreciably within the time a pulse of vitamin D is able to elicit a detectable physiological response..

Avioli *et al.* (1967a) and later Ponchon and DeLuca (1969a) observed a consistent time-related rebound of radioactivity into the plasma of man and rats, respectively, corresponding to a simultaneous decrease in liver radioactivity. This rebound from the liver (Fig. 8) has subsequently been shown to result from the release or "secretion" of 25-HCC into the systemic circulation likely bound to the α-globulin carrier (DeLuca, 1969).

TABLE I
TISSUE LOCALIZATION OF RADIOACTIVITY AFTER AN INTRAJUGULAR DOSE
OF 1,2-³H-LABELED VITAMIN D₃[a,b]

Tissue	At 4 hours after dose	
	Percent of dose	Relative incorporation[c]
Spleen	1.04 ± 0.17	3,620 ± 292
Lung	1.72 ± 0.49	2,739 ± 732
Heart	0.71 ± 0.20	1,409 ± 353
Intestine (large)	0.35 ± 0.03	813 ± 80
Intestine (small)	1.73 ± 0.07	2,305 ± 502
Intestinal mucosa[d]	—	7,113
Kidney	2.35 ± 0.19	2,201 ± 441
Blood[e]	12.92 ± 1.96	2,472 ± 413
Muscle[f]	8.61 ± 2.75	244 ± 70
Liver	28.59 ± 2.04	5,958 ± 893
Bone[g]	26.78 ± 3.8	501 ± 73
Bone cells[h]	—	12,525
Small intestinal contents	5.62 ± 1.05	2,831 ± 545
Large intestinal contents + feces	3.17 ± 0.38	1,010 ± 277
Total (%)	93.6	—

[a] Reproduced from Neville and DeLuca (1966) with the kind permission of the American Chemical Society.

[b] Rats were fed a vitamin D-deficient diet for 3 weeks before being used. Each deficient rat received an intrajugular injection of 10.7 IU of 1,2-³H vitamin D₃ in 0.2 ml of Tween-NaCl solution. Values ± the standard deviation are averages of 3 rats for 4 hours.

[c] Relative incorporation expressed as disintegrations per minute per 100 mg dry weight.

[d] Calculated on the assumption that small intestine is made up of 30% mucosa and 70% muscle, connective tissue, etc. (on dry weight basis), and that smooth muscle has the same relative incorporation as skeletal muscle.

[e] This assumes that blood is 6% of body weight.

[f] This assumes that muscle is 30% of body weight.

[g] This assumes that skeleton is 15% of body weight.

[h] This assumes that bone is 4% cells on a dry weight basis and all vitamin D is located in these cells. Activity expressed as dpm per 100 mg dry weight of bone cells.

D. 25-HCC—ISOLATION

Using the methods mentioned in a preceding section, Lund and DeLuca (1966) demonstrated that a polar vitamin D metabolite fraction is as active in curing rickets as is vitamin D itself. This fraction was later shown to be heterogeneous (Ponchon and DeLuca, 1969b), and

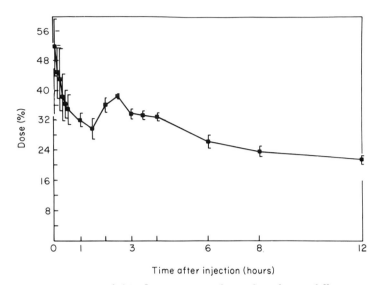

FIG. 8. Time course of ^{3}H disappearance from the plasma following 0.25 μg [1,2-^{3}H]-vitamin D$_3$ given intravenously. Vertical bars represent ±SEM. [Taken from Ponchon and DeLuca (1969a) with the permission of the publisher.]

the amount of biologically active metabolite could be increased to some degree by increased doses of vitamin D (Lund and DeLuca, 1966). These experiments provided the first experimental evidence that vitamin D is converted into an "active" form prior to physiological action. This hypothesis had been suggested earlier (Raoul and Gounelle, 1958); however, these workers incorrectly suggested the adrenal gland in some way mediated the transformation.

The major plasma metabolite designated as peak IV can be elevated to approximately 18 IU/ml (DeLuca, 1970b) by feeding large doses of vitamin D$_3$ to hogs. Thus the plasma of 4 hogs fed large doses of vitamin D$_3$ for 26 days was used as the source of peak IV. The chloroform-methanol extracts of the ammonium sulfate precipitated hog plasma proteins combined with that from a pig which received labeled vitamin D were then applied to a silicic acid column. The impure peak IV was next subjected to liquid–liquid partition column chromatography which yielded 1.3 mg of pure metabolite (Blunt et al., 1968a). Ultraviolet, nuclear magnetic resonance, and mass spectrometry plus gasliquid chromatographic characteristics established the peak IV metabolite as 25-HCC (Fig. 9). This compound has been synthesized by three different methods (Blunt and DeLuca, 1969) for further investigational studies. 25-Hydroxycholecalciferol from human plasma has also been

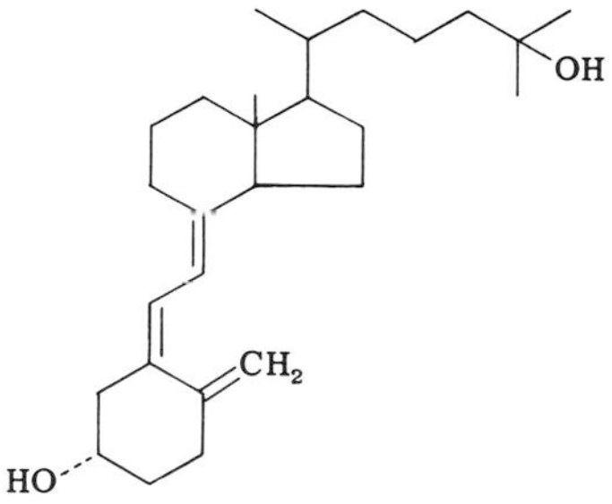

FIG. 9. Structure of 25-HCC.

isolated and identified (Holick and DeLuca, 1971b). Shortly thereafter, using identical experimental techniques, DeLuca and associates (Suda *et al.*, 1969) isolated and identified the peak IV metabolite from vitamin D_2 as 25-hydroxyergocalciferol (25-HEC).

The physiological actions of these metabolites are discussed in the following sections where data will be presented to show that the 25-hydroxylated derivatives are the "circulating active" forms of vitamin D but are not the final metabolically active forms per se, at least in intestine.

E. 25-HCC—BIOSYNTHESIS

The hepatic formation of 25-HCC is of considerable interest in light of its importance in overall vitamin D metabolism. Ponchon *et al.* (1969) demonstrated that functionally hepatectomized rats are unable to form 25-HCC (peak IV) (Fig. 10). These data in conjunction with the plasma rebound phenomenon demonstrate the liver is probably the major if not sole site of conversion. It has also been possible to demonstrate that livers of rats continuously perfused with [^{3}H]-vitamin D_3-containing plasma were able to produce a more polar metabolite which had the same chromatographic and antirachitic properties as 25-HCC (Horsting and DeLuca, 1969) (Fig. 11).

Homogenates of liver hydroxylate vitamin D_3. This enzyme system was found to be heat sensitive and to have an optimum pH of 6.9. The reaction requires reduced pyridine nucleotide and molecular oxygen and was not detected in kidney or intestinal mucosal homogenates. The reaction was not inhibited by DPPD (diphenylparaphenylenediamine) or carbon monoxide, thus indicating the production of 25-HCC was neither by a free radical mechanism (lipid peroxidation system) nor by a typical steroid hydroxylase system requiring cytochrome P450.

Predosing of vitamin D–deficient rats with nonradioactive vitamin D

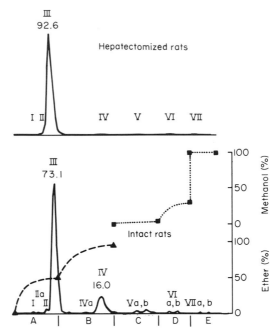

Fig. 10. Chromatographic profiles of lipid extracts of plasma from hepatectomized and intact rats 4 hours after administration of 0.25 μg of [1,2-³H]-vitamin D₃: (———) radioactivity, (- - -) ether in Skelly B, and (. . .) methanol in ether. [Taken from Ponchon *et al.* (1969) with the permission of the publisher.]

markedly reduced the production of 25-HCC from [³H]-vitamin D₃ *in vivo* and *in vitro*. Furthermore, the 25-hydroxylase system is strongly inhibited by the product, 25-HCC. These results suggest that the synthesis and secretion of 25-HCC into the plasma is tightly controlled by product inhibition. The fact that the inhibition can be overcome by giving large amounts of vitamin D suggests that the inhibition plays a major role in the conservation of vitamin D on one hand and in preventing vitamin D toxicity on the other in the face of widely varying intakes of the vitamin from diet or irradiation of skin.

It has been well established that vitamin D₃ is much more effective than DHT at physiological dose levels in mobilizing bone mineral. However, at pharmacological doses as used in the treatment of hypoparathyroidism the reverse is true. Horsting and DeLuca (1971) found that product inhibition is not evident when 25-hydroxydihydrotachysterol, the probable active form of DHT, replaces 25-HCC in the reaction mixture. This suggests that DHT hydroxylation is not subject to product

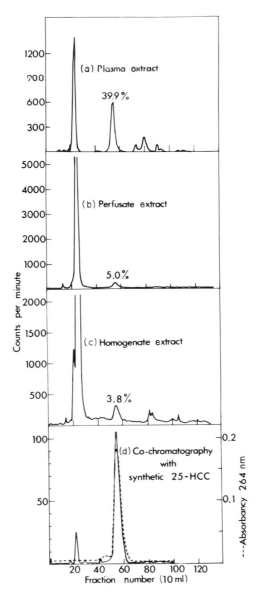

Fig. 11. Silicic acid column chromatography of extracts from: (a) plasma of rats dosed 24 hours previously with 0.25 μg of [1,2-³H]-vitamin D₃, (b) perfusate from normal rat liver after 4 hours of continuous perfusion with 0.15 μg of [1,2-³H]-vitamin D₃, (c) homogenates incubated for 4 hours with 0.15 μg of [1,2-³H]-vitamin D₃, and (d) co-chromatography of metabolite formed in homogenate incubation with standard 25-HCC. (——) Radioactivity and (- - -) O.D. at 264 nm. [Taken from Horsting and DeLuca (1969) with the permission of the publisher.]

inhibition and DHT is hydroxylated to completion by the liver which may account for the effectiveness of DHT at high dose levels.

The characteristics of vitamin D 25-hydroxylase in the liver makes it indeed likely that this system is probably the controlling mechanism for the secretion of 25-HCC into the plasma. Vitamin D has long been considered a dietary essential as a direct result of civilization. The regulated nature of 25-HCC formation supports the belief that vitamin D or more likely 25-HCC is a hormone, by the classic definition, which is synthesized in the liver and secreted into the plasma in a controlled fashion to produce its effects on the target tissues, i.e., intestine and bone.

F. 25-HCC—METABOLISM

Vitamin D_3, when administered as a pulse to deficient animals, circulates as a variety of metabolites including those more polar on silicic acid chromatography than either vitamin D or 25-HCC (Ponchon and DeLuca, 1969b) as well as a less polar metabolite (peak I). Peak I, which possesses limited biological activity, has been identified as an ester of vitamin D and long chain fatty acids (Lund *et al.*, 1967).

The metabolites discussed thus far in this review appear ubiquitous *in vivo;* however, 25-HCC is the "metabolic or hormonal" form, at least at the organ level, responsible for the physiological action of vitamin D_3. In view of this information it becomes clear that functional metabolism in target tissues, as opposed to general overall metabolism, must be studied at the level of the active form rather than the dietary form of the vitamin. Moreover, with the exception of peak I, all metabolites of vitamin D_3 whose structures have been identified thus far are 25-hydroxyl derivatives and hence are undoubtedly derived from 25-HCC. It should be noted that under normal dietary situations the body tissues undoubtedly are in a steady state containing a mixture of metabolites including 25-HCC. Following administration of 0.25 μg (14 IU) of 26,27-^{3}H-labeled 25-HCC (peak IV) to deficient rats, unchanged 25-HCC is the major form circulating in the blood within a 3-hour period (Cousins *et al.*, 1970a). The intestinal mucosal cells, a D vitamin target tissue, within this time period contains primarily metabolites more polar than 25-HCC. When these cells are ruptured and separated into nuclear, mitochondrial, microsomal, and cytoplasmic (105,000 g supernatant) fractions by differential centrifugation, the nuclear fraction within 1 hour contains two major new metabolites, peak V and VI (Fig. 12), both of which are as yet unidentified. The cytoplasm, however, contains over 90% 25-HCC. On the basis of these data and the kinetic behavior

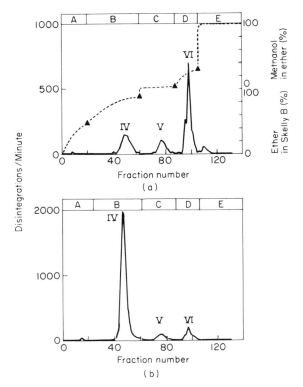

FIG. 12. Silicic acid chromatography of lipid extracts of nuclear and cytoplasmic fractions of intestinal mucosal cells after administration of 0.25μg of [26,27-³H]-25-HCC (Peak IV) to vitamin D-deficient rats. (a) Nuclei: 60 minutes; (b) cytoplasm, 60 minutes. (——) Radioactivity and (- - -) gradient. [Taken from Cousins *et al.* (1970a) with the permission of the publisher.]

of these metabolic interrelationships the hypothesis was proposed that the nucleus is the site of 25-HCC metabolism (Cousins and DeLuca, 1970; Cousins *et al.*, 1970a). The peak V metabolite has subsequently been shown to originate in the kidney (Fraser and Kodicek, 1970; Gray *et al.*, 1971) and will be discussed later. These metabolic events are especially important since they occur before any physiological manifestation of 25-HCC action. Lawson and associates (1969a,b) and Myrtle and associates (1970) have obtained similar results with chicks given [³H]-vitamin D₃, and recently Fraser and Kodicek (1970) and Gray *et al.* (1971) have confirmed these results with chicks using ³H-labeled 25-HCC. Lawson and co-workers (1969b) noted a nearly complete loss of ³H in a metabolite (designated as peak P) localized in intestinal mucosal cell nuclei which is more polar than 25-HCC formed following administration of a mixture of [4-^{14}C]- and [1-^{3}H]-vitamin D$_3$. They have proposed the ^{3}H loss and increased polarity of peak *P* indicates the addition of one oxygen function at the C$_1$ of the A ring and a C$_1$ ketone derivative of 25-HCC has been suggested as a probable structure (Kodicek, 1971). While several molecular structures and rearrangements could account for the tritium loss, the phenomenon has been verified by Haussler *et al.* (1970) and Omdahl *et al.* (1971).

It has been established (Ponchon and DeLuca, 1969b) that the circulating level of 25-HCC in rats after a 10 IU pulse of vitamin D$_3$ is approximately 1 IU; hence, further metabolic experiments were conducted with 0.025 μg (1.4 IU) of [^{3}H]-25-HCC. In these experiments the mucosal cell nuclei (Fig. 13) show *in vivo* accumulation of the polar peak V metabolite as early as 1 hour after administration of ^{3}H 25-HCC. An interesting aspect of these experiments is that an even more polar metabolite (peak VI) appears rapidly then decreases as peak V accumulates (Cousins *et al.*, 1970b). As an explanation of these data the hypothesis was advanced that 25-HCC constitutes the circulating or hormonal form of vitamin D while polar metabolites are the metabolically active forms (Cousins and DeLuca, 1970a; Cousins *et al.*, 1970b).

If the above hypothesis is tenable metabolites derived from 25-HCC should exist in bone, a second target of action, as well as intestine.

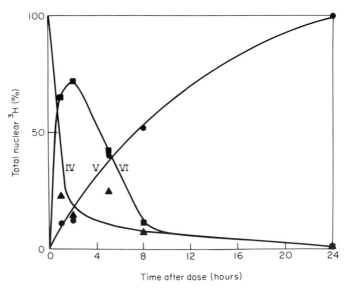

FIG. 13. Appearance of metabolites in intestinal mucosal nuclei following administration of 0.025 μg of [26,27-^{3}H]-25-HCC (Peak IV) to vitamin D-deficient rats. [Taken from Cousins *et al.* (1970b) with the permission of the publisher.]

Fresh marrow-free bone (femur and tibia) was found to contain such a metabolite (peak V) (Fig. 14) as well as a nonpolar metabolite (peak I) (Cousins *et al.*, 1970b).

Peak I is undoubtedly an ester of 25-HCC. Esters of vitamin D have been found in bone and possibly 25-HCC is also a substrate for the enzyme system involved in this formation. The significance of esterification in bone is not known, but vitamin D esters are biologically active and may contribute to overall utilization and storage of the D vitamins (Fraser and Kodicek, 1969).

A peak VI metabolite has not been detected in the chloroform phase of bone extractions as was observed in the intestine. Alternate bone extraction methods have also failed to yield such a metabolite (Cousins and DeLuca, 1970b). The reason for this difference is not known at the present time. Nevertheless, the appearance of peak V in bone in response to 0.025 μg of 25-HCC well before bone mobilization is induced in hypocalcemic rats with a 2.5 μg dose is evident and indicates the peak V could be of functional significance.

Peak V metabolites have also been found in plasma, liver, and kidney; however, products of 25-HCC metabolism are most evident at early time periods in the intestine (Cousins *et al.*, 1970b). Fraser and Kodicek (1970) have recently suggested the functional, more polar metabolites

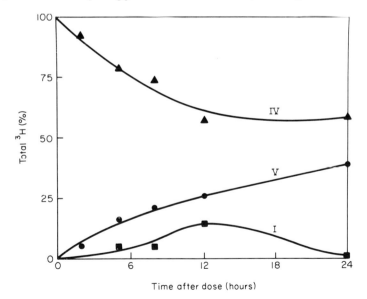

FIG. 14. Appearance of metabolites, peak I and peak V, in bone from vitamin D-deficient rats administered a 0.025-μg dose of [26,27-³H]-25-HCC (Peak IV). [Taken from Cousins *et al.* (1970b) with the permission of the publisher.]

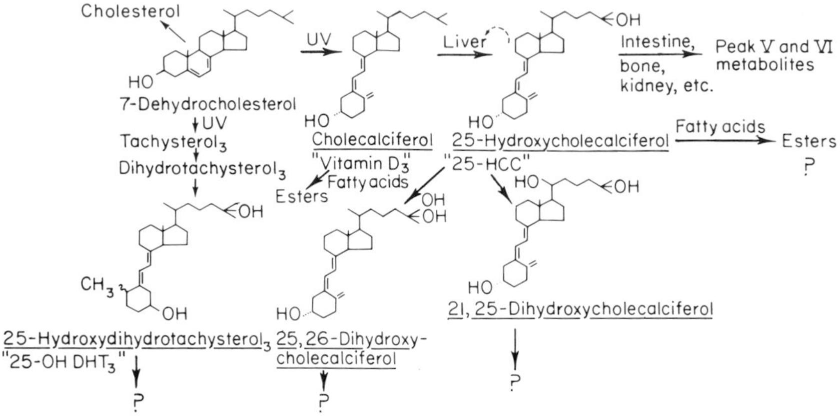

FIG. 15. Chemical and biosynthetic relationships of the D vitamins derived from 7-dehydrocholesterol. Underlined name indicates the structure has vitamin D activity. Heavy arrows indicate a known or probable metabolic conversion. Light arrows indicate a known chemical synthetic sequence. The broken arrow indicates an *in vivo* product inhibition.

in intestine are made in the kidney and are then taken up by the intestine from the plasma. Clearly the intestinal polar metabolite is formed in the kidney (Gray *et al.*, 1971), but the other peak V metabolites found elsewhere may originate elsewhere.

Recently, the peak V component of the plasma from hogs fed high levels of vitamin D_3 has been resolved into three major fractions; peaks Va, Vb, and Vc. Peaks Va and Vc have been identified as 21,25-dihydroxycholecalciferol (21,25-DHCC) (Suda *et al.*, 1970b) and 25,26-dihydroxycholecalciferol (25,26-DHCC) (Suda *et al.*, 1970c), respectively. The exact significance of these compounds is as yet unknown; however, recent data to be discussed in later sections indicate these two metabolites are formed in response to large doses of vitamin D and 25-HCC, but are not the major peak V components in bone and intestinal mucosa at physiological doses. However, it is of some interest that the 21,25-DHCC has preferential biological activity in the mobilization of bone whereas the 25,26-DHCC acts preferentially on intestinal calcium transport. Figure 15 illustrates the known biosynthetic and synthetic interrelationships of the D vitamins derived from 7-dehydrocholesterol.

G. VITAMIN D_2 AND DIHYDROTACHYSTEROL

The D vitamins derived from 7-dehydrocholesterol have received the most intensive study since these are the compounds of animal origin.

However, several irradiation products of ergosterol, a fungal and plant steroid are biologically active and are of considerable interest since for reasons of economy they now supply a large portion of the dietary intake of vitamin D for domestic animals and man. The major compound in this category is ergocalciferol (vitamin D_2) which has full biological activity in mammals but is only 10% as active as vitamin D_3 in chickens. This discrimination phenomenon in chicks has recently been studied in detail by Drescher *et al.* (1969). They found that a peak IV metabolite is formed in response to injected vitamin D_2 as in following administration of vitamin D_3; however, this metabolite is rapidly eliminated and hence is unavailable to the tissues. Peak IV derived from vitamin D_2 has been identified as 25-HEC and has a bioactivity of 60 IU/μg (Suda *et al.*, 1969, 1970a) in the rat. Assuming then that 25-HEC is the "circulating active" form of D_2 then the discrimination in chickens is explained simply as an extremely short plasma half-life of 25-HEC apparently caused by an accelerated metabolism and excretion rate (Drescher *et al.*, 1969).

Dihydrotachysterol$_2$ and dihydrotachysterol$_3$ (DHT$_2$ and DHT$_3$), irradiation and reduction products of D vitamin precursors ergosterol and 7-dehydrocholesterol, respectively, are of great importance as therapeutic agents in hypoparathyroidism, but their metabolism has not been studied

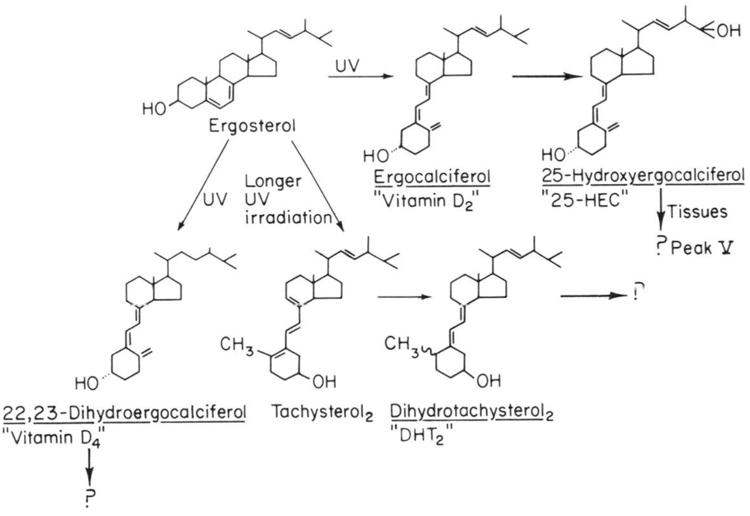

Fig. 16. Chemical and biosynthetic relationships of the D vitamins derived from ergosterol. Underlined name indicates the structure has vitamin D activity. Heavy arrows indicate a known or probable metabolic conversion. Light arrows indicate known chemical synthetic sequence.

extensively. Recently, 25-hydroxy-dihydrotachysterol$_3$ (25-OH-DHT$_3$) was synthesized (Suda *et al.*, 1970d) and found to be markedly effective on bone mobilization but ineffective as an antirachitic agent, a characteristic response to the dihydrotachysterols. Moreover, it is indeed likely that the 25-hydroxylated metabolite will be found to occur *in vivo* in response to DHT and may be the active form of both DHT$_2$ and DHT$_3$.

The low biological activity of vitamin D$_4$ and other analogs of ergosterol and 7-dehydrocholesterol plus the general lack of experimental evidence makes further consideration of them fruitless especially since many excellent monographs and reviews are available on the subject (Fieser and Fieser, 1959; DeLuca, 1970a). We have illustrated the various known biosynthetic and synthetic interrelationships of the D vitamins derived from ergosterol in Fig. 16.

VI. Mechanism of Vitamin D Action on Calcium Absorption

A. Dose–Response Time Lag

DeLuca (1967, 1969) has repeatedly emphasized a lag of at least 10 hours exists between intravenous administration of vitamin D$_3$ and a measurable stimulation of calcium transport (Morii *et al.*, 1967). Since the complete physiological mechanism involved in vitamin D-induced calcium absorption by the small intestine is not known, the reasons for the lag are only partially known.

The time lag cannot be explained by a delay in uptake of the vitamin by the small intestine (Neville and DeLuca, 1966), since ^{3}H-vitamin D, administered either orally or intravenously, is rapidly taken up by the intestine and retained there at a nearly constant level for at least 30 hours. The prerequisite for the metabolic transformation of vitamin D into 25-hydroxylated derivatives prior to physiological action does, however, partially explain the lag (Fig. 17), but, nevertheless, 3–4 hours are still required for 25-HCC to induce active transport.

As stated in an earlier section, the most widely accepted model for the vitamin D-stimulated process is the assembly of an active, carrier-mediated transport system. Harrison and Harrison (1965) have suggested vitamin D merely increases the permeability of the small intestine making the calcium available to a carrier transport system. The fact that actinomycin D blocks the calcium transport effect of vitamin D but not its effect on calcium permeability (Harrison and Harrison, 1966; Zull *et al.*, 1966) suggests protein synthesis is involved. The isolation of a calcium-binding protein (CaBP) from intestinal mucosal cells by

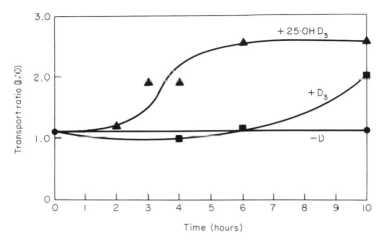

Fɪɢ. 17. Intestinal calcium transport response to 0.25 μg of either vitamin D₃ or 25-HCC.

Wasserman and co-workers (1968) indeed argues in favor of a requirement for protein synthesis. However, Drescher and DeLuca (1971a,b) have reported CaBP production in response to vitamin D is actually the conversion of a pre-CaBP to CaBP and does not require protein synthesis per se. This assembly phenomenon is undoubtedly time-consuming and therefore could add to the lag period. In this regard it should be emphasized that actinomycin D can block the conversion of 25-HCC into peak V (Tanaka and DeLuca, 1971). These data argue strongly in favor of peak V being the vitamins' "active form" in the intestine and that protein synthesis at the level of the transport system is not involved. Since peak V production is actinomycin D-sensitive, both RNA and protein synthesis are necessarily involved in this conversion step and thus would contribute to the time lag.

At this time the time lag in response to vitamin D appears attributable to four factors: (1) the absorption of dietary vitamin D by the small intestine; (2) conversion of vitamin D to its 25-hydroxy analog; (3) conversion of 25-HCC to peak V, which requires RNA and protein synthesis; and (4) the assembly of the components of the calcium transport system.

B. Calcium Absorption *in vitro*

Olson and DeLuca (1969) found that perfused intestine from a vitamin D–deficient rat maintains a low rate of calcium transport while that from a rat given vitamin D 24 hours previously transports calcium

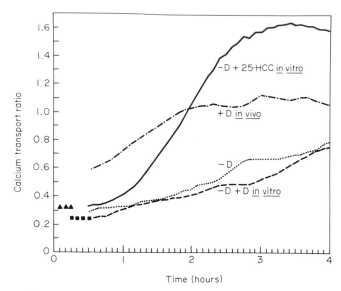

FIG. 18. Calcium transport response of isolated perfused intestine to 2.5 μg of 25-HCC or 250 μg of vitamin D₃. [Taken from Olson and DeLuca (1969) with the permission of the publisher.]

rapidly. When the vitamin is administered *in vitro* via the mesenteric artery, as much as 250 μg has little or no effect on calcium transport, while 2.5 μg of 25-HCC raises transport to +D *in vivo* levels (Fig. 18). In view of the new information available on the peak V metabolites, the calcium response *in vitro* induced by 25-HCC must also be considered as pharmacological. It is possible that large and unphysiological doses of 25-HCC may substitute directly for the peak V metabolite in the intestinal system.

Reports of a direct *in vitro* effect of unmodified vitamin D on loops of isolated small intestine have appeared (Schachter, 1963). The extremely large levels of vitamin D added to the incubations in these studies essentially preclude drawing definite conclusions as to possible physiological significance.

C. ACTINOMYCIN D INHIBITION AND RNA SYNTHESIS

A lag of 2–3 hours exists between 25-HCC administration and initiation of calcium transport. Actinomycin D given prior to, but not after, vitamin D blocks this response (Zull *et al.*, 1965, 1966; Norman, 1965). The antibiotic does not interfere with the absorption or distribution of vitamin D nor does it inhibit PTH action or cause mucosal cell damage (Zull *et al.*, 1966). This work led to the natural conclusion that the antibiotic was functioning in the expected manner, i.e., binding to the guanosine moieties of DNA (Goldberg and Reich, 1964) thus blocking the synthesis of messenger RNA (mRNA) being made in response to vitamin D.

Short-term (pulse) labeling of RNA with ^{3}H-orotic acid demonstrated that in the intestinal mucosa, nuclear, but not ribosomal, RNA synthesis was markedly enhanced by prior administration of vitamin D to deficient rats. This enhancement was maximal 3 hours after the dose (Stohs *et al.*, 1967), well before calcium transport. Similar experiments have been conducted in the chick (Norman, 1966). Ribonucleic acid synthesis was also stimulated by 25-HCC (Cousins *et al.*, 1970a). The template activity (RNA-synthesizing ability) of chromatin isolated from the intestinal mucosa of rats was shown to be stimulated when vitamin D was administered *in vivo* (Hallick and DeLuca, 1969). It was suggested that vitamin D *in vivo* "unmasks" a specific section of the DNA carrying the code for components of the calcium transport system. Recently, Tanaka and DeLuca (1971) have demonstrated that the actinomycin D-sensitive process in vitamin D action is at the level of 25-HCC metabolism rather than on the transport system per se. This was discussed before and will be again in the following section. Therefore, the exact biological reason for the stimulation of RNA synthesis in the intestine is unknown.

The subcellular localization of ^{3}H in intestinal mucosal cells from physiological doses of [^{3}H]-vitamin D_3 showed that the nucleus is the major site of accumulation. Stohs and DeLuca (1967) demonstrated with carefully purified nuclei that the outer membrane of the nucleus was the actual association site. The subcellular location of [^{3}H]-25-HCC supports this hypothesis (Cousins *et al.*, 1970a). Haussler and Norman (1969) concluded, in contrast, that the chromatin was the actual site. Both groups postulated that receptor molecules were responsible for the accumulation phenomenon. The possibility that steroid hormones bind to a specific site in target tissues, first shown experimentally by Jensen and Jacobson (1962), provided the model for the vitamin D receptor. Vitamin D analogs such as dihydrotachysterol and vitamin D itself were found to compete *in vivo* for the "receptor." The dichotomy as to the exact site of the "receptor" was finally resolved and the nuclear membrane appears to be the specific location (Chen *et al.*, 1970). Previous reports of a chromosomal receptor were ascribed to highly impure chromatin preparations. However, the physiological meaning of the subcellular location data is now uncertain since the function of the active peak V metabolite does not involve genetic machinery.

D. Metabolism of 25-HCC

The metabolism of 25-HCC in the intestinal mucosa has been considered in detail in a previous section. Numerous studies on the metabolism of [^{3}H]-vitamin D demonstrated that the metabolites more polar than the former are present in certain tissues and blood following physiological doses of the radioactive vitamin (Haussler *et al.*, 1968; Ponchon and DeLuca, 1969b; Lawson *et al.*, 1969a). Because the production of 25-HCC is closely regulated the use of [^{3}H]-25-HCC for metabolic studies beyond 25-HCC is a distinct advantage. Studies with [^{3}H]-25-HCC in two species, rat and chick, and at numerous dose levels have demonstrated that in intestine the peak V and VI metabolites appear in the mucosal cell nuclei (Cousins *et al.*, 1970a; Gray and DeLuca, 1971) much earlier than they appear in other major organs, blood serum and the cytoplasm (105,0000 g supernatant) of the mucosa. The production of peak V from 25-HCC as well as vitamin D$_3$ is blocked by prior administration of actinomycin D (Tanaka and DeLuca, 1971). Moreover, peak V is able to evoke a stimulation of intestinal calcium transport in actinomycin D-treated animals (Tanaka *et al.*, 1971). Clearly, therefore, the actinomycin D-sensitive step in the inhibition of calcium transport is at the level of the production of peak V which by analogy must be the functional metabolite (tissue active form) in this target tissue. The kidney has recently been proposed as the site of peak V production by Fraser and Kodicek (1970). These investigators found nephrectomy completely abolished the appearance of peak P (essentially synonomous with peak V) in blood plasma and intestinal mucosa. Moreover, the metabolic transformation of 25-HCC into peak P could only be detected *in vitro* in homogenates of kidney. Numerous preparations from small intestine and other tissues apparently failed to show this conversion. In the authors' laboratory, the synthesis of peak V has been clearly shown to take place in kidney tissue in confirmation of the work of Fraser and Kodicek (Gray *et al.*, 1971).

While the functional significance of the polar metabolites in vitamin D action is under study, it must be recognized that renal disease is associated with a dysfunction in calcium metabolism. Chronic renal failure, for example, has been shown to markedly affect vitamin D metabolism (Avioli *et al.*, 1968), and renal osteodystrophy (renal rickets) is characterized by hypocalcemia, a failure of bone calcification (McLean and Urist, 1968) and a failure in calcium absorption. Recently, it has been suggested that in chronic renal disease there is a failure of synthesis of peak V, the metabolite of vitamin D responsible for intestinal calcium transport, while 25-HCC, the active form in bone mineral mobilization, is made normally. Thus, the lowered calcium absorption results in transient hypocalcemia and secondary hyperparathyroidism. There is then both a failure of calcification (osteomalacia) and bone erosion by the secondary hyperparathyroidism (Gray *et al.*, 1971).

E. Calcium Absorption and Transport

There is abundant evidence that calcium is transported against an electrochemical potential gradient (Wasserman, 1963; Schachter, 1963; Martin and DeLuca, 1969a). Schachter and co-workers believed that vitamin D participates in this system by stimulating the transfer of calcium across the brush border surface of mucosal cells and also across the serosal surface. Harrison and Harrison, on the other hand, believed that the vitamin is involved only in carrier mediated permeability of intestine to calcium. Martin and DeLuca (1969a) have provided evidence that sodium ions are required for the transfer of calcium across the serosal surface while vitamin D is involved in the transfer of calcium across the mucosal surface. The latter process appears dependent upon metabolic energy and is cation oriented.

The action of vitamin D or rather its very polar metabolite (peak V) on intestine does not involve RNA synthesis but does involve the activation or assembly of calcium transport machinery.

Wasserman and Taylor (1966) demonstrated a CaBP present in the supernatant fraction of mucosal cells from vitamin D-treated chicks which was absent in rachitic chicks. This protein, which is apparently part of the calcium carrier mechanism, has been purified and studied in great detail (Wasserman and Taylor, 1968; Wasserman *et al.*, 1968). Its molecular weight is 24,000–28,000 and it selectively binds one calcium ion per protein molecule. The formation constant is highest for calcium; however, other divalent cations are able to replace calcium although less efficiently. Harmeyer and DeLuca (1969) have questioned the relationship of CaBP and calcium absorption since they found CaBP formation lags several hours behind calcium absorption. Recently, the Cornell group has reported CaBP is detectable in the goblet cells prior to calcium absorption when a sensitive immunoassay technique is employed (Taylor and Wasserman, 1969). Drescher and DeLuca (1971a,b) have isolated from rat intestine the CaBP which has a molecular weight of 8,200. Its formation in response to vitamin D appears to involve conversion of a preexisting protein to the CaBP.

A calcium-dependent adenosinetriphosphatase (ATPase) appears in the brush borders of intestinal mucosa from rats and chicks given vitamin D (Martin *et al.*, 1969; Melancon and DeLuca, 1970). Moreover, there is a good correlation between appearance of the Ca-ATPase and calcium absorption (Melancon and DeLuca, 1970). The presence of this enzyme would presumably couple the energy of ATP to the transport process (Martin and DeLuca, 1969a). The exact relationship of the CaBP, ATPase, and other intestinal enzymes reportedly stimulated by vitamin D (Taylor and Wasserman, 1970; Nagode *et al.*, 1970) in the transport mechanism is as yet unknown, but very likely the CaBP and ATPase are in some way intimately associated in the transport process.

F. Model of Vitamin D Action in the Intestine

Figure 19 diagrammatically summarizes the current working model of the action of vitamin D in bringing about its physiological action in the intestine. Vitamin D_3, derived either from ultraviolet irradiation of 7-dehydrocholesterol in the skin or directly from the diet, is hydroxylated at the C-25 position in the liver via a product-inhibited enzymic system. This step is an important control site responsible for the secretion of 25-HCC into the plasma. The exact metabolic fate of 25-HCC as it circulates in the plasma bound to a specific protein(s) is not fully delineated. The best evidence suggests it is picked up by virtually all tissues; however, the kidney is able to convert it into a polar metabolite (peak V) which loses a ^{3}H when labeled in the carbon-1 position. This metabolite is sequestered by the mucosal cells of the small intestine. This polar metabolite (presumably the tissue active form of vitamin D in calcium transport) then triggers the steps leading to calcium transport. The peak V metabolite is able to elicit a positive calcium absorptive response in actinomycin D-treated animals suggesting

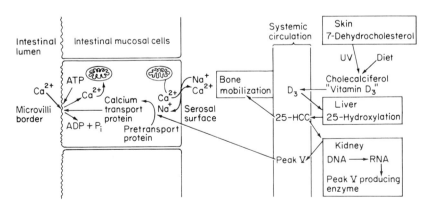

FIG. 19. Model of vitamin D action on the calcium transport system in the intestinal mucosa.

(1) RNA synthesis is not directly involved and the metabolite actually induces an assembly of transport components, and (2) the actinomycin D-sensitive step is in the conversion of 25-HCC to the polar metabolite by the kidney.

The transport protein or proteins appear at the brush border surface of the intestinal cell. Adenosine triphosphate then energizes the transfer of calcium from the intestinal lumen across the plasma membrane to the cell cytoplasm. Presumably the calcium-dependent ATPase system is involved at this step. Calcium ion interacts with the mitochondria in the area of the cytoplasm adjacent to the mucosal surface while calcium ion leaves the mitochondria near the serosal surface because of the low calcium concentration in this region. At the serosal surface a sodium gradient brings about the expulsion of calcium into the extracellular fluid in exchange for sodium. The sodium-potassium ATPase system maintains the high extracellular sodium concentration necessary for the transfer.

The model proposed in Fig. 19, which has changed dramatically in less than a year, will undoubtedly be drastically modified in the future, but nevertheless it is the most logical concept consistent with all the data available to us.

VII. Mechanism of Vitamin D Action on Bone Mineral Metabolism

A. GENERAL CONSIDERATIONS

The mechanism of vitamin D action on bone has not received the widespread attention afforded the intestinal system. Undoubtedly, the difficulty in obtaining homogeneous cell populations from calcified tissues is a major handicap in this area of investigation. The effect of vitamin D on the mobilization of bone mineral at a physiological level is clear; however, an effect on enhanced deposition of mineral into bone lacks firm experimental evidence.

B. VITAMIN D METABOLISM IN BONE

Bone mineral resorption lags at least 8 hours after administration of vitamin D_3 to deficient rats on a low calcium diet (DeLuca, 1969). As has been stated earlier, physiological doses of [³H]-vitamin D_3 are quickly taken up by virtually all tissues including bone (Neville and DeLuca, 1966). Vitamin D or metabolites thereof have been detected in bone very rapidly following [³H]-vitamin D administration (Neville and DeLuca, 1966), demonstrating that the lag could not result from a lag in transport and assimilation of the vitamin. Since the time lag is 4 hours shorter when 25-HCC is given instead of vitamin D, at least a portion of the lag following vitamin D results from the necessity for hepatic catalyzed synthesis of 25-HCC (Fig. 20) (Blunt *et al.*, 1968b).

Lipid extracts of minced marrow-free bone yield many polar metabolites of vitamin D_3 and 25-HCC as well as esters of both compounds (Ponchon and DeLuca, 1969b). After administration of [^{3}H]-25-HCC to hypocalcemic rats a peak V metabolite fraction appears (Cousins *et al.*, 1970b), which is now known to be a mixture of metabolites including 21,25-DHCC and the unidentified metabolite also present in the intestine (Holick and DeLuca, 1971b). Lawson and co-workers (1969a) found that in rachitic chick bone the ^{3}H:^{14}C ratio of a metabolite (peak *P*) in the peak V region was one-half that of the [1-^{3}H,4-^{14}C] vitamin D_3 administered. This partial loss of ^{3}H at the 1-carbon is most logically the result of a mixture of peak V metabolites in bone as mentioned above. The possible functional nature of these metabolites is not known; however, the peak V metabolite from intestine has less biological activity than 25-HCC in bone mineral mobilization (Omdahl *et al.*, 1971). In view of the finding that Fraser and Kodicek (1970) were unable to detect *in vitro* formation of polar metabolites from [^{3}H]-25-HCC with intestinal homogenates but could with kidney homogenates, it is interest-

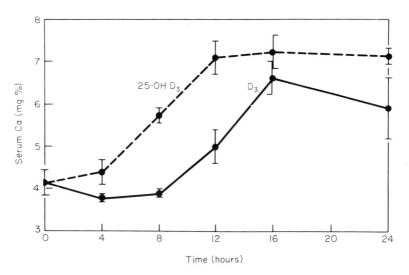

FIG. 20. Response of serum calcium level of rats on a vitamin D-deficient, low calcium diet to either 2.5 μg of vitamin D_3 or 2.5 μg of 25-HCC. [Taken from Blunt *et al.* (1968b) with the permission of the publisher.]

ing that repeated attempts to achieve the *in vitro* conversion of [³H]-25-HCC into peak V with several bone preparations also was unsuccessful (Cousins and DeLuca, 1970b).

It has been demonstrated by Carlsson and Lindquist (1955) that mobilization of bone mineral is a linear function of dose In contrast to calcium absorption which is asymptotic. Interestingly, the production of peak V bone metabolites is a dose-related phenomenon suggesting that they may play a functional role.

C. Bone Mobilization *in vitro*

It has been suggested that vitamin D is necessary for expression of PTH action on bone on the basis of the fact that vitamin D deficiency severely limits the bone resorption response to PTH thus producing hypocalcemia (Rasmussen *et al.*, 1963) with concomitant secondary hyperparathyroidism (Au and Raisz, 1965).

Using isolated cultures of fetal rat bone, Raisz (1965) found the resorption in response to PTH is reduced in medium containing serum from vitamin D-deficient animals rather than serum from normal animals. Of importance, however, is the fact that large amounts of vitamin D added directly to the cultures have given inconsistent resorption responses (Raisz, 1965; Goldhaber, 1963).

Trummel *et al.* (1969) found that resorption (measured by the release of ⁴⁵Ca previously incorporated into bone shafts of 19-day fetal bones) in response to vitamin D_2 or vitamin D_3 added directly to the cultures by several methods was not obvious during the first 3 days of culture, but there was a partial, although inconsistent, enhancement of resorption in the last half of a 6-day culture period. The media from the cultures treated with vitamin D_3 was biologically inactive in fresh cultures indicating a chemical transformation of the vitamin had not taken place in this period. However, 25-HCC (peak IV), an active metabolite of vitamin D_3 which has been shown to occur in bone (Lund and DeLuca, 1966), does induce a substantial stimulation of bone resorption (Table II). The resorption response to 25-HCC is qualitatively comparable to purified PTH (Fig. 21). When 25-HCC and PTH are both added to cultures in amounts below which they normally are effective a synergistic resorption response is clearly observed (Table III) (Raisz and Trummel, 1971). The concentration of either 25-HCC or PTH had to be increased tenfold to manifest an equivalent response. The synergistic effect suggests that the two agents act at different cellular sites as was suggested previously (DeLuca *et al.*, 1968). Raisz and Trummel (1971) found brief exposure of the bone cultures to PTH or 25-HCC induced pro-

TABLE II
Effect of Crystalline Vitamin D₃ and 25-HCC
on Bone Resorption[a,b]

	Cumulative ^{45}Ca release (treated/control ratio)	
Treatment	0–3 days	0–6 days
Vitamin D₃		
40 IU/ml	0.91 ± 0.06	0.93 ± 0.06
320 IU/ml	0.99 ± 0.07	1.24 ± 0.17
25-HCC		
9 IU/ml	1.31 ± 0.10^{c}	1.43 ± 0.10^{c}
18 IU/ml	1.33 ± 0.12^{c}	1.65 ± 0.21^{c}

[a] The shafts of the radius and of the ulna were dissected from 19-day fetal rats taken from mothers that had been injected with 0.5 mCi of ^{45}Ca on the previous day. The bones were cultured at 37°C in a chemically defined medium [BGJ with 1 mg/ml bovine serum albumin (fraction V)] and gassed with 5% CO_2, 20% O_2, and 75% N_2. 25-HCC and crystalline vitamin D₃ were added in ethanol, and test and control media were adjusted to contain 1% ethanol. Values are given as mean ± SE for four pairs of cultures.

[b] Reproduced from Raisz and Trummel (1971) with the kind permission of the University of Wisconsin Press.

[c] Significantly different from 1.0, $P < 0.05$.

longed resorptive responses indicative of osteoclastic or fibroblastic proliferation. These workers reasoned that since similar cell changes occur in response to both agents, which presumably act at different sites, a common secondary factor may be involved. Cyclic 3′,5′-adenosine monophosphate production (Raisz et al., 1968) and calcium ion translocation (Raisz and Trummel, 1971) have both been suggested as the intermediary factor. The latter phenomenon, which had been suggested previously (Zull et al., 1966), is most attractive. Calcitonin which inhibits PTH-induced in vitro resorption also blocks 25-HCC-induced resorption (Fig. 22) (Trummel et al., 1969); however, preliminary evidence suggests hydrocortisone inhibits PTH-induced but not 25-HCC-induced resorption (Raisz and Trummel, 1971).

Bone, when perfused by an in vivo technique has been shown to respond to high doses of vitamin D (Van Nguyen and Jowsey, 1970). Bone formation was found to be markedly increased while resorption remained essentially unchanged in response to 500 μg of vitamin D₃

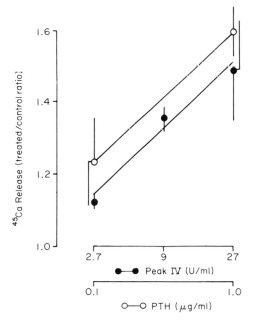

Fig. 21. Effect of 25-HCC (Peak IV) or parathyroid hormone on ^{45}Ca release from fetal rat bone in tissue culture.

TABLE III

SYNERGISTIC EFFECT OF LOW DOSES OF PTH AND 25-HCC
ON BONE RESORPTION[a,b]

Treatment	Cumulative ^{45}Ca release (treated/control ratio)	
	0–2 days	0–4 days
PTH (0.03 μg/ml)	1.03 ± 0.13	1.04 ± 0.05
25-HCC (0.015 μg/ml)	0.96 ± 0.04	0.96 ± 0.07
PTH (0.03 μg/ml) + 25-HCC (0.015 μg/ml)	1.45 ± 0.16[c]	1.75 ± 0.28[c]

[a] For procedure, see footnote a to Table II. Values are given as mean ± SE for four pairs of cultures.

[b] Reproduced from Raisz and Trummel (1971) with the kind permission of the University of Wisconsin Press.

[c] Significantly different from 1.0, $P < 0.05$.

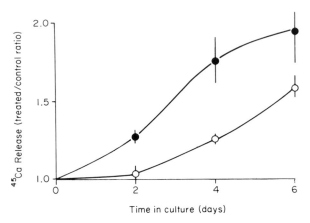

Fɪɢ. 22. Effect of purified calcitonin (CT) on the stimulation of ^{45}Ca release from fetal rat bone by 25-HCC (peak IV) in tissue culture: (●) 9 IU/ml/control and (○) 9 IU/ml plus TCT 0.3 μg/ml control. [Taken from Trummel *et al.* (1969) with the permission of the publisher.]

per kilogram of body weight infused over a 4-hour period. The use of high, unphysiological doses in this experiment precludes any hypothesis regarding the possible role of unmodified vitamin D in bone formation although this has been suggested (Raisz and Trummel, 1971).

D. Enzyme Changes and Vitamin D Deficiency

Numerous investigators have proposed that various enzymatic changes in bone are directly controlled by vitamin D or are in some way involved in the vitamins' mode of action. Meyer and Kunin (1969) have proposed that the glycolytic enzymes of rat epiphyseal cartilage are regulated by vitamin D *in vivo*. Bone alkaline phosphatase activity is enhanced in deficient animals administered vitamin D (Wergedal, 1969; Menzel *et al.*, 1970). Collagen biosynthesis has also been reported to be stimulated *in vivo* by administration of vitamin D (Canas *et al.*, 1969). As yet, however, the enzymic changes brought on by vitamin D deficiency have been generally considered to be secondary rather than primary effects.

E. Model for Vitamin D Action on Bone

It is difficult to provide a model broad enough to encompass all available experimental data involving vitamin D and bone. The effect of

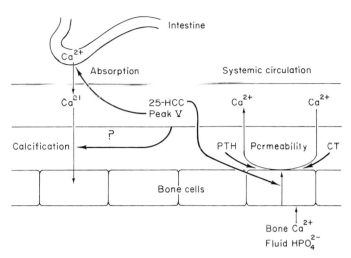

Fig. 23. Model of vitamin D action on the mechanisms that regulate the mineralization of bone.

the vitamin and its metabolites on bone mineral mobilization is clear. It undoubtedly involves specific protein synthesis of some step inasmuch as mobilization is blocked by prior administration of actinomycin D. Numerous metabolites of vitamin D including 25-HCC, 21,25-DHCC, and an unidentified peak V metabolite are all present in bone extracts. Thus, the "active" metabolite in bone is not as yet known although more than one metabolite may be involved in synergistic mechanisms within bone cells. Parathyroid hormone and CT act to increase and decrease, respectively, the bone extracellular fluid permeability barrier. The direct participation of vitamin D in the calcification process is not supported experimentally but has not been ruled out either. The model shown in Fig. 23 is speculative in nature but attempts to explain existing data on the molecular basis of vitamin D action on bone.

References

Albright, F., Butler, A. M., and Bloomberg, E. (1937). *Amer. J. Dis. Child.* **54**, 529.

Arnaud, C., Rasmussen, H., and Arnast, C. (1966). *J. Clin. Invest.* **45**, 1955.

Askew, F. A., Bourdillon, R. B., Bruce, H. M., Jenkins, R. G., and Webster, T. A. (1930). *Proc. Roy. Soc., Ser. B* **107**, 76.

Association of Official Analytical Chemists (1966). "Official Methods of Analysis," Ass. Offic. Anal. Chem., Washington, D.C.

Au, W. Y., and Raisz, L. G. (1965). *Amer. J. Physiol.* **206**, 637.

Avioli, L. V., and Lee, S. W. (1966). *Anal. Biochem.* **16**, 193.

Avioli, L. V., Lee, S. W., McDonald, J. E., Lund, J., and DeLuca, H. F. (1967a). *J. Clin. Invest.* **46**, 983.

Avioli, L. V., Williams, T., Lund, J., and DeLuca, H. F. (1967b). *J. Clin. Invest.* **46**, 1907.

Avioli, L. V., Birge, S., Lee, S. W., and Slatopolsky, E. (1968). *J. Clin. Invest.* **47**, 2239.

Balsan, S. (1970a). Personal communication.

Balsan, S. (1970b). *Calcif. Tissue Res.* **4**, Suppl., 45.

Bauer, G. C., Carlsson, A., and Lindquist, B. (1955). *Kgl. Fysiogr. Sallsk. Lund, Foerh.* **25**, 1.

Baylink, D., Stauffer, M., Wergedal, J., and Rich, C. (1970). *J. Clin. Invest.* **49**, 1122.

Bligh, E. G., and Dyer, W. J. (1959). *Can. J. Biochem. Physiol.* **37**, 911.

Blunt, J. W., and DeLuca, H. F. (1969). *Biochemistry* **8**, 671.

Blunt, J. W., DeLuca, H. F., and Schnoes, H. K. (1968a). *Biochemistry* **7**, 3317.

Blunt, J. W., Tanaka, Y., and DeLuca, H. F. (1968b). *Proc. Nat. Acad. Sci. U. S.* **61**, 1503.

Bringe, A. N., Jorgenson, N. A., and DeLuca, H. F. (1970). Unpublished results.

Bronner, F. (1964). *In* "Mineral Metabolism" (C. L. Comar and F. Bronner, eds.), Vol. 2, Part 2A, p. 342. Academic Press, New York.

Canas, F., Brand, J. S., Neuman, W. F., and Terepka, A. R. (1969). *Amer. J. Physiol.* **216**, 1092.

Carlsson, A. (1952). *Acta Physiol. Scand.* **26**, 212.

Carlsson, A., and Lindquist, B. (1955). *Acta Physiol. Scand.* **35**, 53.

Chen, T. C., Weber, J. C., and DeLuca, H. F. (1970). *J. Biol. Chem.* **245**, 3776.

Cousins, R. J., and DeLuca, H. F. (1970a). *In* "Symposium Proceedings—The Biochemistry, Metabolism and Chemical Analysis of Vitamin D and Related Compounds," pp. 21–37. Ass. Vitam. Chem., Chicago, Illinois.

Cousins, R. J., and DeLuca, H. F. (1970b). Unpublished results.

Cousins, R. J., DeLuca, H. F., Suda, T., Chen, T., and Tanaka, Y. (1970a). *Biochemistry* **9**, 1453.

Cousins, R. J., DeLuca, H. F., and Gray, R. W. (1970b). *Biochemistry* **9**, 3649.

Crowfoot, D., and Dunitz, J. D. (1948). *Nature (London)* **162**, 608.

DeLuca, H. F. (1967). *Vitam. Horm. (New York)* **25**, 315.

DeLuca, H. F. (1969). *Fed. Proc., Fed. Amer. Soc. Exp. Biol.* **28**, 1678.

DeLuca, H. F. (1970a). *In* "The International Encyclopedia of Pharmacology and Therapeutics" (H. Rasmussen, ed.), pp. 101–329. Pergamon, Oxford.

DeLuca, H. F. (1970b). *In* "Symposium Proceedings—The Biochemistry, Metabolism and Chemical Analysis of Vitamin D and Related Compounds," pp. 1–20. Ass. Vitam. Chem., Chicago, Illinois.

DeLuca, H. F., and Avioli, L. V. (1970). *Arch. Intern. Med.* **126**, 896.

DeLuca, H. F., Morii, H., and Melancon, M. J. (1968). *In* "Parathyroid Hormone and Thyrocalcitonin (Calcitonin)" (R. V. Talmage and L. F. Bélanger, eds.), Int. Congr. Ser. No. 159, p. 448. Excerpta Med. Found., Amsterdam.

Drescher, D., and DeLuca, H. F. (1971a). *Biochemistry* **10**, 2302.

Drescher, D, and DeLuca, H. F. (1971b). *Biochemistry* **10**, 2308.

Drescher, D., DeLuca, H. F., and Imrie, M. H. (1969). *Arch. Biochem. Biophys.* **130**, 657.

Earp, H. S., Ney, R. L., Gitelman, H. J., Richman, R., and DeLuca, H. F. (1970). *N. Engl. J. Med.* **283**, 627.

Edlund, D. O., Aufinsen, J. R., Filippini, F. A., and Hendershot, W. F. (1970). *In* "Symposium Proceedings—The Biochemistry, Metabolism and Chemical Analysis of Vitamin D and Related Compounds," pp. 44–65. Ass. Vitam. Chem., Chicago, Illinois.

Fanconi, G. (1950). *Bone Struct. Metab., Ciba Found. Symp.*, 1955 p. 187.

Fieser, L. F., and Fieser, M. (1959). *In* "Steroids," pp. 90–169. Reinhold, New York.

Folch, J., Lees, M., and Sloan-Stanley, G. H. (1957). *J. Biol. Chem.* **226**, 497.

Fourman, P., Royer, P., Level, M. J., and Morgan, D. B. (1968). "Calcium Metabolism and the Bone." Blackwell, Oxford.

Fraser, D. R., and Kodicek, E. (1969). *Brit. J. Nutr.* **23**, 135.

Fraser, D. R., and Kodicek, E. (1970). *Nature (London)* **228**, 764.

Funk, C. (1912). *J. State Med.* **20**, 341.

Glisson, F. (1650). "DeRachitide." London.

Goldberg, I. H., and Reich, E. (1964). *Fed. Proc., Fed. Amer. Soc. Exp. Biol.* **23**, 958.

Goldhaber, P. (1963). *In* "Mechanisms of Hard Tissue Destruction," Publ. No. 75, p. 609. Amer. Ass. Advance, Sci., Washington, D.C.

Goldstein, A., Aronow, L., and Kalman, S. M. (1968). "Principles of Drug Action." Harper, New York.

Graham, J. B., McFalls, V. W., and Winters, R. W. (1959). *Amer. J. Hum. Genet.* **11**, 311.

Gran, F. C. (1960). *Acta Physiol. Scand.* **50**, 132.

Gray, R. W., and DeLuca, H. F. (1971). *Arch. Biochem. Biophys.* **145**, 276.

Gray, R. W., Boyle, I., and DeLuca, H. F. (1971). *Science* **172**, 1232.

Greaves, J. D., and Schmidt, C. L. (1933). *J. Biol. Chem.* **102**, 101.

Guyton, A. C. (1966). "Textbook of Medical Physiology," 3rd ed. Saunders, Philadelphia, Pennsylvania.

Hallick, R. B., and DeLuca, H. F. (1969). *Proc. Nat. Acad. Sci. U. S.* **63**, 528.

Harmeyer, J., and DeLuca, H. F. (1969). *Arch. Biochem. Biophys.* **133**, 247.

Harris, L. J. (1956). *In* "The Biochemistry and Physiology of Bone" (G. H. Bourne, ed.), 1st ed., p. 608. Academic Press, New York.

Harrison, H. E., and Harrison, H. C. (1941). *J. Clin. Invest.* **20**, 47.

Harrison, H. E., and Harrison, H. C. (1960). *Amer. J. Physiol.* **199**, 265.

Harrison, H. E., and Harrison, H. C. (1961). *Amer. J. Physiol.* **201**, 1007.

Harrison, H. E., and Harrison, H. C. (1964). *Metab., Clin. Exp.* **13**, 952.

Harrison, H. E., and Harrison, H. C. (1965). *Amer. J. Physiol.* **208**, 370.

Harrison, H. E., and Harrison, H. C. (1966). *Proc. Soc. Exp. Biol. Med.* **121**, 312.

Harrison, H. E., Harrison, H. C., and Park, E. A. (1958). *Amer. J. Physiol.* **192**, 432.

Harrison, H. E., Lifshitz, F., and Blizzard, R. M. (1967). *N. Engl. J. Med.* **276**, 894.

Haussler, M. R., and Norman, A. W. (1969). *Proc. Nat. Acad. Sci. U. S.* **62**, 155.

Haussler, M. R., Myrtle, J. F., and Norman, A. W. (1968). *J. Biol. Chem.* **243**, 4055.

Haussler, M. R., Littledike, E. T., Boyce, D. W., and Rasmussen, H. (1970). *Fed. Proc., Fed. Amer. Soc. Exp. Biol.* **29**, 368 (abstr.).

Hess, A. F., and Weinstock, M. (1924). *J. Biol. Chem.* **62**, 301.

Hess, A. F., Weinstock, M., and Helman, F. D. (1925). *J. Biol. Chem.* **63**, 305.

Heymann, W. (1937). *J. Biol. Chem.* **122**, 249.

Hioco, D., Miravet, L., and Bordier, P. (1970). *Calcif. Tissue Res.* 4 Suppl., 47.

Holick, M., and DeLuca, H. F. (1970). Unpublished data.

Holick, M., and DeLuca, H. F. (1971a). *J. Lipid Res.* **12**, 460.

Holick, M., and DeLuca, H. F. (1971b). Manuscript in preparation.

Hopkins, F. G. (1912). *J. Physiol. (London)* **44**, 425.

Horsting, M., and DeLuca, H. F. (1969). *Biochem. Biophys. Res. Commun.* **36**, 251.

Horsting, M., and DeLuca, H. F. (1971). Manuscript in preparation.

Howland, J., and Kramer, B. (1921). *Amer. J. Dis. Child.* **22**, 105.

Huldschinsky, S. (1919). *Deut. Med. Wochenschr.* **45**, 712.

Jensen, E. V., and Jacobson, H. I. (1962). *Recent Progr. Horm. Res.* **18**, 387.

Kodicek, E. (1955). *Biochem. J.* **60**, XXV.

Kodicek, E. (1959). *Proc. Int. Congr. Biochem., 4th, 1958* Vol. 1, p. 198.

Kodicek, E. (1971). *In* "The Fat Soluble Vitamins" (H. F. DeLuca and J. W. Suttie, eds.), pp. 81–91. Univ. of Wisconsin Press, Madison.

Kodicek, E., and Thompson, G. A. (1965). *In* "Structure and Function of Connective and Skeletal Tissue" (S. F. Jackson *et al.*, eds.), pp. 369–372. Butterworth, London.

Lawson, D. E., Wilson, P. W., and Kodicek, E. (1969a). *Nature (London)* **222**, 171.

Lawson, D. E., Wilson, P. W., and Kodicek, E. (1969b). *Biochem. J.* **115**, 269.

Lengemann, F. W., Wasserman, R. H., and Comar, C. L. (1959). *J. Nutr.* **68**, 443.

Lund, J., and DeLuca, H. F. (1966). *J. Lipid Res.* **7**, 739.

Lund, J., DeLuca, H. F., and Horsting, M. (1967). *Arch. Biochem. Biophys.* **120**, 513.

McCollum, E. V., and Davis, M. (1913). *J. Biol. Chem.* **15**, 167.

McCollum, E. V., Simmonds, N., Shipley, P. G., and Park, E. A. (1922a). *J. Biol. Chem.* **51**, 41.

McCollum, E. V., Simmonds, N., Becker, J. E., and Shipley, P. G. (1922b). *J. Biol. Chem.* **53**, 253.

McCollum, E. V., Simmonds, N., Becker, J. E., and Shipley, P. G. (1922c). *Johns Hopkins Hosp., Bull.* **33**, 229.

McLean, F. C., and Urist, M. R. (1968). "Bone," 3rd ed. Univ. of Chicago, Press, Chicago.

Malm, O. J. (1963). *In* "The Transfer of Calcium and Strontium Across Biological Membranes" (R. H. Wasserman, ed.), p. 143. Academic Press, New York.

Martin, D. L., and DeLuca, H. F. (1969a). *Arch. Biochem. Biophys.* **134**, 139.

Martin, D. L., and DeLuca, H. F. (1969b). *Amer. J. Physiol.* **216**, 1351.

Martin, D. L., Melancon, M. J., and DeLuca, H. F. (1969). *Biochem. Biophys. Res. Commun.* **35**, 819.

Maynard, L. A., and Lossli, J. K. (1962). "Animal Nutrition," 5th ed. McGraw-Hill, New York.

Melancon, M. J., and DeLuca, H. F. (1970). *Biochemistry* **9**, 1658.

Mellanby, E. (1919a). *J. Physiol. (London)* **52**, lili.

Mellanby, E. (1919b). *Lancet* **196**, 407.

Menzel, J., Eilon, G., Klien, T., and Tishbee, A. (1970). *Calcif. Tissue Res.* **4**, Suppl., 51.

Meyer, W. L., and Kunin, A. S. (1969). *Arch. Biochem. Biophys.* **129**, 438.

Morii, H., and DeLuca, H. F. (1967). *Amer. J. Physiol.* **213**, 358.

Morii, H., Lund, J., Neville, P., and DeLuca, H. F. (1967). *Arch. Biochem. Biophys.* **120**, 508.

Murty, T. K., Day, K. D., and Kodicek, E. (1966) *Biochem. J.* **98**, 293.

Myrtle, J. F., Haussler, M. R., and Norman, A. W. (1970). *J. Biol. Chem.* **245**, 1190.

Nagode, L. A., Haussler, M. R., Boyce, D. W., Pechet, M., and Rasmussen, H. (1970). *Fed. Proc., Fed. Amer. Soc. Exp. Biol.* **29**, 368 (abstr.).

Nair, P. P., and deLeon, S. (1968). *Arch. Biochem. Biophys.* **128**, 663.

Neuman, W. F. (1958). *AMA Arch. Pathol.* **66**, 204.

Neuman, W. F., and Neuman, M. W. (1958). "The Chemical Dynamics of Bone Mineral." Univ. of Chicago Press, Chicago.

Neville, P. F., and DeLuca, H. F. (1966). *Biochemistry* **5**, 2201.

Nicolaysen, R. (1937). *Biochem. J.* **31**, 122.

Nicolaysen, R., and Eeg-Larsen, N. (1953). *Vitam. Horm. (New York)* **11**, 29.

Nicolaysen, R., and Eeg-Larsen, N. (1956). *Bone Struct. Metab., Ciba Found. Symp., 1955* pp. 175–184.

Norman, A. W. (1965). *Science* **149**, 185.

Norman, A. W. (1966). *Biochem. Biophys. Res. Commun.* **23**, 335.

Norman, A. W., and DeLuca, H. F. (1963). *Biochemistry* **2**, 1160.

Olson, E. B., and DeLuca, H. F. (1969). *Science* **165**, 405.

Omdahl, J., Holick, M., Suda, T., Tanaka, Y., and DeLuca, H. F. (1971). *Biochemistry* **10**, 2935.

Orr, W. J., Holt, L. E., Jr., Wilkens, L., and Boone, F. H. (1923). *Amer. J. Dis. Child.* **26**, 362.

Osborne, T. B., and Mendel, L. B. (1913a). *J. Biol. Chem.* **15**, 311.

Osborne, T. B., and Mendel, L. B. (1913b). *J. Biol. Chem.* **16**, 423.

Oser, B. L. (1965). "Hawk's Physiological Chemistry," 14th ed. McGraw-Hill, New York.

Pak, C. Y., DeLuca, H. F., Chavez de los Rios, J. M., Suda, T., Ruskin, B., and Delea, C. S. (1970). *Arch. Intern. Med.* **126**, 239.

Palm, T. A. (1890). *Practitioner* **45**, 270.

Pechet, M. M., Bobadilla, E., Carroll, E. L., and Hesse, R. H. (1967). *Amer. J. Med.* **43**, 696.

Ponchon, G., and DeLuca, H. F. (1969a). *J. Clin. Invest.* **48**, 1273.

Ponchon, G., and DeLuca, H. F. (1969b). *J. Nutr.* **99**, 157.

Ponchon, G., Kennan, A. L., and DeLuca, H. F. (1969). *J. Clin. Invest.* **48**, 2032.

Potts, J. T., and Deftos, L. J. (1969). *In* "Duncan's Diseases of Metabolism" (P. K. Bondy and L. E. Rosenberg, eds.), 6th ed., Vol. 2, p. 957. Saunders, Philadelphia, Pennsylvania.

Raisz, L. G. (1965). *J. Clin. Invest.* **44**, 103.

Raisz, L. G., and Trummel, C. L. (1971). *In* "The Fat Soluble Vitamins" (H. F. DeLuca and J. W. Suttie, eds.), pp. 93–99. Univ. of Wisconsin Press, Madison.

Raisz, L. G., Brand, J. S., Au, W. Y., and Niemann, I. (1968). *In* "Parathyroid Hormone and Thyrocalcitonin (Calcitonin)" (R. V. Talmage and L. F. Bélanger, eds.), Int. Congr. Ser. No. 159, p. 370. Excerpta Med. Found., Amsterdam.

Raoul, Y., and Gounelle, J. C. (1958). *C. R. Acad. Sci.* **247**, 161.

Rasmussen, H., DeLuca, H. F., Arnaud, C., Hawker, C., and von Stedingk, M. (1963). *J. Clin. Invest.* **42**, 1940.

Rikkers, H., and DeLuca, H. F. (1967). *Amer. J. Physiol.* 213, 380.
Rikkers, H., Kletzien, R., and DeLuca, H. F. (1969). *Proc. Soc. Exp. Biol. Med.* 130, 1321.
Rosenheim, O., and Webster, T. A. (1925). *Lancet* 1, 1025.
Schachter, D. (1963). *In* "The Transfer of Calcium and Strontium Across Biological Membranes" (R. H. Wasserman, ed.), pp. 197–210. Academic Press, New York.
Schachter, D., and Rosen, S. M. (1959). *Amer. J. Physiol.* 196, 357.
Schachter, D., Kimberg, D. V., and Shenker, H. (1961). *Amer. J. Physiol.* 200, 1263.
Schachter, D., Finkelstein, J. D., and Kowarski, S. (1964). *J. Clin. Invest.* 43, 787.
Schenk, F. (1937). *Naturwissenschaften* 25, 159.
Sebrell, W. H., Jr., and Harris, R. S., eds. (1954). "The Vitamins," 1st ed., Vol. 2, pp. 131–266. Academic Press, New York.
Seely, J. R., and De Luca, H. F. (1970). Unpublished results.
Shipley, P. G., Kramer, B., and Howland, J. (1925). *Amer. J. Dis. Child.* 30, 37.
Shipley, P. G., Kramer, B., and Howland, J. (1926). *Biochem. J.* 35, 304.
Siegmund, O. H., ed. (1961). "The Merck Veterinary Manual," 2nd ed., pp. 538–541. Merck and Co., Rahway, New Jersey.
Steenbock, H. (1924). *Science* 60, 224.
Steenbock, H., and Black, A. (1924). *J. Biol. Chem.* 61, 405.
Steenbock, H., and Black, A. (1925). *J. Biol. Chem.* 64, 263.
Steenbock, H., and Hart, E. B. (1913). *J. Biol. Chem.* 14, 59.
Steenbock, H., and Herting, D. (1955). *J. Nutr.* 57, 449.
Stohs, S. J., and DeLuca, H. F. (1967). *Biochemistry* 6, 3328.
Stohs, S. J., Zull, J. E., and DeLuca, H. F. (1967). *Biochemistry* 6, 1304.
Suda, T., DeLuca, H. F., Schnoes, H. K., and Blunt, J. W. (1969). *Biochemistry* 8, 3515.
Suda, T., DeLuca, H. F., and Tanaka, Y. (1970a). *J. Nutr.* 100, 1049.
Suda, T., DeLuca, H. F., Schnoes, H. K., Ponchon, G., Tanaka, Y., and Holick, M. F. (1970b). *Biochemistry* 9, 2917.
Suda, T., DeLuca, H. F., Schnoes, H. K., Tanaka, Y., and Holick, M. F. (1970c). *Biochemistry* 9, 4776.
Suda, T., Hallick, R. B., DeLuca, H. F., and Schnoes, H. K. (1970d). *Biochemistry* 9, 1651.
Tanaka, Y., and DeLuca, H. F. (1971). *Proc. Nat. Acad. Sci. U. S.* 68, 605.
Tanaka, Y., DeLuca, H. F., Omdahl, J., and Holick, M. (1971). *Proc. Nat. Acad. Sci. U. S.* 68, 1286.
Taylor, A. N., and Wasserman, R. H. (1969). *Fed. Proc., Fed. Amer. Soc. Exp. Biol.* 28, 759 (abstr.).
Taylor, A. N., and Wasserman, R. H. (1970). *Fed. Proc., Fed. Amer. Soc. Exp. Biol.* 29, 368 (abstr.).
Thomas, J. W., Okamoto, M., and Moore, L. A. (1954). *J. Dairy Sci.* 37, 1220.
Trummel, C. L., Raisz, L. G., Blunt, J. W., and DeLuca, H. F. (1969). *Science* 163, 1450.
U. S. Pharmacopoeia, (1955). 14th rev., pp. 889–892. Mack Publ., Easton, Pennsylvania.
U. S. Pharmacopoeia, (1965). 17th rev., pp. 891–894. Mack Publ., Easton, Pennsylvania.

Van Nguyen, V., and Jowsey, J. (1970). *J. Bone Joint Surg., Amer. Vol.* **52**, 1041.

Waddell, J. (1934). *J. Biol. Chem.* **105**, 711.

Wasserman, R. H. (1963). *In* "The Transfer of Calcium and Strontium Across Biological Membranes" (R. H. Wasserman, ed.), pp. 211–228. Academic Press, New York.

Wasserman, R. H. (1971). *In* "The Fat Soluble Vitamins" (H. F. DeLuca and J. W. Suttie, eds.), pp. 21–37. Univ. of Wisconsin Press, Madison.

Wasserman, R. H., and Taylor, A. N. (1966). *Science* **152**, 792.

Wasserman, R. H., and Taylor, A. N. (1968). *J. Biol. Chem.* **243**, 3987.

Wasserman, R. H., Corradino, R. A., and Taylor, A. N. (1968). *J. Biol. Chem.* **243**, 3978.

Wergedal, J. E. (1969). *Calcif. Tissue Res.* **3**, 67.

Whistler, D. (1645). "The Rickets," Thesis.

Windaus, A., Linsert, O., and Weidlick, G. (1932). *Juytus Liebigs Ann. Chem.* **492**, 226.

Windaus, A., Schenk, F., and von Werder, F. (1936). *Hoppe-Seyler's Z. Physiol. Chem.* **241**, 100.

Zull, J. E., Czarnowska-Misztal, E., and DeLuca, H. F. (1965). *Science* **149**, 182.

Zull, J. E., Czarnowska-Misztal, E., and DeLuca, H. F. (1966). *Proc. Nat. Acad. Sci. U. S.* **55**, 177.

CHAPTER 8

Calcitonin

D. HAROLD COPP

I. Introduction

Ionic calcium plays an important role in many cellular processes, and its concentration in body fluids is regulated with remarkable precision in higher vertebrates. The importance of the parathyroid glands in controlling this level was first postulated in 1909 (MacCallum and Voegtlin, 1909). In contrast, the existence of calcitonin, a second factor in calcium regulation, was not recognized until 1961 (Copp et al., 1961), and its association with the ultimobranchial gland was first clearly demonstrated

in 1967 (Copp *et al.*, 1967a). The progress in this field over the past
five years has been remarkably rapid. For more details concerning these
advances, reference should be made to recent reviews (Copp, 1969a,b,
1970; Hirsch and Munson, 1969; Potts and Deftos, 1969; Rasmussen
and Tenenhouse, 1970). Much valuable information is also available in
the published proceedings of the third parathyroid conference held in
1967 (Talmage and Bélanger, 1968), and of two international symposia
on calcitonin held in London, England in 1967 and 1969 (Taylor, 1968,
1970). The fourth parathyroid conference dealing with parathyroid hormone and the calcitonins was held at Chapel Hill, North Carolina in
1971 (Talmage and Munson, 1972).

II. Historical Developments

The early history of the field has been reviewed by Copp (1967),
who pointed to certain evidence prior to 1961 which indicated active
hormonal control of hypercalcemia. One such experiment carried out
in 1958 is illustrated in Fig. 1. A series of 8 dogs was perfused for
8 hours with 1 USP unit of parathyroid extract per kilogram per hour.

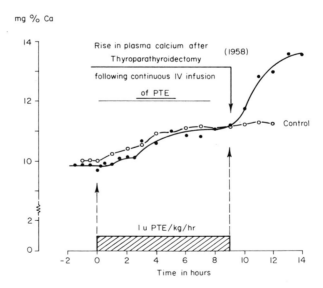

Fig. 1. Early evidence for calcitonin. Change in plasma calcium during infusion of
1 USP unit parathyroid extract (PTE)/kg/hour in dogs. Note the rapid increase in
plasma calcium which occurred after thyroparathyroidectomy (indicated by the solid
arrow). After Copp (1963).

Plasma calcium rose 1 mg% and remained at this level for several hours
after the perfusion was stopped. When the experiment was repeated
on a second series of 10 dogs and the thyroid and parathyroid glands
were removed at the end of the 6-hour perfusion of parathyroid extract
(PTE), plasma calcium rapidly rose to almost 14 mg%, suggesting that
removal of the glands had impaired control of the parathormone-induced
hypercalcemia (Copp, 1963). A similar experiment was that of Sanderson
et al. (1960). They observed that the plasma calcium returned to pre-
injection levels within a few hours after infusion of 10 mg Ca/kg/hr
into intact dogs. However, when they repeated this procedure in thyro-
parathyroidectomized dogs, the plasma calcium returned to the preinfu-
sion level very slowly, indicating impairment of the normal control.

The significance of these observations became apparent the following
year when Copp *et al.* (1961, 1962) presented evidence for a hypocalcemic hormone which was released when the isolated thyroid–parathyroid gland complex in dogs was perfused with hypercalcemic blood.
They named the hormone *calcitonin* since it was evidently involved
in regulating the level or "tone" of calcium in the body fluids. These
experiments were confirmed by Kumar *et al.* (1963). Originally thought
to come from the parathyroids, it soon became apparent that the hormone was produced primarily by cells present in the mammalian thyroid.
Hirsch *et al.* (1963, 1964) had observed that parathyroidectomy by the
Erdheim technique of hot-wire cautery caused a greater fall in plasma
calcium than that which occurred following surgical removal of the
glands. They felt that this might have resulted from release of a calci-
tonin-like substance when the glands were cauterized. They also found
that extraction of minced rat or hog thyroid with N/10 HCl isolated
a substance which had a very potent hypocalcemic and hypophos-
phatemic effect when injected into young rats. They tentatively proposed
the name *thyrocalcitonin* for this substance to indicate its thyroid origin
and possible identity with calcitonin, as indeed proved to be the case.
The importance of this work cannot be overemphasized, for it opened
the way to chemical characterization of the hormone and to its use
in physiological studies.

The thyroid origin of calcitonin was confirmed in the goat (Foster
et al., 1964a), pig (Care, 1965), and rat (Talmage *et al.*, 1965). However, it soon became apparent that the cells in the thyroid which responded to hypercalcemia were not the colloid-containing follicular cells
but were distinctive mitochondrion-rich cells (Foster *et al.*, 1964b)
which corresponded to the argyrophilic parafollicular cells described by
Nonidez (1932). Bussolati and Pearse (1967) demonstrated the localization of calcitonin in these cells by immunofluorescent techniques, and

they proposed that they be called "C" cells to indicate their role in calcitonin production. Calcitonin and C cells have subsequently been demonstrated in human thymus and parathyroid (Galante et al., 1968). Using specific staining techniques, Pearse and Carvalheira (1967) demonstrated that the C cells of the mouse thyroid were derived from the ultimobranchial body of the embryo. While these cells become embedded in the thyroid (and often in parathyroid IV) in mammals, in other vertebrates they are found in a distinct and separate ultimobranchial gland. Calcitonin is absent from the thyroid but is present in high concentrations in the ultimobranchial glands of chickens, turkeys (Copp et al., 1967a; Tauber, 1967), and dogfish sharks (Copp et al., 1967b). It is essentially an ultimobranchial hormone which is found in the thyroid and parathyroids of mammals only because of the presence within these glands of cells of ultimobranchial origin.

III. Ultimobranchial Glands and C Cells

The ultimobranchial is older than the parathyroid phylogenetically, for it is found in all jawed vertebrates including sharks and bony fishes, while the parathyroid appears first in amphibia when they change from an aquatic to a terrestrial environment (Copp, 1969c). The name *ultimobranchialer Körper* proposed by Greil (1905) is logical, for the ultimobranchial gland develops from the terminal (ultimate) branchial pouch. As shown in Fig. 2, the parathyroids develop from a similar

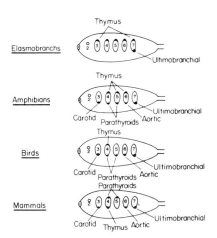

FIG. 2. Diagrammatic representation of the glandular derivatives of the branchial pouches in various classes of vertebrates. After Smith (1960).

location in the third and fourth pouch. The comparative anatomy of these structures has been reviewed by Watzka (1933), and in representative species of all classes of vertebrates they have been found to contain substantial amounts of calcitonin (Copp and Parkes, 1968).

In the thyroid, the C cells are larger than the regular follicular cells. They do not contain colloid nor free or bound iodine, nor do they respond to thyroid stimulating hormone (TSH). Many secretory granules can be demonstrated by electron micrography, and these decrease in number after a period of hypercalcemia (Matsuzawa and Kurosumi, 1967). The C cells have a number of histochemical properties in common with other cells which produce polypeptide hormones, e.g., the insulin-secreting β cells of the pancreatic islets and the adrenocorticotropic hormone- (ACTH)-producing cells of the pituitary. These properties include a high content of α-glycerophosphate dehydrogenase and cholinesterase, and the ability to synthesize and concentrate 5-hydroxytryptamine (Pearse, 1966). Pearse (1970) has suggested that these cells may all have a common origin from neuroectodermal cells of the neural crest of the embryo.

IV. Standards and Assay

Reliable standards and assay methods are essential for following hormone purification and for quantitative physiological studies. The original assay procedure of Hirsch *et al.* (1964) was based on the hypocalcemic effect 1 hour after subcutaneous injection of the preparation into young male rats of the Holtzman strain which had been fed a low calcium diet for 4 days. One Hirsch unit was defined as the activity of a standard preparation of hog thyroid (10 μg) which produced a fall of 1 mg% in the plasma calcium of the test rats.

As interest in the field began to increase in 1965, the Division of Biological Standards of the National Institute for Medical Research, Mill Hill, London, England provided investigators with an international reference standard, Thyroid Calcitonin Research Standard A. One (MRC, Medical Research Council) unit was defined as the activity in 40 mg of this crude preparation of hog thyroid. It is approximately equivalent to 100 Hirsch units. Research Standard A has now been replaced by Thyroid Calcitonin Research Standard B prepared with partially purified porcine calcitonin, and standards for human and salmon calcitonin are now available from the same source.

Improvements in the original assay of Hirsch *et al.* (1964) have been proposed by Cooper *et al.* (1967). The sensitivity of the assay is in-

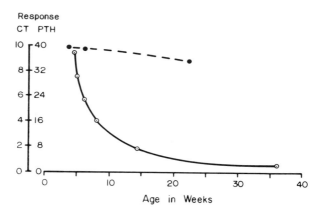

Fig. 3. Effect of age on the response to intraperitoneal injection of 165 mU (MRC) bovine calcitonin (CT) or 80 USP units bovine parathormone (PTH) per 100 g body weight in rats. After Copp and Kuczerpa (1968).

creased by simultaneous administration of phosphate and is decreased by a low phosphate regimen (Copp and Kuczerpa, 1968). As shown in Fig. 3, age of the test animals is also a major factor in sensitivity to the hormone, the response being far less dramatic in older animals. The most sensitive bioassay is that of Sturtridge and Kumar (1968) based on the fall in plasma calcium 30 minutes following intravenous injection of the test preparations into very young 50–60 g rats. With this assay, it is possible to detect 0.25 mU (MRC) of porcine or salmon calcitonin. This represents 0.1 ng of pure salmon hormone. There are substantial species differences in response, the mouse, for example, being 65 times as sensitive to chicken calcitonin as it is to an equivalent dose in MRC milliunits of Research Standard B of porcine calcitonin (Parsons and Reynolds, 1968).

Very sensitive radioimmunoassays have been developed for porcine calcitonin (Deftos *et al.,* 1968; Arnaud *et al.,* 1968; Tashjian, 1969). These are based on competition between radioiodine-labeled pure hormone and the unlabeled hormone present in the unknown or standard sample for binding sites on the antibody. The most sensitive of these can measure as little as 1 pg (10^{-12} g) and can detect the hormone in normal circulating plasma.

V. Chemistry

The original extraction method of Hirsch *et al.* (1964) consisted of homogenizing 1 g of fresh minced hog thyroid with 1 liter of N/10

HCl followed by incubation at room temperature for 30 minutes. The preparation was then centrifuged at 600 g for 30 minutes in a refrigerated centrifuge, the active factor recovered with the supernate retaining its potency for up to 6 months when freeze-stored. Progress in purification was rapid, and within 4 years, pure porcine calcitonin had been isolated and its primary structure had been determined in several laboratories (Potts *et al.*, 1968; Franz *et al.*, 1968; Kahnt *et al.*, 1968). It is a straight-chain peptide containing 32 amino acid residues, with a molecular weight of 3500 and a biological activity of 100 MRC units/mg. Its primary structure has certain distinctive features. There is an intrachain disulfide bridge at the N terminus between the cysteines at positions 1 and 7. There is also an amide (prolinamide) at the C terminus. These features are also distinctive of the structures of Vasopressin and oxytocin.

Pure human calcitonin has been isolated from medullary thyroid carcinoma tissue—a tumor of the ultimobranchial C cells. The amino acid sequence has been determined (Riniker *et al.*, 1968) and the hormone has been synthesized (Sieber *et al.*, 1968). It exists as a relatively inactive dimer (calcitonin-D) and the active monomer (calcitonin-M). A third calcitonin has been isolated from 200 pounds of ultimobranchial glands collected from over a million Pacific salmon. Within a few months of the commencement of processing this material, pure salmon calcitonin was isolated (O'Dor *et al.*, 1969), the amino acid sequence was determined (Niall *et al.*, 1969) and the hormone was synthesized (Guttman *et al.*, 1969). The amino acid sequences of porcine, bovine, human, and salmon calcitonin are shown in Fig. 4. All the calcitonins which have been characterized have the same basic structure, containing 32 amino acids, with a seven-membered disulfide ring at the N terminus and prolinamide at the C terminus. There is also an aromatic amino acid (tyrosine or phenylalanine) at position 22 and glycine at position 28. However, there are great differences between porcine, salmon, and human calcitonin in the intermediate amino acids. There is only one amino acid difference between porcine and human insulin, but there are 18 differences between the respective calcitonins. The entire molecule appears to be essential, for removal of the amide group at the C terminus or shortening the chain by a single amino acid results in almost complete loss of biological activity.

The mammalian calcitonins (bovine, porcine, and human) all have similar biological activity in the rat (100 MRC units/mg), but the activity of salmon hormone is 30–50 times as great in the rat and over 100 times as great in the mouse. Salmon calcitonin is much more stable in plasma and has a prolonged hypocalcemic effect when injected into

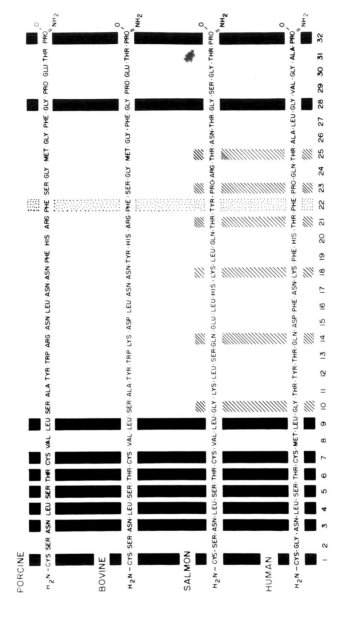

FIG. 4. Amino acid sequences of porcine, bovine, salmon, and human calcitonin. Solid bars indicate common amino acids. From Niall et al. (1969). Reproduced through the courtesy of the National Academy of Sciences, U. S.

rabbits (Copp, 1970). De Luise *et al.* (1970) observed that porcine calcitonin was rapidly inactivated by rat liver and liver supernatants, while salmon calcitonin was much less susceptible to such inactivation.

VI. Action

In young mammals, the most obvious effect of injecting calcitonin is a 20–50% fall in the level of plasma calcium and phosphate. The greatest reduction occurs between 30 minutes and 2–3 hours. The response is obtained in parathyroidectomized rats (Tashjian, 1965); thus, it cannot be explained solely on the basis of suppression of the action of parathyroid hormone. The hypocalcemic effect has been observed in eviscerate (Aliopoulios and Munson, 1965) and nephrectomized rats (Hirsch *et al.*, 1964), and since there were no significant changes in the calcium content of soft tissues (Kenny and Heiskell, 1965), it is logical to assume that the primary action of calcitonin is on bone.

A. On Bone

In cultures of limb-bone rudiments from 15-day-old mouse embryos, Gaillard (1967) observed that addition of 0.5–1.0 mU/ml of porcine calcitonin to the medium reduced the number of osteoclasts and increased the number of typical osteoblasts. He concluded that the hormone shifted the balance from bone resorption to bone absorption. It also abolished the osteolytic effect of parathyroid extracts. Similar effects were observed by Aliopoulios *et al.* (1966a) and by Friedman and Raisz (1965). Using half calvaria from 4-day-old mice prelabeled with ^{45}Ca, Reynolds (1968) showed that both porcine and chicken calcitonin inhibited calcium release resulting from stimulation of bone resorption with vitamin A. Reynolds *et al.* (1970) found that the calcitonins from ultimobranchial glands of nonmammals (chicken, salmon, and dogfish shark) were much more effective in inhibiting bone resorption and calcium release from the prelabeled calvaria than were porcine and human calcitonin. Indeed, a concentration of 5000 ng/ml of porcine calcitonin (CT) was much less effective than 0.8 ng/ml of salmon CT (Minkin *et al.*, 1971). The latter appeared to completely suppress cell-mediated calcium release (bone resorption) for at least 20 hours.

The observations *in vitro* have been supported by experiments *in vivo*. Foster *et al.* (1966) observed that administration of porcine calcitonin four times daily to young parathyroidectomized rats for 4 weeks produced heavier bones with more trabeculae than in similar animals injected with vehicle. The number of bone-resorbing osteoclasts was also reduced to one-third the number present in the untreated group. In patients with Paget's disease, Bijvoet et al. (1970) observed a significant reduction in urinary excretion of hydroxyproline when calcitonin was administered, indicating reduction in bone resorption. Jowsey (1969) reported that daily administration of 0.5 and 5.0 MRC units/kg of porcine calcitonin for 5 months to adult cats fed a low calcium diet prevented the bone resorption and mineral loss observed in the control cats fed the same diet. There is also some evidence that calcitonin may increase bone formation. Wase et al. (1967) found increased amounts of new cortical bone in calcitonin-treated rats as measured by tetracycline labeling. Further evidence that the hormone increases net retention of calcium in bone is provided by experiments of MacIntyre et al. (1967). They found that addition of CT to blood perfusing an isolated cat tibia resulted in an arteriovenous difference of $+5\%$ in calcium concentration. Kinetic studies with ^{45}Ca by Milhaud and Moukhtar (1966) indicated that 3 days of calcitonin treatment reduced the index of bone catabolism, V_{0-}, from 56.1 mg/day to 9.4 mg/day.

B. On Gut and Kidney

Cramer et al. (1969) failed to find any effect of porcine and chicken calcitonin on the absorption of calcium from Thiry-Vella intestinal loops, and it is generally assumed that any increase in calcium absorption during chronic administration of calcitonin results from secondary stimulation of the parathyroids by the calcitonin-induced hypocalcemia. However, there is substantial evidence that calcitonin does have an effect on kidney. Robinson et al. (1966) reported a phosphaturic effect of calcitonin when administered to parathyroidectomized rats, and Pak et al. (1970) observed an increase in the renal clearance of calcium. Aldred et al. (1970) found that administration of salmon CT in a dose of 0.5 MRC unit/100 g to intact animals produced an alkaline diuresis, natriuresis, hypercalciuria, hyperphosphaturia, and hypomagnesuria. Porcine calcitonin in doses up to 2.0 MRC units/kg did not significantly influence the urinary parameters. Keeler et al. (1971) confirmed these findings and reported that doses of salmon calcitonin of 0.1 μg/kg tripled the sodium excretion in normal rats. Although the effect may not be specific, there is no doubt that under appropriate circumstances, salmon calcitonin is a very potent natriuretic and diuretic agent. Perhaps this may be related to the fact that the hormone and ultimobranchial glands developed at a time when primitive fishes migrated to the sea and were exposed for the first time to the high sodium and calcium concentrations of seawater. In patients with Paget's disease, calcitonin treatment initially increased sodium and calcium excretion (Bijvoet *et al.*, 1970), followed by compensatory increases in aldosterone. After treatment was stopped, retention of sodium, calcium, and water occurred.

C. Other Effects

Parkinson and Radde (1970) have presented evidence that calcitonin stimulates the activity of a Ca^{2+}- and Mg^{2+}-dependent ATPase in red cell membranes which may be involved in actively pumping calcium out of these cells. A more general view has been taken by Rasmussen and Tenenhouse (1970), who have suggested that this may be a fundamental action of calcitonin on cells in general and may serve to reduce the intracellular calcium, counteracting the effects of parathormone. Since the ultimobranchials and calcitonin developed first when primitive fish were exposed to the high calcium concentration of seawater (which has eight times the Ca^{2+} concentration of plasma), the hormone may be acting to protect the cells from excessive calcium. MacManus and Whitfield (1970) have reported that calcitonin inhibits the mitogenic action of parathormone and of dibutyryl cyclic AMP. They suggest that this effect may also be the result of lowering intracellular Ca^{2+}.

Calcitonin stimulates glycosaminoglycan synthesis by embryo calf bone *in vitro* (Martin *et al.*, 1969) suggesting that it may have a role in bone synthesis.

VII. Comparative Studies

Until recently, most of the work on calcitonin has been confined to mammals. However, the recognition of the ultimobranchial origin of calcitonin (Copp *et al.*, 1968) and the isolation of salmon calcitonin (O'Dor *et al.*, 1969) has stimulated interest in the action of the hormone in other vertebrates.

Rasquin and Rosenbloom (1954) observed that hypertrophy of the ultimobranchial glands was associated with confinement of Mexican cave fish in total darkness and with skeletal deformities. They suggested that perhaps the ultimobranchial was a homologue of the parathyroid in land vertebrates. They were correct as far as its association with calcium metabolism, but in fact the two glands have antagonistic actions. In the fish, *Fundulus heteroclitus*, porcine calcitonin had no hypocalcemic effect (Pang and Pickford, 1967). However, in the European eel, *Anguilla anguilla L.*, porcine calcitonin at doses of 10 and 50 mU caused a significant fall in plasma calcium and a rise in plasma phosphorus (D. K. O. Chan et al., 1968). In elasmobranchs, which have a cartilaginous rather than a bony skeleton, the ultimobranchial glands are well developed. High concentrations of calcitonin have been found in dogfish (Copp et al., 1967b). However, the hormone had no significant effect on plasma calcium levels in these animals (Copp, 1969c).

D. R. Robertson has been primarily responsible for the very exciting studies on ultimobranchial function in frogs. In Rana pipiens, he observed (Robertson, 1968) that administration of 200,000 IU of vitamin D and exposure of the animals to an environment containing 0.8% calcium in the water produced a hypercalcemia which was associated with hypertrophy of the ultimobranchial glands. The effect was reversible since the glands returned to normal size after the frogs were kept for 3 weeks in low calcium water. Following ultimobranchialectomy in frogs, there was a period of hypercalcemia and depletion of the calcium stores in the paravertebral lime sacs (Robertson, 1969). Histological examination revealed decreased numbers of osteoblasts and increased osteoclast counts.

In turtles, Clark (1968) demonstrated calcitonin activity in ultimobranchial glands (but not in thyroid extracts). However, she was unable to show any hypocalcemic effect in turtles when porcine calcitonin was injected.

In domestic fowl, most workers have failed to find any significant change in plasma calcium when various calcitonins were injected. This may result from the very rapid response of the parathyroid glands in birds. Kraintz and Intscher (1969) did observe a hypocalcemic effect when the hormone was injected into parathyroidectomized birds. A. S. Chan et al. (1969) observed hyperplasia and hypertrophy of the C cells of the chicken ultimobranchial gland when the birds were exposed to a high calcium diet which increased the plasma calcium from 10.4 to 13.9 mg%. In ultimobranchialectomized chickens, Brown et al. (1969) found that the control of hypercalcemia following infusion of parathyroid hormone was impaired, as is the case in mammals. In young turkeys, Copp et al. (1970a) reported that ultimobranchialectomy performed during infusion of 10 mg Ca/kg/hr resulted in an immediate and dramatic increase in plasma calcium (see Fig. 5). In newly hatched cockerels given daily injections of salmon calcitonin (1 MRC unit/bird) for 14 weeks, microradiographs revealed complete suppression of bone resorption and a condition in the cortical bone which resembled osteopetrosis (Copp et al., 1970b).

There seems little doubt that in some nonmammals calcitonin is involved in calcium regulation and does inhibit bone resorption.

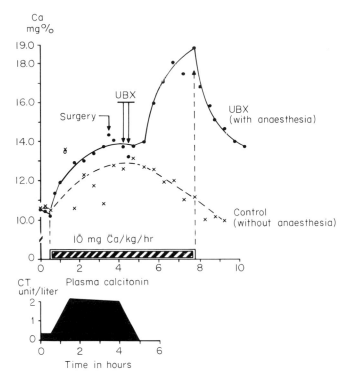

Fig. 5. Effect of ultimobranchialectomy during calcium infusion in a young turkey (4.5 kg, male). From Copp *et al.* (1970a). Reproduced through the courtesy of Heinemann Medical Books, London.

VIII. Clinical Implications

Calcitonin has been extracted from human thyroid glands, but the concentration (0.1–2 MRC units/g) is low compared with that in the thyroids of other animals (Aliopoulios *et al.*, 1966b). One of the problems is that the C cells in humans are located in and around the superior parathyroid (parathyroid IV) and are frequently left behind when the surgeon performs a partial thyroidectomy. Very high levels (143–488 MRC units/g) have been reported in medullary carcinoma of thyroid (Melvin *et al.*, 1970). This is recognized as a tumor of the C cells (Williams, 1970). The effects of this congenital condition have been reviewed by Potts and Deftos (1969) and may include secondary hyperparathyroidism, along with a number of associated endocrinopathies.

Because the hypocalcemic effect of calcitonin is the result of suppression of osteolysis and is manifest prominently only in young animals

with a high rate of bone turnover, it is not surprising that calcitonin
has very little hypocalcemic effect in normal adults. However, the effect
is quite striking in cases of osteolytic bone disease, and it may indeed
be of value in diagnosing and evaluating this condition. Currently, calcitonin is being used to treat hypercalcemic conditions resulting from
excessive bone breakdown, including hyperparathyroidism, osteolytic
bone tumors, immobilization osteoporosis, and Paget's disease. It is particularly useful in the last condition (Bijvoet et al., 1970; Potts and
Deftos, 1969) where it produces remissions and relief of bone pain,
maintaining its effect for several weeks after treatment has been stopped.
It is perhaps significant that many patients with Paget's disease have
been so convinced of the value of calcitonin treatment that they have
continued self-medication.

With regard to the very important condition of senile osteoporosis,
there is still only meager evidence as to the possible beneficial effects
of calcitonin. Jowsey (1969) has shown that chronic administration of
porcine calcitonin inhibited the loss of bone mineral in cats resulting
from a low calcium regimen. Baud et al. (1970) has claimed that such
treatment may be useful in human senile osteoporosis. However, very
convincing proof is necessary before it may be concluded that calcitonin
is of real value in this important disease.

IX. Control of Secretion

There is substantial evidence that hypercalcemia stimulates hyperplasia and hypersecretion of the C cells in the mammalian thyroid and
in the ultimobranchial glands of other vertebrates. In cultures of C
cells from dog thyroid, a high level of calcium in the medium caused
discharge of the secretory granules (Bussolati et al., 1969). In the classic
experiments of Copp et al. (1962), which led to the recognition of
the existence of calcitonin, it was shown that its release was stimulated
by hypercalcemia without the mediation of the nervous system or the
anterior pituitary. The sensitive methods of bioassay made it possible
for Care et al. (1968) to demonstrate the effect of the level of calcium
in blood perfusing the pig thyroid on the rate of secretion or release
of calcitonin. This is shown in Fig. 6, where it is compared with the
rate of secretion of parathormone (PTH) in the cow (Potts and Deftos,
1969). In these short-term studies it is obvious that release of either
hormone is determined by a simple proportional control based on the
level of ionic calcium in blood perfusing the glands. However, there
is evidence that a sudden increase in plasma calcium will trigger release

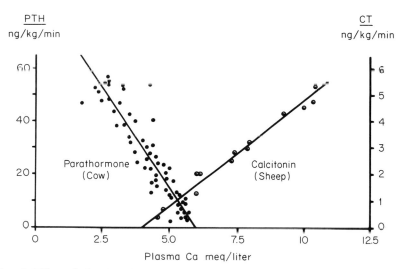

Fig. 6. Effect of plasma calcium concentration on the rate of secretion of calcitonin by a mature sheep (from data of Care *et al.*, 1968) and of parathormone in the cow (from data of Potts and Deftos, 1969).

of a "pulse" of calcitonin (derivative control), while persistent hypercalcemia causes hyperplasia of the C cells (a type of integrative control). It is perhaps significant that the PTH and CT secretion lines intersect at the normal calcium level of 10.3 mg%. The relationship can be expressed by the equation: $dCT/dt = 0.36$ ($P_{Ca} - 12$) ng/kg/minute, where P_{Ca} = the plasma calcium in mg%. Care *et al.* (1970) have shown that adenyl cyclase and cyclic 3'5'-adenosine monophosphate are involved in calcitonin release, which is stimulated by pancreozymin, glucagon, and dibutyryl cAMP.

X. Role in Homeostasis

There is ample evidence that thyroparathyroidectomy impairs the ability of an animal to control hypercalcemia. This has been demonstrated following calcium infusion in dog (Sanderson *et al.*, 1960; Copp, 1964), rat (Sturtridge and Kumar, 1967), and man (O'Brien and McIntosh, 1967). This was also demonstrated (Copp *et al.*, 1970a) when ultimobranchialectomy was performed during calcium infusion in young turkeys (see Fig. 5). Similar impairment has been demonstrated following administration of excessive doses of parathyroid extract to dogs (Copp, 1964) and rats (Hirsch, 1967). The experiment of Copp *et al.* (1962)

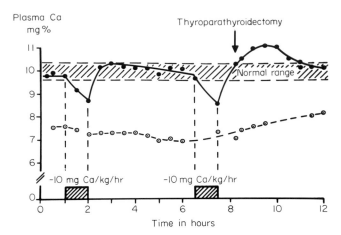

Fig. 7. Example of calcium regulation in a young dog. Recovery from ethylene-diaminetetraacetate- (EDTA) induced hypocalcemia with intact glands and following total thyroparathyroidectomy as indicated by the arrow. (From Copp, 1962; reproduced through the courtesy of Yearbook Publishers, Chicago.)

illustrated in Fig. 7 indicates the efficient homeostatic control in the presence of intact thyroids and parathyroids, and the hypercalcemic overshoot which occurs when these glands have been removed. However, in all these conditions, the hypercalcemic challenge was artificially induced.

Gray and Munson (1969) showed that administration of a large dose of calcium by stomach tube, or rapid consumption of a high calcium meal, had no significant effect on the plasma calcium of rats with intact thyroids. However, when these experiments were repeated in thyroidectomized rats with functional parathyroid transplants, an episode of hypercalcemia occurred. They concluded that the calcitonin-producing C cells had an important function in preventing such periods of hypercalcemia. It is significant that Cooper and Deftos (1970) observed a dose-related increase in plasma calcitonin levels when calcium was given orally, even though there was no significant change in plasma calcium. This could be mediated by secretion of pancreozymin which Care *et al.* (1970) found stimulated calcitonin release from the pig thyroid. Thus calcium release from bone could be reduced at a time that calcium was being absorbed from the gut, thus obscuring changes in plasma calcium.

Another experiment demonstrating a normal physiological function of calcitonin has been carried out by Lewis *et al.* (1971) on parathyroidectomized rats with functional parathyroid transplants. They found that removal of the thyroid glands while the animals were on a low calcium diet resulted in a significant reduction in calcium absorption and bone calcium in pregnant and lactating rats. They concluded that the C cells and calcitonin had an important role in protecting the skeleton from the effects of calcium stress in these conditions.

XI. Summary

Calcitonin is a very potent hypocalcemic hormone produced by C cells in the mammalian thyroid and in the ultimobranchial glands of other jawed vertebrates. It has an important role in controlling induced hypercalcemia by inhibiting cell-mediated calcium release from bone. It may prove of value in diagnosing and treating osteolytic bone disease as well as other calcium disorders.

Acknowledgments

The author would like to express appreciation to Mrs. Mary Forsyth and Mrs. Valerie Walker for assistance in preparing the manuscript, Kurt Henze for preparation of diagrams, and the Medical Research Council of Canada for support of some of the experimental work reported here.

References

Aldred, J. P., Kleszynski, R. R., and Bastian, J. W. (1970). *Proc. Soc. Exp. Biol. Med.* 134, 1175.
Aliopoulios, M. A., and Munson, P. L. (1965). *Surg. Forum* 16, 55.
Aliopoulios, M. A., Goldhaber, P., and Munson, P. L. (1966a). *Science* 151, 330.
Aliopoulos, M. A., Voelkel, E. F., and Munson, P. L. (1966b). *J. Clin. Endocrinol. Metab.* 26, 897.
Arnaud, C. D., Littledike, T., Tsao, H. S., and Kaplan, E. L. (1968). *Mayo Clin. Proc.* 43, 496.
Baud, C. A., de Siebenthal, J., Langer, B., Tupling, M. R., and Mach, R. S. (1970). *In* "Calcitonin 1969" (S. Taylor, ed.), pp. 540–546. Heinemann, London.
Bijvoet, A. L. M., van der Sluys Veer, J., Wildiers, J., and Smeenk, D. (1970). *In* "Calcitonin 1969" (S. Taylor, ed.), pp. 531–539. Heinemann, London.
Brown, D. M., Perey, D. Y. E., Dent, P. B., and Good, R. A. (1969). *Proc. Soc. Exp. Biol. Med.* 130, 1001.
Bussolati, G., and Pearse, A. G. E. (1967). *J. Endocrinol.* 37, 205.
Bussolati, G., Naovne, R., Gasparri, G., and Monga, G. (1969). *Experientia* 25, 641.
Care, A. D. (1965). *Nature (London)* 205, 1289.
Care, A. D., Cooper, C. W., Duncan, T., and Orimo, H. (1968). *In* "Parathyroid Hormone and Thyrocalcitonin (Calcitonin)" (R. V. Talmage and L. F. Bélanger, eds.), Int. Congr. Ser. No. 159, pp. 417–427. Excerpta Med. Found., Amsterdam.
Care, A. D., Bates, R. F. L., and Gitelman, H. J. (1970). *J. Endocrinol.* 48, 1.

Chan, A. S., Cipera, J. D., and Bélanger, L. F. (1969). *Rev. Can. Biol.* **28**, 19.

Chan, D. K. O., Chester Jones, I, and Smith, R. N. (1968). *Gen. Comp. Endocrinol.* **11**, 243.

Clark, N. B. (1968). *Endocrinology* **83**, 1145.

Cooper, C. W., and Deftos, L. J. (1970). *Fed. Proc., Fed. Amer. Soc. Exp. Biol.* **29**, No. 2, 253 (abstract No. 37).

Cooper, C. W., Hirsch, P. F., Toverud, S. U., and Munson, P. L. (1967). *Endocrinology* **81**, 610.

Copp, D. H. (1962). *In* "Yearbook of Endocrinology, 1961–2 Series" G. S. Gordan, ed.), pp. 10–18. Yearbook Publ., Chicago, Illinois.

Copp, D. H. (1963). *Oral Surg., Oral Med., Oral Pathol.* **16**, 872.

Copp, D. H. (1964). *Recent Progr. Horm. Res.* **20**, 59–88.

Copp, D. H. (1967). *Amer. J. Med.* **43**, 648.

Copp, D. H. (1969a). *In* "Mineral Metabolism" (C. L. Comar and F. Bronner, eds.), Vol. 3, pp. 453–513. Academic Press, New York.

Copp, D. H. (1969b). *J. Endocrinol.* **43**, 137.

Copp, D. H. (1969c). *In* "Fish Physiology" (W. S. Hoar and D. J. Randall, eds.), Vol. 2, pp. 377–398. Academic Press, New York.

Copp, D. H. (1970). *Annu. Rev. Physiol.* **32**, 61.

Copp, D. H., and Kuczerpa, A. (1968). *In* "Calcitonin" (S. Taylor, ed.), pp. 18–24. Heinemann, London.

Copp, D. H., and Parkes, C. O. (1968). *In* "Parathyroid Hormone and Thyrocalcitonin (Calcitonin)" (R. V. Talmage and L. F. Bélanger, eds.), Int. Congr. Ser. No. 159, pp. 74–84. Excerpta Med. Found., Amsterdam.

Copp, D. H., Davidson, A. G. F., and Cheney, B. (1961). *Proc. Can. Fed. Biol. Soc.* **4**, 17.

Copp, D. H., Cameron, E. C., Cheney, B., Davidson, A. G. F., and Henze, K. G. (1962). *Endocrinology* **70**, 638.

Copp, D. H., Cockcroft, D. W., and Kueh, Y. (1967a). *Can. J. Physiol. Pharmacol.* **45**, 1095.

Copp, D. H., Cockcroft, D. W., and Kueh, Y. (1967b). *Science* **158**, 924.

Copp, D. H., Cockcroft, D. W., Kueh, Y., and Melville, M. (1968). *In* "Calcitonin" (S. Taylor, ed.), pp. 306–321. Heinemann, London.

Copp, D. H., Brooks, C. E., Low, B. S., Newsome, F., O'Dor, R. K., Parkes, C. O., Walker, V., and Watts, E. G. (1970a). *In* "Calcitonin 1969" (S. Taylor, ed.), pp. 281–294. Heinemann, London.

Copp, D. H., Low, B. S., and Bélanger, L. F. (1970b). *Program 52nd Meet. Endocrin. Soc., U. S.* p. 123.

Cramer, C. F., Parkes, C. O., and Copp, D. H. (1969). *Can. J. Physiol. Pharmacol.* **47**, 181.

Deftos, L. J., Lee, M. R., and Potts, J. T., Jr. (1968). *Proc. Nat. Acad. Sci. U. S.* **60**, 293.

de Luise, M., Martin, T. J., and Melick, R. A. (1970). *J. Endocrinol.* **48**, 181.

Foster, G. V., Baghdiantz, A., Kumar, M. A., Slack, E., Soliman, H. A., and MacIntyre, I. (1964a). *Nature (London)* **202**, 1303.

Foster, G. V., MacIntyre, I., and Pearse, A. G. E. (1964b). *Nature (London)* **203**, 1029.

Foster, G. V., Doyle, F. H., Bordier, P., and Matrajt, H. (1966). *Lancet* **2**, 1428.

Franz, J., Rosenthaler, J., Zehnder, K., Doepfer, W., Huguenin, R., and Guttman, S. (1968). *Helv. Chim. Acta* **51**, 218.

Friedman, J., and Raisz, L. G. (1965). *Science* **150**, 1465.

Gaillard, P. J. (1967). *Proc., Kon. Ned. Akad. Wetenschap., Ser. C* **70**, 309.

Galante, L., Gudmundsson, T. V., Matthews, E. D., Tse, A., Williams, E. D., Woodhouse, N. J. Y., and MacIntyre, I. (1968). *Lancet* **2**, 537.

Gray, T. K., and Munson, P. L. (1969). *Science* **166**, 512.

Greil, A. (1905). *Anat. Hefte (Wiesbaden)* **29**, 445.

Guttman, S., Pless, J., Huguenin, R. L., Sandrin, E., Bossert, H., and Zehnder, K. (1969). *Helv. Chim. Acta* **52**, 1789.

Hirsch, P. F. (1967). *Endocrinology* **80**, 539.

Hirsch, P. F., and Munson, P. L. (1969). *Physiol. Rev.* **49**, 548.

Hirsch, P. F., Gauthier, G. F., and Munson, P. L. (1963). *Endocrinology* **73**, 244.

Hirsch, P. F., Voelkel, E. F., and Munson, P. L. (1964). *Science* **146**, 412.

Jowsey, J. (1969). *Endocrinology* **85**, 1196.

Kahnt, F. W., Riniker, B., MacIntyre, I., and Neher, R. (1968). *Helv. Chim. Acta* **51**, 214.

Keeler, R., Walker, V., and Copp, D. H. (1971). *Can. J. Physiol. Pharmacol.* (in press).

Kenny, A. D., and Heiskell, C. A. (1965). *Proc. Soc. Exp. Biol. Med.* **120**, 269.

Kraintz, L., and Intscher, K. (1969). *Can. J. Physiol. Pharmacol.* **47**, 313.

Kumar, M. A., Foster, G. V., and MacIntyre, I. (1963). *Lancet* **2**, 480.

Lewis, P., Rafferty, B., Shelley, M., and Robinson, C. J. (1971). *J. Endocrinol.* **49**, ix.

MacCallum, W. G., and Voegtlin, C. (1909). *J. Exp. Med.* **11**, 118.

MacIntyre, I., Parsons, J. A., and Robinson, C. J. (1967). *J. Physiol. (London)* **191**, 393.

MacManus, J. P., and Whitfield, J. F. (1970). *Endocrinology* **86**, 934.

Martin, T. J., Harris, G. S., Melick, R. A., and Fraser, J. R. E. (1969). *Experientia* **25**, 375.

Matsuzawa, T., and Kurosumi, K. (1967). *Nature (London)* **213**, 927.

Melvin, K. E. W., Voelkel, E. F., and Tashjian, A. H., Jr. (1970). In "Calcitonin 1969" (S. Taylor, ed.), pp. 487–496. Heinemann, London.

Milhaud, G., and Moukhtar, M. S. (1966). *Proc. Soc. Exp. Biol. Med.* **123**, 207.

Minkin, C., Reynolds, J. J., and Copp, D. H. (1971). *Can. J. Physiol. Pharmacol.* (in press).

Niall, H. D., Keutmann, H. T., Copp, D. H., and Potts, J. T., Jr. (1969). *Proc. Nat. Acad. Sci. U. S.* **64**, 771.

Nonidez, J. F. (1932). *Amer. J. Anat.* **49**, 479.

O'Brien, M. M., and McIntosh, H. W. (1967). *Can. Med. Ass. J.* **97**, 941.

O'Dor, R. K., Parkes, C. O., and Copp, D. H. (1969). *Can. J. Biochem.* **47**, 823.

Pak, C. Y. C., Ruskin, B., and Casper, A. (1970). In "Calcitonin 1969" (S. Taylor, ed.), pp. 154–160. Heinemann, London.

Pang, P. K. T., and Pickford, G. E. (1967). *Comp. Biochem. Physiol.* **21**, 573.

Parkinson, D. K., and Radde, I. C. (1970). In "Calcitonin 1969" (S. Taylor, ed.), pp. 466–471. Heinemann, London.

Parsons, J. A., and Reynolds, J. J. (1968). *Lancet* **1**, 1067.

Pearse, A. G. E. (1966). *Vet. Rec.* **79**, 587.

Pearse, A. G. E. (1970). In "Calcitonin 1969" (S. Taylor, ed.), pp. 125–140. Heinemann, London.

Pearse, A. G. E., and Carvalheira, A. F. (1967). *Nature (London)* **214**, 929.
Potts, J. T., Jr., and Deftos, L. J. (1969). *In* "Duncan's Diseases of Metabolism" (P. K. Bondy and L. E. Rosenberg, eds.), 6th ed., Vol. 2, pp. 904–1082. Saunders, Philadelphia, Pennsylvania.
Potts, J. T., Jr., Niall, H. D., Keutmann, H. T., Brewer, H. B., Jr., and Deftos, L. J. (1968)'. *Proc. Nat. Acad. Sci. U. S.* **59**, 1321.
Rasmussen, H., and Tenenhouse, A. (1970). *In* "Biochemical Actions of Hormones" (G. Litwack, ed.), Vol. 1, pp. 365–413. Academic Press, New-York.
Rasquin, P., and Rosenbloom, L. (1954). *Bull. Amer. Mus. Natur. Hist.* **104**, 359.
Reynolds, J. J. (1968). *Proc. Roy. Soc., Ser. B* **170**, 61.
Reynolds, J. J., Minkin, C., and Parsons, J. A. (1970). *Calcif. Tissue Res.* **4**, 350.
Riniker, B., Neher, R., Maier, R., Kahnt, F. W., Byfield, P. G. H., Gudmundsson, T. V., Galante, L., and MacIntyre, I. (1968). *Helv. Chim. Acta* **51**, 1738.
Robertson, D. R. (1968). *Z. Zellforsch. Mikrosk. Anat.* **85**, 441.
Robertson, D. R. (1969). *Gen. Comp. Endocrinol.* **12**, 479.
Robinson, C. J., Martin, T. J., and MacIntyre, I. (1966). *Lancet* **2**, 83.
Sanderson, P. H., Marshall, F., III, and Wilson, R. E. (1960). *J. Clin. Invest.* **39**, 662.
Sieber, P., Brugger, M., Kamber, B., Riniker, B., and Rittel, W. (1968). *Helv. Chim. Acta* **51**, 2057.
Smith, H. (1960). "Evolution of Chordate Structure," p. 1297. Holt, New York.
Sturtridge, W. C., and Kumar, M. A. (1967). *Endocrinology* **81**, 1287.
Sturtridge, W. C., and Kumar, M. A. (1968). *J. Endocrinol.* **42**, 501.
Talmage, R. V., and Bélanger, L. F., eds. (1968). "Parathyroid Hormone and Thyrocalcitonin (Calcitonin)," Int. Congr. Ser. No. 159. Excerpta Med. Found., Amsterdam.
Talmage, R. V., and Munson, P. L., eds. (1972). "Calcium, Parathyroid Hormone and the Calcitonins," Excerpta Medica Foundation, Amsterdam. (in press)
Talmage, R. V., Neuenschwander, J., and Kraintz, L. (1965). *Endocrinology* **76**, 103.
Tashjian, A. H., Jr. (1965). *Endocrinology* **77**, 375.
Tashjian, A. H., Jr. (1969). *Endocrinology* **84**, 140.
Tauber, S. D. (1967). *Proc. Nat. Acad. Sci. U. S.* **58**, 1684.
Taylor, S., ed. (1968). "Calcitonin. Proceedings of a Symposium on Thyrocalcitonin and the C Cells." Heinemann, London.
Taylor, S., ed. (1970). "Calcitonin 1969." Heinemann, London.
Wase, A. W., Solewski, J., Rickes, E., and Seidenberg, J. (1967). *Nature (London)* **214**, 388.
Watzka, M. (1933). *Z. Mikrosk.-Anat. Forsch.* **34**, 485.
Williams, E. D. (1970). *In* "Calcitonin 1969" (S. Taylor, ed.), pp. 483–487. Heinemann, London.

CHAPTER 9

Pathological Calcification

REUBEN EISENSTEIN

I. Introduction

The problem of calcification, whether it be normal or pathological, ultimately resolves itself into an aspect of physical chemistry. This is so because in both instances the end result which defines the problem is the deposition of crystalline or amorphous calcium salts in tissues. Normally these salts are deposited in the skeleton. In the case of pathological calcifications, they are deposited in abnormal sites where they are usually of little clinical consequence, but, can, if located in strategic sites such as cardiac valves or if very extensive as in calcinosis universalis, be of serious clinical significance. In addition, reactions of the body to the presence of calcium salts in abnormal sites may predispose to or alter tissue responses to other insults, and this appears to be one of the most significant clinical aspects of this process.

Although it would be expected that the factors contributing to the precipitation of calcium salts from solutions resembling body fluids would be well worked out by now, this is not yet true, partly because this is apparently not a simple problem in physical chemistry (Neuman and Neuman, 1958) and partly because ions other than calcium or phosphate such as lead, iron, or silicates may alter ion interactions (Schiffman *et al.*, 1966). Even if this problem were solved, cells metabolize calcium, phosphates, and carbonates, the ions primarily involved in calcifications. They secrete and sequester these ions and produce materials which alter pH and accelerate or inhibit precipitation. They produce organic matrices with characteristics such that they favor calcification and others which probably retard it.

This will not be an exhaustive review of this subject. Rather, it will focus on certain aspects of the problem and will begin with a brief discussion of the chemistry of calcification, proceed to a discussion of some types of abnormal calcification with special reference to arterial calcification, then consider the consequences of this process, concluding with a discussion of the difficulties involved in developing a unified theoretical formulation from the available data. It will not consider abnormal ossification, which is a distinctly different phenomenon.

II. Chemical Principles

The ionic composition of the intercellular fluid is normally supersaturated with respect to calcium and phosphate in the sense that these fluids will lose ions to a crystal or precipitate of calcium phosphate (Posner, 1969). The partition of serum inorganic phosphate has been discussed by Walser (1962). Its concentration in the plasma, in the presence of an adequate diet, is largely regulated in the kidney where parathyroid hormone regulates its tubular reabsorption. There is also evidence that vitamin D may affect the intestinal absorption of this ion, probably secondary to its effect on calcium (Kowarski and Schacter, 1969).

Blood calcium is not completely ionized, a sizable proportion being complexed to proteins, largely albumin, and to smaller organic ions such as citrate. The critical physiological measurement is the ionized calcium, since only this form of calcium can form inorganic precipitates or crystals. This measurement, at present, cannot be easily made. Aside from availability in the diet, serum calcium levels are largely regulated by two polypeptide hormones, parathyroid hormone and calcitonin, and a sterol, vitamin D. Parathyroid hormone has, as its prime target organ, bone where it induces resorption and the kidney where it decreases the reabsorption of phosphate. It also, at least in experimental situations, affects calcium transport in other cells, including HeLa cells in culture (Borle, 1968). Calcitonin, a secretion of the medullary cells of the thyroid gland, inhibits bone resorption in experimental situations; but there is little evidence in man that it has a measurable effect on calcium metabolism, perhaps because too few studies have been done in young children in whom calcium metabolism is more labile than in adults. Calcium, calcitonin, and parathyroid hormone are interrelated in a complex three-way feedback mechanism, since the levels of the two hormones are controlled at least partly by the ionic concentrations in the body fluids and they, in turn, affect the level of serum calcium.

Vitamin D, which can be produced by ultraviolet irradiation of the skin, is largely obtained from the diet. It is absorbed in the intestine and transported to the liver where it is converted to an active metabolite, 25-OH cholecalciferol (Ponchon and DeLuca, 1969). One of its effects is to induce protein synthesis (Eisenstein and Passavoy, 1964), including the synthesis of a calcium-carrying protein (Taylor and Wasserman, 1967). It seems to have its primary effect in regulating the absorption of calcium from the gut, although there is evidence that it may have direct effects on bone and other tissues (Canas *et al.*, 1969) and may also affect the absorption of phosphate from the gut (Kowarski and Schachter, 1969).

Most calcific deposits whether normal or pathological consist of crystalline calcium phosphates in the form of apatite, although calcite, whitlockite, aragonite, and calcium carbonates and sulfates are found in unusual circumstances (Frondel and Prien, 1942; Cogan *et al.*, 1958). Although it is now orthodox teaching that crystal formation is the initial event, the question of whether this is so or whether amorphous calcium phosphates form first with subsequent crystallization is still unsettled (Posner, 1969). As in bone and cartilage, there are only two generally considered theories of calcium salt formation. The first states that a high enough local ionic concentration of calcium and phosphate somehow must accumulate for precipitation to occur. The second states that some organic component, collagen in the case of bone, has properties mimicking those of apatite crystals. Since the extracellular fluid is supersaturated and metastable with respect to calcium and phosphate, such an organic structure could act as a seed crystal and thus as a starting point for a self-propagating process (Glimcher, 1960). Currently, opinion is developing that both situations may occur concurrently.

Regardless of which or either of these theories is correct, there are complex effects on local concentrations of the involved ions mediated by the immediate effects of cell metabolism and of the products of cells. As has so often been emphasized in the past, it must be reemphasized here that these effects are local. Though related to general body metabolism, they are quantitatively and perhaps qualitatively altered by local factors which promote, inhibit, or resorb calcification. It is to these factors that most of this essay will be directed.

III. Dystrophic Calcification

Dystrophic calcification, which occurs without any generalized derangement of calcium metabolism, is one of the very common reactions of the body to injury. It is an almost universal sequel of several types of granulomatous inflammation, and patterns of calcification occur in several types of tumors to the extent that they are useful in radiologic diagnosis.

There are a number of theoretical approaches to the problem of dystrophic calcification, but before discussing them, it might be worthwhile to describe the morphological setting in which they occur. These deposits are found in and near injured or dying cells. It has been stated that those types of necrosis which leave behind some orderly tissue structure including recognizable cell or connective tissue structure predispose to calcification, while those which result in complete tissue dissolution do not (Hass, 1956; Eisenstein *et al.*, 1960). This was based on the observations that caseation and coagulative necrosis frequently calcified while liquefactive necrosis did not and that amorphous extracellular deposits such as amyloid and certain types of hyalin did not while elastic fibers, basement membranes, and other more ordered extracellular structures frequently did. As the electron microscope has become more widely used in the study of pathological processes, this generalization requires revision, for amyloid and hyaline have been shown to be organized, even crystalline fibrils, and recognizable cell fragments including organized membranes can be found after almost any type of cell death. Perhaps a more modern generalization would be that with regard to intracellular calcification, those cells which die slowly enough to maintain enzymic activity though disordered, remaining in place long enough for them to accumulate significant amounts of mineral before they are swept away by repairative processes, are those which tend to calcify; while those which are destroyed explosively and are rapidly digested, as occurs in suppuration, rarely calcify.

A second generalization is that in mammals at least there are some tissues which calcify and others which do so only under exceptional circumstances. Thus, liver and brain are highly resistant to calcification, except where tissue not normally present (e.g., metastatic tumors or parasites) is found. On the other hand, the kidney, heart, certain arteries, the spleen, some portions of the gastrointestinal tract and lung readily calcify under appropriate conditions. On a gross level, two examples may be cited. The umbilical cord practically never calcifies while the placenta almost universally undergoes focal calcification at term. In the gastrointestinal tract, the beds of gastric and, less frequently, duodenal peptic ulcers may calcify while ulcerative lesions of the lower intestine almost never do except for certain neoplasms. In addition, if the parenchymal cells of an organ have a tendency to calcify, the stroma of that organ including its intrinsic vasculature does also (Hass *et al.*, 1958). An exception to this may be the lenticulostriate artery branches, but here the mineral is apparently largely iron. The reverse is also true. Whether this similarity in susceptibility of stroma and parenchyma is related to the metabolic activity of parenchymal cells is problematical. In such tissues, the arterial vasculature rather than the venous one is most readily calcifiable, thus suggesting that the varying calcifiability of arterial systems is more related to intrinsic anatomic and metabolic factors, very likely developmental in nature. The subject of calcification of tumors is descriptively complex and will not be discussed in any detail here, nor will stones in body cavities be discussed.

Students of this subject have frequently noted a hierarchy of susceptibility to mineralization of anatomic sites within any locus. Thus, in arteries the first elective site of calcification is usually the inner elastic lamella, with subsequent spread to other lamellae, then smooth muscle cells, then nonfibrillar extracellular space, and, finally, collagen fibrils. At any time in this sequence, calcium salts may be removed from one of the early sites of deposition while it is being accumulated in one of the sites lower in the hierarchy of susceptibility (Hass, 1956; Eisenstein *et al.*, 1960). Aside from this, the anatomic picture is rendered even more complex by the elaboration of new cells and connective tissue in response to the calcific injury, some of which in turn may calcify. Nevertheless, the spread of calcification is obviously limited or our homes as well as our parks would rapidly become populated with stone statues.

Among the connective tissues, some structures tend to calcify more than others. In contrast to bone, tendon, and cartilage, the order of susceptibility seems to be elastin, nonfibrillar extracellular space, basement membranes, and collagen in that order. Even within susceptible cells, some foci seem to have a greater predilection for calcification than others. This will be taken up more fully in the discussion of metastatic calcification where it has been more extensively studied. Suffice it to say at this point that mitochondria have a great tendency to accumulate calcium.

IV. Pathogenetic Factors

A. Polysaccharides

As in bone and cartilage, most authors on the subject of the role of polysaccharides in abnormal calcification have implicitly accepted the idea that two things are required for mineralization: a high enough local concentration of calcium and phosphate or carbonate and a calcifiable matrix. As in science in general, the advent of new techniques, particularly if they are simple, has spawned new ideas. Thus, the development of histochemical techniques for the demonstration of acid and neutral polysaccharides in sections of fixed tissue led to their application to studies of abnormal calcification. It was found that such deposits were almost invariably accompanied by these materials which are in part responsible for the deep basophilia which pathologists usually use to identify calcification. In keeping with ideas then current among investigators of skeletal mineralization, the idea developed that these accumulations of polysaccharides were important in the genesis of abnormal calcifications as well and might even be the calcifiable matrix (Levine *et al.*, 1949). The observation that the umbilical cord and certain types of cartilage are resistant to calcification argues against this thesis. A series of experiments in which it was shown that these compounds accumulate in sites of calcification only after calcium phosphate salts are present argues strongly that they represent a reaction to the presence of calcium salts (Konetzki *et al.*, 1962; Eisenstein *et al.*, 1965). Such a thesis is strengthened when it is recalled that calcium phosphates have a high affinity for negatively charged molecules, among which acid mucopolysaccharides are included, to the degree that they are useful in the chromatography of nucleic acids (Main and Cole, 1957). The rejection of this idea does not imply that these complex anions may not play a secondary role, perhaps supplying a new calcifiable matrix, or in stabilizing a calcific deposit, or as protection against a spreading lesion. The observation that in calcifying cartilage there is present a polysaccharide which inhibits normal mineralization may lend more credence to this notion (Howell *et al.*, 1969). The reactivity of polysaccharides with calcium may also be altered by the cationic protein, lysozyme, which has recently been shown to be present in at least some calcified sites rich in acid mucopolysaccharides (Kuettner *et al.*, 1968; Eisenstein *et al.*, 1970).

A comparison between polysaccharide matrices and calcification in cartilage and abnormal sites provides interesting contrasts. In cartilage, where the bulk of the extracellular materials are polysaccharide in nature, calcification occurs in this milieu. Here, biochemical data of some detail are becoming available, and it is apparent that the types of polysaccharides present near the calcifying front in this tissue are quite different from those elsewhere in cartilage (Lindenbaum and Kuettner, 1967; Howell *et al.*, 1969). In kidney, at least, the protein–polysaccharide content is relatively low, particularly in renal tubular cells where mineralization begins. Stainable polysaccharides do, however, appear after calcification has begun, presumably secondarily bound to apatites, but adequate biochemical data are not yet available as to their composition (Konetzki *et al.*, 1962). It will be of interest if they are similar to the protein–polysaccharides of calcifying cartilage where the temporal relationships to mineralization are so different.

B. Tissue Alkalinity

It is well known that calcium phosphate salts are more soluble at low pH than at more alkaline ones. This, together with the predilection of organs which secrete hydrogen ions such as kidney, stomach, and lung to calcification in hypercalcemic states, has led to the idea that local tissue alkalinity is responsible for these sites of predilection and may indeed play an important role in pathological calcification. This notion is strengthened by the observation that alkalinizing diets enhance calcification (Mulligan and Stucker, 1948). This thesis, however appealing, loses much of its force on more careful scrutiny, even from an anatomic point of view. Thus, in the stomach, the smooth muscle cells of the gastric wall and the vascularization they encompass—both of which may be several millimeters away from the acid secreting cells—calcify as well as the acid-secreting cells (Hass *et al.*, 1958). Complete transection of both vagus nerves, which inhibits gastric secretion, does not prevent calcification if the appropriate stimulus is applied. And, in dying liver cells, the intracellular pH is said to fall (Majno *et al.*, 1960).

Nevertheless, the idea of local alkalinity favoring calcification should not be discarded lightly. The critical experiments which are needed in this area are measurements of pH at specific anatomic sites in intact

tissues. Now that microelectrode techniques have advanced to the point
that accurate intracellular pH determination is feasible, this aspect of
the problem should be soluble.

C. METABOLIC THEORIES

It is an often ignored truism that, except perhaps for certain genetic
disorders, all pathologic processes are quantitative or topographic alterations of normal body constituents. This dictum, which is simply a modern
restatement of Virchow's ancient concept of cellular pathology, is rein-
forced when it is recalled that with the exception of exogenous or virus-
induced materials, possibly amyloid, and some genetic disorders, no
pathological material has been demonstrated which is not normally
present in the body. Thus, although Robison's theory of alkaline phosphatase (Robison, 1923) has failed to withstand the test of time in
its original form, it has the great merit of being perhaps the first rational
chemical approach to this problem which considered things other than
ions meandering through the body fluids until they collected to form
precipitates. With the passage of time and the accumulation of knowledge, it has become apparent that a number of substances are normally
present which influence the solubility of calcium, the availability of
inorganic phosphate, and the crystallizability of calcium phosphates.

One such compound that has received attention is citric acid, a normal
intermediate in carbohydrate metabolism, which chelates calcium in a
nonionic form. It accumulates in the lysing bones of animals injected
with parathyroid extract (Neuman *et al.*, 1956). Diamox, a diuretic
which results in a decrease in renal citrate concentration, causes nephrocalcinosis if it is given to rats (Harrison and Harrison, 1955). In the
nephrocalcinosis caused by hypervitaminosis D, renal citrate levels fall
as calcification begins (Eisenstein *et al.*, 1965). Other dicarboxylic acids
are present, but citric acid, as the most common of these organic compounds, has received the most attention.

Another group of compounds which is almost certainly of physiological
importance are pyrophosphate salts which normally circulate in small
amounts. These compounds are apatite crystal poisons which probably
affect the surface properties of the crystals. Their presence, the demonstration of pyrophosphatases which split them so they lose the ability
to inhibit nucleation, and the fact that injections of these compounds
inhibit calcification (Bisaz *et al.*, 1968; Fleisch *et al.*, 1960; Irving *et
al.*, 1966) provide strong evidence that they play a role in the regulation
of calcification. Most important from a practical point of view is that
phosphonyl compounds which are not rapidly biodegradable have now

been synthesized. This offers hope for the prevention of abnormal calcifications and therefore their sequelae (Francis *et al.*, 1969).

With regard to phosphate, most ideas have invoked enzymes which split organic phosphates to increase the local concentration of inorganic phosphates and thus favor calcification. Thus, almost every phosphate and phosphatase has been implicated at some time or other from adenosine triphosphate (ATP) (Leonard and Scullin, 1969) to the phosphatases of lysosomes.

One thought presented by Hass in a previous edition of this volume may prove to have validity (Hass, 1956). It is becoming increasingly clear that metabolic pathways are not only chemically but also structurally intimately associated. This has been particularly well demonstrated in the work on the arrangement of mitochondrial enzymes. If such an integrated mechanism were disrupted by cell injury, acceptor enzymes for inorganic ions split from their organic radicals conceivably might not be available and thus could act in a manner analogous to Robison's suggestion for alkaline phosphatase. The role of lipids, which have been found at calcifying fronts, remains enigmatic (Wuthier, 1968; Irving and Wuthier, 1968), but the notion that calcium soaps are of importance does not seem tenable (Wells, 1914).

V. Metastatic Calcification

Metastatic calcification connotes calcification of soft tissues which occur in hypercalcemic states such as hypervitaminosis D and hyperparathyroidism. Other clinical situations in which this may occur include sarcoidosis, the milk alkali syndrome which occurs in patients with peptic ulcerations who ingest large amounts of milk and bicarbonates, and massive osteolysis from several causes including immobilization, metastatic tumors, and several bone diseases of obscure nature such as Paget's disease. In current clinical practice the commonest conditions in which widespread metastatic calcification occurs are hyperparathyroidism secondary to chronic renal failure, especially in patients undergoing prolonged dialysis to maintain life, and in patients with osseous metastases, especially from breast cancer.

These two conditions are of particular interest because they illustrate how complex the metabolic interrelationships may be in these conditions. The kidneys of patients with several diseases fail to secrete phosphate and thus develop high serum phosphate levels. These patients are acidotic as well and have low total and ionized serum calcium levels. Since parathyroid hormone secretion is controlled by the calcium concentration in extracellular fluid, more of this hormone is secreted and the glands themselves undergo a secondary hyperplasia. The cycle is made even more vicious by the metabolic acidosis which enhances bone resorption and the relatively immobility of these sick patients. Now that chronic dialysis for the treatment of renal failure has become common, it has been noted that pathological calcification is particularly widespread and severe. In some patients there is evidence that raising the level of serum calcium does not suppress production of the hormone. These two observations, together with the fact that these people have normal serum electrolytes at least part of the time, have given rise to the idea that constant stimulation of parathyroid hormones may ultimately give rise to a situation in which the glands behave like neoplasms in that they are no longer responsive to the physiological regulation of the serum calcium level. The term *tertiary hyperparathyroidism* has been used to describe this state (Katz *et al.*, 1969).

In metastatic breast carcinoma inhibition of motion caused by bone pain and hypercalcemia-induced lethargy aggravate the osteolytic process caused by the tumor cells. In addition, there is evidence that these tumors produce vitamin D–like steroids. Hypervitaminosis D itself is no longer as frequent a cause of overt metastatic calcification as in the days when large amounts were used to treat tuberculosis. There is evidence, however, that overdosages in pregnancy can cause a peculiar syndrome characterized by abnormalities of the facial bones, cardiac defects, and coarctation of the aorta, most likely related to abnormal mineralization of these sites *in utero* (Friedman and Mills, 1969). The discovery of this relationship has once again raised the question of whether the vitamin D ingested in foods to which it has been added and in one or two vitamin pills a day may contribute to the arterial calcification so common in adults. Evidence on this question is not adequate to form an opinion but it is of interest that in certain experimental situations a very small dose of the vitamin, acting in synergy with other insults such as hypercholesterolemia and nicotine injections, can result in extensive arterial calcification (Hass *et al.*, 1966, 1969).

An interrelationship of still another type is seen in patients with medullary carcinomas of the thyroid gland which produce large amounts of thyrocalcitonin. Among other things, these patients may develop hyperfunctioning parathyroid glands with resultant hypercalcemia. Whether the parathyroid lesion is an adaptive response to the one in the thyroid gland or is induced by the same aberration which induces the thyroid tumor is still an open question.

Some hypercalcemic states are only unusually accompanied by metastatic calcification. One of these is multiple myeloma, a malignant proliferation of plasma cells accompanied by increased amounts of circulating globulins produced by these cells. It is thought that here much of the calcium is combined with serum proteins much like what occurs in the serum of egg-laying birds (Ericson *et al.*, 1955).

An additional type of experimental calcification described by Selye and his collaborators should be mentioned, calciphylaxis. This subject has been extensively reviewed elsewhere (Selye, 1962) and will therefore not be discussed here in any detail. Briefly, the method consists of applying a physical or chemical insult, termed a *challenger*, to an animal which has received an agent such as dihydrotachysterol, a vitamin D–like sterol, or parathyroid extract, termed a *sensitizer*, at a specific time after the sensitizer has been given. The result is a severe, but remarkably localized calcification, with the locus of calcification depending largely on the nature of the challenger. A dramatic example is the administration of the sensitizer and simple skin trauma. The result is severe cutaneous calcinosis. This type of experimental approach provides an investigator with an opportunity to study remarkably localized calcifications, e.g., in the vagus nerves.

As Scarpelli has pointed out (Scarpelli, 1965), the distinction between dystrophic and metastatic calcification is probably in part artificial, because hypercalcemia itself may result in cell injury. There is also mounting evidence that the localization of calcium in a given tissue is not simply a consequence of hypercalcemia but the result of local metabolic effects of the agent which induces the hypercalcemia. In this regard it is instructive to compare the renal lesions induced in three types of rodent hypercalcemia. In hypervitaminosis D, an early site of calcification is in tubular mitochondria, and this is accompanied by uncoupling of oxidative phosphorylation (Scarpelli, 1965). Hyperparathyroidism results in a similar anatomic distribution (Caulfield and Schrag, 1964). If hypercalcemia is induced by calcium gluconate injections, calcium salts in the form of carbonates are virtually restricted to basement membranes (Schneider *et al.*, 1960; Caulfield and Schrag, 1964). In magnesium deficiency, renal cellular calcification may be extensive, but it spares the mitochondria with apatite crystals appearing randomly in tubular cell cytoplasm and as calcified casts (Battifora *et al.*, 1966). The calcification of magnesium deficiency is also remarkable in that in the heart there is uncoupling of oxidative phosphorylation and mitochondria are the first demonstrable site of calcification (Hettgveit *et al.*, 1964; Vitale *et al.*, 1957), while in the kidney mitochondrial metabolism is apparently normal and these organelles do not calcify (Battifora *et al.*, 1966).

In recent years, considerable electron microscopic and biochemical effort has been expended in studying the role of mitochondria in calcification, both normal and pathological. Before this discussion is begun, however, it should be pointed out that there is now evidence that both parathyroid hormone and vitamin D have direct effects on calcium metabolism in a variety of cells outside bone, kidney, and gut, at least in pharmacological doses. With the advent of simple, routine techniques for electron microscopy, attention has been directed at intracellular sites of calcification. Examination of the literature reveals a remarkable propensity for mitochondria to accumulate calcium salts in response to a variety of injuries including toxic injury to the heart, liver, and kidney (Hettgveit *et al.*, 1964; Caulfield and Schrag, 1964; Reynolds, 1965). Indeed, amorphous calcium phosphates have been described in a variety of normal cells. Isolated mitochondria have the ability to actively transport calcium and other ions across their membranes (DeLuca and Engstrom, 1961), and excess calcium salts within these organelles seem to induce uncoupling of oxidative phosphorylation which Scarpelli (1965) has shown increases the accumulation of calcium salts in vitamin D–induced nephrocalcinosis. The demonstration of calcium salts in their biologic site by electron microscopy is a matter of some difficulty, since the fixing procedure may result in loss, accretion, or translocation of these materials. Fixatives enriched with calcium or which employ phosphate buffers demonstrate larger amounts of calcium salts. The question, therefore, arises as to whether the numerous lovely micrographs which have shown calcium salts in mitochondria are an artifact of preparation, i.e., do they demonstrate sites of enhanced calcium binding, sites in which altered metabolic states permit rapid mineral accretion from the fixing solution or adjacent cytoplasm, or actual biologic sites of mineral? The other question which these observations, not only on mitochondria but also in increasingly numerous other sites, raises is where the line between normal and abnormal should be drawn. The importance of these two questions is particularly relevant to the work of Matthews and his collaborators (J. M. Martin and Matthews, 1969; Matthews *et al.*, 1968). These investigators have demonstrated within calcifying tissues that calcium laden mitochondria are present within cells, and move across cells, apparently acting as transporters of calcium in packaged form. Whether these packages actually represent calcium within the cell or calcium binding sites which vary in their effectiveness and location remains unsettled. This is, of course, a broader metabolic question than the one to which this review is addressed. Another, similar type of observation has been made on the kidney of hypercalcemic rats. Here, in tissue fixed in phosphate-buffered osmic acid, electron dense deposits have been seen in specific cytoplasmic sites (Biava *et al.*, 1969). A reasonable explanation for these observations is that there are sites in the cell which are either normally rich in calcium ions or are sites of calcium transport. It would be expected that in injured cells it is these sites in which ionic calcium would first accumulate. In a hypercalcemic animal, if one wishes to indulge in semantics, such an accumulation could not yet be considered pathologic. However, as *in vitro* studies of mitochondrial metabolism have shown, excessive calcium ions do lead to metabolic derangements, which should interfere with normal barriers to ion translocation within cells. Since extracellular fluid is supersaturated with respect to calcium phosphates, further growth of the mineral should occur and this is indeed what happens. This sort of approach which views the initial, critical phases of an abnormal process as an overloading of a normal metabolic pathway may perhaps form the basis of a rational biological theory of abnormal calcification.

VI. Arterial Calcification

Throughout this review there has been an implicit idea that students of normal and pathological calcification have much to learn from each other. To illustrate this, let us take as a text, Fig. 1, a hematoxylin-eosin stained section of a calcified aorta of a rabbit with hypervitaminosis D. Similar lesions can be found in aged breeder rats, human peripheral muscular arteries, and a number of other natural and experimental diseases associated with both hyper- and normocalcemia. The media of the artery is extensively calcified, with calcific deposits encrusting all the elements of the arterial media. Note, however, that between the lumen and the calcified area is a layer of cells and stroma, somewhat analogous to osteoid, very similar to that of the normal artery wall. There are differences, the most obvious being that these cells and their surrounding stroma are not as precisely organized. Note too that these areas, which have newly formed over the calcified area, are not calcified and, indeed, are extremely resistant to calcification, much like rachitic osteoid in bone. The calcified areas in the media, like bone, can undergo considerable reorganization through cellular mechanisms. Figure 2 illustrates one such mechanism in which multinucleated giant cells bearing a superficial anatomic, but rather precise functional, similarity to osteoclasts are resorbing the calcified tissues. In Fig. 3 (p. 372) a capillary plexus is seen excavating the medial calcification in a manner reminiscent of the capillaries in the vascular epiphyseal growth plate. The newly formed fibrocellular intimal cushion and cellular resorbtive elements are reactions to the stimulus of calcification and considerably modify arterial responses to other insults such as hypercholesterolemia. If nothing else,

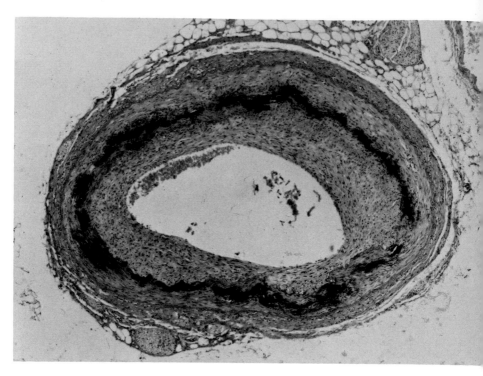

Fig. 1. Low power micrograph of the aorta from a rabbit with hypervitaminosis D. In the midportion of the arterial wall is a circumferential band of darkly staining calcification. Deep to the area of calcification is relatively normal media; overlying it is a mass of newly formed cells and stroma, similar to the underlying media in composition but less regularly organized. It is not calcified.

the figures illustrate striking analogies with bone, although the function, structure, chemical composition, and types of mechanical stress are obviously quite different.

The final section of this review will be an analysis of this lesion as exemplified primarily in experimental hypervitaminosis D. The initial gross site of calcification is the arch of the aorta, with subsequent centrifugal spread down the aorta and out its branches. The relative amount of elastin also diminishes peripherally. The arterial branches show definite patterns of calcification: some like the renal, gastric, splenic, duodenal, muscular, and distal colic arteries calcify readily while others such as the cerebral, hepatic, adrenal, and proximal colic arteries are extremely resistant. The microscopic and biochemical discussion will be restricted to the aorta, since analysis has been most detailed in this vessel and since its branches are primarily muscular and therefore ana-

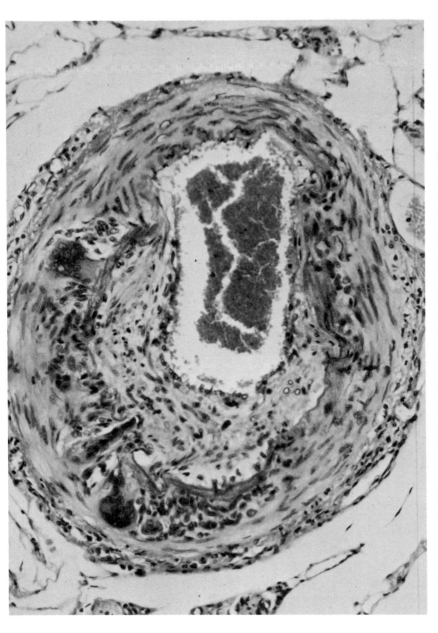

FIG. 2. In this artery, also from a rabbit with hypervitaminosis D, multinucleated giant cells are seen excavating an area of calcification.

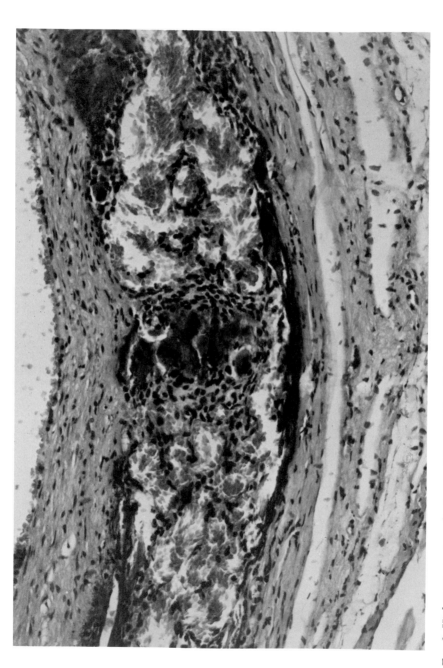

FIG. 3. Higher power view of artery wall from rabbit with hypervitaminosis D. Note the capillary plexus excavating the darkly stained calcified masses.

tomically different. In the aorta, the initial mineralization occurs in the inner elastic lamellae which, for a time, appear to act as a barrier to spread of the process.

From analogous experiments with kidney it seems that before histologically recognizable calcifications can be seen, calcium begins to accumulate in the vessel wall, and phosphate begins to accumulate shortly thereafter (Eisenstein *et al.*, 1970; Dahl and Dole, 1952). By contrast, phosphate appears to collect first in calcifying meningiomas (Bennington *et al.*, 1970). At about this time, electron microscopy of tissues fixed in ionic enriched solutions reveals large amounts of mineral within mitochondria of smooth muscle cells (Matthews, 1970). The first extracellular site in which mineral crystals appear is within and on the surface of the inner elastic lamellae, and here they seem to be relatively more densely packed within the fibrillar component of elastin (Eisenstein and Zeruolis, 1964). Shortly after calcium phosphates accumulate, both chemical analysis (Konetzki *et al.*, 1962) and staining with metachromatic dyes indicate that acid mucosubstances are present in sites of calcification. Data from other tissues indicate that these materials are secondarily bound to mineral crystals (Eisenstein *et al.*, 1965). As the process of mineralization spreads through the arterial wall, it involves other elastic lamellae, necrotic smooth muscle cells, and, to a much lesser extent, collagen. The reasons why collagen, which is so susceptible to mineralization in bone, is so resistant in most soft tissue are not completely clear. It is, however, becoming clear that collagens from different sites may vary.

In the advanced lesion (Fig. 4), the mineral deposits are arranged in a number of morphological patterns, depending on the site in which they occur, and individual crystals may grow to relatively large size. Within elastic fibers, however, they remain quite small. This failure of crystals to grow in size seems to be a feature in common with other mineralizing matrices which have the ability to nucleate apatite from metastable solutions of calcium phosphate. In response to the medial calcification, a proliferation of cells and stroma occurs over the calcified mass which is morphologically similar in its composition to that of normal arterial wall but less well organized. These newly formed elements are quite resistant to mineralization.

If calcified arteries are homogenized in sucrose, and subcellular fractions assayed for calcium and phosphate, large amounts are found in a rapidly sedimentable fraction containing heavily mineralized material. Mitochondria contain somewhat more calcium and PO_4 than those of control aortas, microsomes still more, while the greatest increment is found in the nonsedimentable supernatant. Analyses of similar subcellu-

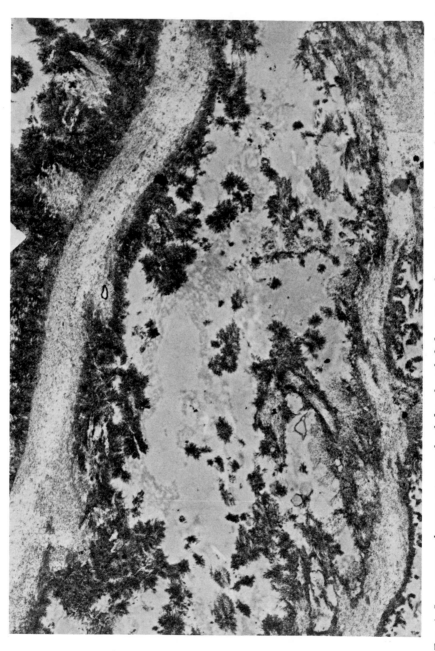

FIG. 4. Low power electron micrograph of densely calcified aorta similar to Fig. 1 (approximately ×5000). The dark material represents calcium, which is present within elastic fibers and is heavily encrusted on their surfaces. The crystals are larger in the tissue distant from elastic tissue where once smooth muscle cells were present.

lar fractions for lysosomal enzymes reveal that the activity of several of the acid hydrolases is increased above normal. One of these enzymes, lysozyme, is markedly different from the others in its distribution. In cell particulates it sediments with the rapidly sedimentable heavily calcified fraction and histochemically appears to be particularly active in heavily calcified areas (Eisenstein *et al.*, 1970). Lysozyme is a small, highly cationic protein which has a high affinity for the anionic mucopolysaccharide molecules, but it has no known substrate in mammalian tissue which it can catalytically degrade (Kuettner *et al.*, 1968). It is felt that when lysosomes rupture, they release all their enzymes but that lysozyme, because of its cationic properties, is secondarily bound to the acid mucopolysaccharides at calcified sites. Since it has been suggested that lysozyme may function to regulate the reactivity of acid polysaccharides (Kuettner *et al.*, 1968), this secondary binding may be biologically significant. The activities of alkaline phosphatase and 5'-nucleotidase increase while that of nonspecific carboxylesterase decreases (Zemplenyi, 1968).

The known sequence of materials accumulated in mineralizing sites thus appears to be calcium, then phosphate, then acid mucopolysaccharides, then lysozyme, with each substance binding the next one in the sequence, probably largely on the basis of ionic interactions. On the basis of these morphological and biochemical analyses, the two structures in the arterial wall which play a critical role in calcification are smooth muscle cells and elastin. In the smooth muscle cell, the role of mitochondria has already been alluded to, and the importance of calcium fluxes in smooth muscle is well known and need not be discussed here. It is of importance that ionic transport in the aorta has both active and passive components, and that the active one is altered by experimental interventions (Hudgkins and Weiss, 1969; Garrahan *et al.*, 1965). The calcium and phosphate, must, of course, cross the endothelial cell layer to reach the calcifying sites.

The elastic fiber itself is basically a two component system (Ross and Bornstein, 1969), the bulk of which is made up of an isotropic protein, elastin, which stains faintly with acid dyes, is resistant to digestion by trypsin or chymotrypsin, is only slowly solubilized by such strong reagents as dilute NaOH or concentrated formic acid, but is digestible with elastase. It is amorphous when viewed in the electron microscope and has an undetermined substructure. Although it is doubtful that it has yet been isolated pure and undenatured, it seems to contain about 1% hydroxyproline, large amounts of proline, glycine, alanine, and valine and smaller amounts of aspartic and glutamic acids, threonine, serine, and cystine. It is virtually unique in containing desmosine and iso-

desmosine which are thought to be involved in cross-linking of the molecule that should perhaps best be regarded as a macromolecular gel
cross-linked by these compounds (Ayer, 1964). Aged human aortic
elastin, which contains and binds more calcium than that from younger
people, has a higher proportion of dicarboxylic amino acids (Lansing
et al., 1950, 1951; Eisenstein *et al.*, 1964). The fiber swells and shrinks
considerably, depending on the pH and ionic strength (Ayer, 1964),
and binds more calcium in the stretched than the relaxed state. A second
component of the fiber is a smaller (110 Å diam) cylindrical microfibril
which is digestable by trypsin or chymotrypsin and solubilized by di-
thiothreitol; but, like elastin, it is resistant to collagenase and hyaluronidase. It is solubilized by formic acid. It is thought to be formed
before elastin and may determine its anatomic orientation (Ross and
Bornstein, 1969).

Elastin is an effective nucleator of apatite *in vitro* (Sobel, 1966).
It has also been shown that rat arterial elastin calcifies if incubated
in calcifying solutions including aged serum (G. R. Martin *et al.*, 1963).
This model has been extensively analyzed, and specific sites containing
iron have been found to be critical in this process (Schiffman *et al.*,
1964, 1966; Schiffman, 1969). Indeed, iron salts of amino acids have
also been found to be effective nucleators.

The role of various components of the serum has also been analyzed.
If segments of rat arteries are incubated in serum, they accumulate
more calcium from the serum of rats with hypervitaminosis D than
from normal rats. Addition of vitamin D alone or calcium alone to normal
serum does not affect calcium accumulation, but addition of both induces
greater calcium binding. Thus, high levels of calcium and vitamin D
in the serum appear to act synergistically (Eisenstein *et al.*, 1969).

Nevertheless, even if the details of how elastic tissue calcifies were
completely solved in isolated systems, the problem of arterial calcification
would not be. The elastin which calcifies when it is isolated does not
do so normally in the intact animal. The arterial wall, like bone, cartilage,
and every other tissue is a functionally integrated structure.

The inner portion of the media, where calcification begins, is nourished
through a complete layer of endothelial cells which are attached by
watertight seals. These cells, however, are frequently damaged, which
may alter their filtering properties. Once past the endothelial cell, the
extracellular fluid, whose ionic composition and distribution is still incompletely known, will be affected by the metabolism of smooth muscle
cells as well as by the distribution and ionic properties of the macromolecules of arterial connective tissue. Each of these has specific water
and ion binding properties which will greatly affect ionic compartmen-

talization and reactivity. The whole structure is constantly and rhythmically stretched by pulsatile blood flow, and stretch is known to alter ion binding by at least some polyelectrolytes. Finally, the composition of the blood and the metabolic activities of the cells in the arterial wall are affected by hormonal and other factors. Thus, what started out in this essay as a problem in physical chemistry has been rendered infinitely complex by life. This is not a plea for a return to vitalism, or a denial of the validity for a sound biochemical approach. It is, however, a reminder that, as in the molecular biology of nucleic acids it is a long step from phage genetics to the solution of the problem of metazoan differentiation, it is also a long way from test-tube experiments with isolated macromolecules in defined media to an intact organ in a living animal.

Although calcification is, by our definition, simply precipitation or crystallization of inorganic calcium salts in tissues, the processes which lead to a chemical environment which permits this even may vary depending on the pathogenetic stimulus and the site in which it is applied. The tissue response to calcium deposits will also vary. Thus, although a theoretical formulation of the physical chemistry of calcification may be well within our grasp, a formulation of the factors preceding and following calcification seems to elude us—as much because of the intrinsic variabilities of cells and tissues as because of the incompleteness of our understanding of these living units as functionally integrated entities.

A few very general predictions regarding the results of future investigations do appear possible at this time. It seems likely that such studies will reveal that in most forms of calcification cells play an early central pathogenetic role, primarily related to the transport of ions across membranes, in part, in packaged form such as in mitochondrial granules or other specialized structures. A disturbance of such a transport system, could, in the case of rapidly developing dystrophic calcification, well result from a disturbance in the discriminatory functions of cell membranes so that the rate of calcium influx is increased and that of egress decreased. The excess intracellular mineral, in turn, would lead to further metabolic alterations, within which disorders of cellular metabolism of phosphate may occur with progressive mineral accretion. The rate and extent of accumulation of mineral in extracellular matrices would then depend on the rate of excretion of ions, the ion binding properties of the extracellular matrices, and the composition of extracellular fluid. Metastatic calcification probably differs in that the primary lesion is an overloading of normal metabolic pathways as the initial step in the chain of pathogenesis. Slowly developing dystrophic calcification, such as occurs in human arterial calcification, appears to be most likely primarily an extracellular event related to slow accretion of ions by binding to existing matrices—elastin in the case of the aorta. The fate of the calcific deposits and the changes they induce in the tissues further complicate these processes.

Finally, it should be pointed out that the binding and the degree of solubility of calcium salts, on which calcification ultimately depends, are considerably modulated by a variety of materials ranging in size from macromolecules such as protein–polysaccharides to the hydrogen ion, whose normal physiological roles may be quite unrelated to calcium or phosphate metabolism.

Acknowledgments

The author is grateful to Dr. George M. Hass for his constantly stimulating encouragement. Some of the work described here was supported by U. S. Public Health Service Grant HE-06713.

References

Ayer, J. P. (1964). *Int. Rev. Connect. Tissue Res.* **2**, 33.

Battifora, H., Eisenstein, R., Laing, G., and McCreary, P. (1966). *Amer. J. Pathol.* **48**, 421.

Bennington, J. L., Smith, J. V., and Lagunoff, D. (1970). *Lab. Invest.* **22**, 241.

Biava, C. B., Williams, G. A., Sakai, T., and Harges, C. K. (1969). *Amer. J. Pathol.* **55**, 54a.

Bisaz, S., Russell, R. G., and Fleisch, H. (1968). *Arch. Oral Biol.* **13**, 683.

Borle, A. A. (1968). *J. Cell Biol.* **36**, 567.

Canas, F., Brand, J. S., Neuman, W. F., and Terepka, A. R. (1969). *Amer. J. Physiol.* **216**, 1092.

Caulfield, J. P., and Schrag, P. E. (1964). *Amer. J. Pathol.* **44**, 365.

Cogan, D. G., Hurlbut, C. S., and Kuwabara, T. (1958). *J. Histochem. Cytochem.* **6**, 143.

Dahl, L. K., and Dole, V. P. (1952). *J. Exp. Med.* **95**, 341.

DeLuca, H. F., and Engstrom, G. W. (1961). *Proc. Nat. Acad. Sci. U. S.* **47**, 1744.

Eisenstein, R., and Passavoy, M. (1964). *Proc. Soc. Exp. Biol. Med.* **117**, 77.

Eisenstein, R., and Zeruolis, L. (1964). *Arch. Pathol.* **77**, 27.

Eisenstein, R., Trueheart, R. E., and Hass, G. M. (1960). *In* "Calcification in Biological Systems," Publ. No. 64, p. 281. Amer. Ass. Advance. Sci., Washington, D.C.

Eisenstein, R., Ayer, J. P., Papajiannis, S., Hass, G. M., and Ellis, H. (1964). *Lab. Invest.* **13**, 1198.

Eisenstein, R., Battifora, H., and Ellis, H. (1965). *Amer. J. Pathol.* **47**, 487.

Eisenstein, R., Ellis, H., and Rosato, J. (1969). *Proc. Soc. Exp. Biol. Med.* **132**, 58.

Eisenstein, R., Arsenis, C., Lisk, P., and Kuettner, K. E. (1970). *Fed. Proc., Fed. Amer. Soc. Exp. Biol.* **29**, 553.

Ericson, A. T., Clegg, R. E., and Hein, R. E. (1955). *Science* **122**, 199.

Fleisch, H., Maerki, J., and Russell, R. G. (1960). *Proc. Soc. Exp. Biol. Med.* **122**, 317.

Francis, M. D., Russell, R. G. G., and Fleisch, H. (1969). *Science* **165**, 1264.

Friedman, W. F., and Mills, L. F. (1969). *Pediatrics* **43**, 12.

Frondel, C., and Prien, E. L. (1942). *Science* **95**, 431

Frondel, C., and Prien, E. L. (1946). *Science* **103**, 326.

Garrahan, P., Villamil, M. F., and Zadunaisky, J. A. (1965). *Amer. J. Physiol.* **209**, 955.

Glimcher, M. J. (1960). *In* "Calcification in Biological Systems," Publ. No. 64, p. 421. Amer. Ass. Advance. Sci., Washington, D.C.

Harrison, H. E., and Harrison, H. C. (1955). *J. Clin. Invest.* **34**, 1662.

Hass, G. M. (1956). *In* "The Biochemistry and Physiology of Bone" (G. H. Bourne, ed.), 1st ed., p. 767. Academic Press, New York.

Hass, G. M., Trueheart, R. E., Taylor, C. B., and Stumpf, M. (1958). *Amer. J. Pathol.* **34**, 395.

Hass, G. M., Landerholm, W., and Hemmens, A. (1966). *Amer. J. Pathol.* **49**, 739.

Hass, G. M., Henson, D. E., Scott, R. A., McClain, E., and Hemmens, A. (1969). *Amer. J. Pathol.* **57**, 405.

Hausler, M. R., Myrtle, J. E., and Norman, A. W. (1968). *J. Biol. Chem.* **243**, 4055.

Hettgveit, H. A., Herman, L., and Mishra, R. K. (1964). *Amer. J. Pathol.* **45**, 757.

Howell, D. S., Pita, J. C., Marquez, J. F., and Gatter, R. (1969). *J. Clin. Invest.* **48**, 630.

Hudgkins, P. M., and Weiss, G. B. (1969). *Amer. J. Physiol.* **217**, 1310.

Irving, J., and Wuthier, R. E. (1968). *Clin. Orthop. Related Res.* **56**, 237.

Irving, J. T., Schibler, D., and Fleisch, H. (1966). *Proc. Soc. Exp. Biol. Med.* **122**, 582.

Katz, A. I., Hampers, C. L., and Merrill, J. P. (1969). *Medicine (Baltimore)* **48**, 333.

Konetzki, W., Hyland, R., and Eisenstein, R. (1962). *Lab. Invest.* **11**, 488.

Kowarski, S., and Schachter, D. (1969). *J. Biol. Chem.* **244**, 211.

Kuettner, K. E., Soble, L. W., Eisenstein, R., and Yaeger, J. A. (1968). *Calcif. Tissue Res.* **2**, 93.

Lansing, A. I., Alex, M., and Rosenthal, T. B. (1950). *J. Gerontol.* **5**, 112.

Lansing, A. I., Ramasarma, G. B., Rosenthal, T., and Alex, M. (1951). *Proc. Soc. Exp. Biol. Med.* **76**, 714.

Leonard, F., and Scullin, R. I. (1969). *Nature (London)* **224**, 1113.

Levine, M. D., Rubin, P. S., Follis, R. H., Jr., and Howard, J. E. (1949). *Conf. Metab. Interrelationships, Trans.* **1**, 41.

Lindenbaum, A., and Kuettner, K. E. (1967). *Calcif. Tissue Res.* **1**, 1953.

Lund, J., and DeLuca, H. F. (1964). *J. Lipid Res.* **7**, 27.

Main, R. K., and Cole, J. L. (1957). *Arch. Biochem. Biophys.* **68**, 186.

Majno, G., LaGutta, M., and Thompson, E. T. (1960). *Virchons Arch. Pathol. Anat. Physiol.* **333**, 421.

Martin, G. R., Schiffman, E., Blanden, H. A., and Nylen, M. (1963). *J. Cell Biol.* **16**, 243.

Martin, J. H., and Matthews, J. L. (1969). *Calcif. Tissue Res.* **3**, 184.

Martin, J. H., and Matthews, J. L. (1970). *Clin. Orthop. Related Res.* **68**, 273.
Matthews, J. L. (1970). Personal communication.
Matthews, J. L., Martin, J. H., and Collins, E. J. (1968). *Clin. Orthop. Related Res.* **58**, 213.
Mulligan, R. M., and Stucker, F. L. (1948). *Amer. J. Pathol.* **24**, 451.
Neuman, W. F., and Neuman, M. W. (1958). "The Chemical Dynamics of Bone Material." Univ. Chicago Press, Chicago.
Neuman, W. F., Firschein, P. S., Chen, P. S., Mulryan, B. J., and DiStefano, V. (1956). *J. Amer. Chem. Soc.* **78**, 3363.
Ponchon, G., and DeLuca, H. F. (1969). *J. Clin. Invest.* **48**, 1273.
Posner, A. S. (1969). *Physiol. Rev.* **49**, 760.
Reynolds, E. S. (1965). *J. Cell Biol.* **25**, 53.
Robison, R. (1923). *Biochem. J.* **17**, 286.
Ross, R., and Bornstein, M. (1969). *J. Cell Biol.* **40**, 368.
Scarpelli, D. G. (1965). *Lab. Invest.* **14**, 123.
Schiffman, E. (1969). *Calcif. Tissue Res.* **3**, 125.
Schiffman, E., Martin, E. R., and Corcoran, B. A. (1964). *Arch. Biochem. Biophys.* **107**, 284.
Schiffman, E., Corcoran, B. A., and Martin, G. R. (1966). *Arch. Biochem. Biophys.* **115**, 87.
Schneider, A. F., Reaven, E. P., and Reaven, G. (1960). *Endocrinology* **67**, 733.
Selye, H. (1962). "Calciphylaxis." Univ. of Chicago Press, Chicago.
Sobel, A. E. (1966). *Nature (London)* **211**, 45.
Taylor, A. N., and Wasserman, R. H. (1967). *Arch. Biochem. Biophys.* **119**, 536.
Trummel, C. L., and Raisz, L. G. (1969). *Science* **163**, 1450.
Vitale, J. J., Nakamura, M., and Hegsted, D. M. (1957). *J. Biol. Chem.* **228**, 573.
Walser, M. (1962). *J. Clin. Invest.* **41**, 1454.
Wasserman, R. H., and Taylor, A. N. (1966). *Science* **152**, 791.
Wells, H. G. (1914). "Clinical Pathology," 2nd ed. Saunders, Philadelphia, Pennsylvania.
Wuthier, R. E. (1968). *J. Lipid Res.* **9**, 68.
Zemplenyi, T. (1969). "Enzyme Chemistry of the Arterial Wall," p. 151. Lloyd-Luke, London.

Author Index

Numbers in italics refer to the pages on which the complete references are listed.

Subject Index

A

Acromegaly, 177
    growth hormone and, 179
    osteoporosis in, 188
    rat, symptoms, 179
Adenosine triphosphate, in cartilage, 105
Adrenalectomy, in scurvy, 249
Adrenocorticotropic hormone (ACTH)
    osteogenesis, effect on, 182
    skeletal maturation role, 182–183
Alizarin test, phosphatase determination, 262
Alkaline phosphatase(s)
    activation by vitamin D_2, 81
    bone formation and, 102–115
    embryonic bone, 85–86
    kidney, 80
    in osteoblasts, 87
    in osteocyte cycle, 87
Ameloblasts, 125–137
    amylase incubated, 135
    cytology, 125–129
    glycoprotein in, 129
    Golgi apparatus, 125–129, 135
    Golgi saccules, 127–129, 132, 135
    protein synthesis by, 131
    radioautography, 131–137
        silver grain quantitation, 134
    rough endoplasmic reticulum, 122–123, 131
    secretory, 125–129, 133
    secretory granules, 135–136
    Tomes process, 127
    vesicles, 137

intermediate, 131–132
Apatite, 113
    bone, 105
Arteries
    branches, 370–371
    calcification, 341, 366, 369–378
        collagens and, 373
        elastic fiber, 375–376
        elastin in, 370, 376
        histology, 369–370
        hypervitaminosis D and, 370–372
        process, 373
        serum, role of, 376
Arthritis, caused by growth hormone, 178–179
Articulation, 2
Ascorbic acid, see Vitamin C

B

Barium phosphate, 80
Barium sulfate, perfusion, 8
Blood flow, microscopic study, 9–10
Bone
    blood supply, 2
    citrate content, 108
    density index, 254–255
    diseases, types, 288
    ectopic, formation, 83–84
    formation
        alkaline phosphatase role, 102–115
        phosphate ester role, 103
        in vitro model, 112
    growth apparatus, 163
    healing, essential factors, 41